Praise for
The Nourishing Traditions
Book of Baby & Child Care

The Nourishing Traditions Book of Baby & Child Care will be a cherished reference for many generations to come. Carefully referenced and thoughtfully presented, this important work intelligently weaves traditional wisdom with modern treatments, providing precise instructions useful to parents and practitioners alike. I will recommend that all of my patients read it from cover to cover.

Lindy Woodard, MD
Pediatric Alternatives
Mill Valley, California

I remember so clearly standing in front of the pregnancy and child care section at the bookstore when my husband and I first decided to start a family, trying to figure out which books to buy. My joy and excitement were tempered by confusion and dismay over the excess of conflicting advice. *The Nourishing Traditions Book of Baby & Child Care* is a germane and much needed resource for empowering parents with the necessary instruction to raise a healthy, well balanced child amid the scores of seriously flawed baby and child care books available today.

Sarah Pope
The Healthy Home Economist

I warmly recommend *The Nourishing Traditions Book of Baby and Child Care*. The authors share not only a deep knowledge about food and its value for health, but are also parents and grandparents with great love for children. We live in a world full of misinformation about food and health, the truth is often hard to find. This is one of the true and reliable sources of information for parents on how to bring up healthy children.

Natasha Campbell-McBride, MD
Author of *The Gut & Psychology Syndrome*

An indispensable guide to pregnancy, childbirth and child rearing, informed by common sense, ancestral wisdom and sound science. If every couple read this book prior to becoming pregnant, and followed its nourishing and empowering advice, the future of health care would be profoundly and positively changed.

Kaayla T. Daniel, PhD
Vice President, The Weston A. Price Foundation
Author of *The Whole Soy Story:*
The Dark Side of America's Favorite Health Food

Too often in our modern society we expect to do things right by starting from scratch and assembling our knowledge piecemeal using the scientific method. In *The Nourishing Traditions Book of Baby & Child Care*, the authors show how we have done just that with the art of child rearing, leaving the accumulated wisdom of the ages by the wayside. In the grand tradition of Weston Price, Fallon Morell and Cowan use modern science to explore the wisdom of ancient tradition, providing a firm foundation for a nutritional approach that will nourish both mother and child, allowing each to grasp hold of the gift of radiant and vibrant health.

Chris Masterjohn, PhD
Author of *The Daily Lipid* at
Cholesterol-And-Health.Com

The Nourishing Traditions Book of Baby & Child Care

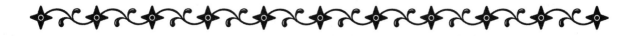

THE
NOURISHING TRADITIONS
BOOK OF BABY & CHILD CARE

Sally Fallon Morell
Thomas S. Cowan, MD

Cover Design by Kim Waters Murray

Published by

NewTrends Publishing, Inc.
Washington, DC 20005

US and Canada Orders (877) 707-1776
www.newtrendspublishing.com   customerservice@newtrendspublishing.com
Available to the trade through
National Book Network (800) 462-6420

Printings: 20,000, 30,000, 25,000, 15,000, 10,000

ISBN
0-9823383-1-7/978-0-9823383-1-5

PRINTED IN THE UNITED STATES OF AMERICA

To Tomorrow's Children

CONTENTS

ACKNOWLEDGEMENTS

This book is the result of many minds and much good advice.

Our sincerest thanks go to our four readers: Lindy Woodard, MD, of Pediatric Alternatives in Mill Valley, California, who gave us the invaluable insights of a holistic pediatrician; Kaayla T. Daniel, PhD, CCN, practicing nutritionist who sees the unhealthy offspring of vegetarians and those following a standard American diet and provided us with guidelines to preconceptual detoxification, along with many other helpful suggestions; Sarah Pope, MGA, the Healthy Home Economist, who shared her experience and wisdom on holistic child care; and, finally, Sarah Fallon, who gave us the insights and example of a young mother on pregnancy, birth and child rearing.

We are indebted to Chris Masterjohn for his research on the fat-soluble activators and the importance of nutrient-dense diets for pregnant women and growing children; some of his inquiries were carried out specifically for this book. Likewise, we are grateful to Jen Allbritton for her contributions on the feeding of babies and growing children. The work of Natasha-Campbell McBride, MD, infuses this book and has provided true healing to thousands of children afflicted with digestive, behavior and learning disorders.

Katherine Czapp did a masterful job with proofreading—far more than catching little errors, but wise advice on many aspects of the manuscript. Thanks also to Leonard Rosenbaum for his expert indexing services.

Others who contributed with ideas, insight and research include Sylvia Onusic, who helped find many references, and David Ayaub, who provided insight on shaken baby syndrome. Thanks also go to Susun Weed, for her material on herbal support for breastfeeding, and Lisa Bianco-Davis who compiled bad advice in modern books on child care. Arabella Forge provided some wonderful recipes for babies.

None of this work would be possible without the presiding genius of Mary G. Enig, PhD, who put together the recipes for the homemade formula and whose wisdom and knowledge on what constitutes a healthy diet for pregnant women and growing children provide the scientific support for the return to traditional diets.

Kim Waters gave us beautiful cover art; and Richard Morris shared his talent in the layout design.

Finally, to our patient and supportive spouses Geoffrey Morell and Lynda Smith Cowan; to our children, who taught us much more than we taught them; and to our grandchildren, who give us surprise and delight.

Sally Fallon Morell
Thomas S. Cowan, MD
January, 2013

Introduction

Childhood as a separate and distinct stage of life is a modern idea; historians who write about trends in child rearing assign this new outlook to the advent of literature on how to raise children. In fact, the appearance of published advice on raising children, starting in the eighteenth century, signals a profound change in western life, one in which the scientific counsel of experts replaces the wisdom of elders and the instincts of parents and grandparents.

Early child rearing literature from Britain and the American colonies displays a distinctly moralistic tone. The writers—who tended to be physicians or ministers—linked child rearing practices with future behavior and character. Whether they wrote from the Calvinist perspective—viewing child rearing as a battle of wills between the inherently sinful child and authoritarian parents—or from the more mellow opinions of enlightenment philosophers like Locke and Rousseau—who advocated a gentle molding of the child, considered innocent at birth—all viewed the family as a microcosm of society and believed that the techniques parents used to raise their children would determine the future character of their community and nation.

During the Enlightenment, with its emphasis on creating a society based on science rather than "superstition," the child no longer appeared as a little adult, but as an impressionable creature that could be molded into a reasonable citizen with the right upbringing, or allowed to develop unsupervised, like an unweeded garden, in haphazard and possibly ruinous fashion.

With the advent of Darwinism and Freudian psychology, the Enlightenment view of the child as a "blank slate" gave way to the notion of the child as inheritor of instincts forged by evolution and of powerful hidden desires. Child rearing experts cautioned against the suppression of these impulses and advised channeling them into activities beneficial to society.

The authoritarian Luther Emmett Holt, author of *The Care and Feeding of Children* (1894), approached the subject as a physician, aiming to put child rearing on a "scientific" basis. He sternly warned new mothers to avoid asking their mothers and grandmothers for advice on how to raise their children. All superstition and baseless traditions of the past must be discarded in favor of an approach forged out of the "scientific method."

Holt was president of the American Pediatric Society, and in this role he presided over crowded pediatric wards where staff was overworked and infant mortality was high. He endorsed bottle feeding using whole milk (milk containing adequate amounts of cream), advocated strict feeding and sleeping schedules, insisted that toilet training

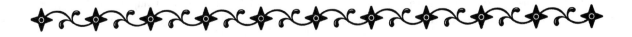

could be achieved by the age of three months and warned mothers not to cuddle or play with their babies, even when they cried. Such treatment over-stimulated them, he said, and gave them germs.

Holt's tome was aimed at the training of mothers and nurses as much as of children; in addition to following lengthy and precise instructions, mothers, like the hospital staff, were expected to keep detailed records of their children's progress.

By the 1920s, books on child rearing couched suggestions in terms of psychology and behaviorism. Following in the authoritarian footsteps of Dr. Holt, John B. Watson considered the programming of children during the first two or three years of life as critical to their future development into manageable workers and citizens. According to Watson, the mature adult was entirely the result of the child's encounter with his environment during the growing years. Like Holt, Watson warned against "too much mother love" and believed that parental detachment helped children develop self control. His book, *Psychological Care of Infant and Child* (1928), sold fifty thousand copies in the first year, and was the force that ushered in the phenomenon of the anxious mother.

More laissez-faire than hardliners like Holt and Watson was Arnold Gesell, author of *Infant and Child in the Culture of Today* (1943). Gesell believed that children should be left alone to go through innately programmed patterns—characterized as innovation, integration and equilibrium—and stages of development. Thus, four-year-olds were "expansive," five-year-olds were "focal" and six-year-olds were "dispersive." But while the child unfolded according to his own internal clock, Gesell enjoined the mother to keep detailed records and fill in color-coded charts so as to spot developmental lags. Even the act of changing diapers called for an entry into the development diary.

THE BITTER LEGACY OF DR. SPOCK

The pediatrician Benjamin Spock believed that writers like Holt and Gesell had created an epidemic of parental "hesitancy" and anxiety. His bestselling book, *The Common Sense Book of Baby and Child Care* (1946)—which has sold fifty million copies—was the first to identify with the feelings of the mothers and opens with the lines: "Trust yourself. You know more than you think you do." Spock offered no theories or charts, acknowledging that the book "really all came out of my head." He argued against feeding schedules and coercive toilet training.

Spock did not demand "unnatural patience" from mothers and although he was not in favor of spanking, he did not consider it a very great evil—it was no worse than "nagging a child for half the day, or trying to make him feel deeply guilty." He felt that children naturally wanted to be good; and he recognized the fact that parents aren't perfect: "We all have our troubles, great or small, and we all take them out on our children to some degree."

Spock sided with mothers, and he also sided with the child: "You sometimes hear it recommended that you should never spank a child in anger, but wait until you have cooled off. That seems unnatural. It takes a pretty grim parent to whip a child when the anger is gone." He warned against punishment that "seems to break a child's heart or. . . break his spirit."

Modern writers have criticized Spock for ushering in an era of permissiveness, but most of today's readers would find his advice on child behavior infused with common sense. "A boy needs a friendly, accepting father," said Dr. Spock, "You can be both firm and friendly."

The bitter legacy of Dr. Spock has less to do with his counsels on the emotional and behavioral aspects of child rearing than with his dietary advice, which if it did not come all out of his head, certainly came out of the early promotional efforts for industrial foods; for Spock was the first child rearing "expert" to endorse processed food for babies, including processed ingredients for infant formula. He was also the first to disparage dietary fats for growing children.

Until Spock published *The Common Sense Book of Baby and Child Care*, pediatricians seeking dietary advice often turned to *Nutrition and Diet Therapy: A Textbook of Dietetics*, by Fairfax T. Proudfit, published throughout the 1930s and 1940s—the eighth edition came out in 1945. Chapter 13, "Artificially Fed Infants," gives us a good example of the collective wisdom of the period: "Nature does not always confer upon a woman the important capacity for nursing her baby, but the women who are able should do so. . . the logical substitute for human milk is cow's milk (or goat's milk)." Proudfit recommended a formula of cow's milk diluted with an equal amount of water and the addition of a small amount of sugar. His first choice for the formula was certified raw milk, "the purest form of raw milk obtainable." He also recommended beef juice, liver and egg yolk as some of baby's first foods. According to Proudfit, baby should receive a few drops of cod liver oil daily, beginning at two weeks, gradually increasing to two teaspoons by the age of three months. However, Proudfit also endorsed infant formula made with pasteurized, sterilized, powdered and condensed milk and suggested introducing cooked cereals at the age of four months.

In *Baby and Child Care*, Spock takes parents much further down the dark alley of processed foods, and he was the first to inculcate a fear of animal fat in infant feeding. He specifically warned against raw milk and, if the milk came from Guernsey cows, suggested pouring off some of the cream. He promoted formula made with evaporated or powdered milk, with sugar added, and skimmed milk when the baby had diarrhea, because "milk is easier to digest when there is no cream in it."[1] He made no mention of cod liver oil but recommended "vitamin drops" to provide vitamins A, C and D.

Empty calories got introduced early in Dr. Spock's regimen, either as orange juice (fresh, frozen or canned) or sugar water given in a bottle. The best weaning food for baby, according to Spock, was cereal, which came before fruit, vegetables, egg yolk and meats.

Baby does not get butter on his vegetables—there is not a single mention of butter in the whole book. Puddings made of milk, egg and starch (tapioca, rice or cornstarch) could be given to baby "for lunch or supper any time after six months. . . supper can be fruit and pudding, or vegetable and pudding."

Spock had nothing against puddings "in jars or cans for babies" except for the fact that "saliva introduced into the container can spoil food rapidly," so baby should not be fed pudding directly out of the can or jar.

Babies could transition to pasteurized milk at nine months, said Spock, but in answer to the question, "When do you change from evaporated to pasteurized milk?" he gave the following startling reply: "The really sensible answer would be 'Never.' Evaporated milk is sterile, cheaper, easier to store, easier to digest, less likely to cause allergy. It's only slightly less convenient to serve. When the baby is off formula, you merely mix equal parts of evaporated milk and boiled water in the cup or bottle just before feeding. . . there's no medical reason why a baby needs to change, so keep him on evaporated milk as long as you are willing to."

Such advice seems incredible today, when even the most conventional books on child rearing warn against highly sugared processed foods for babies, and when the link between diet and behavior in children is emerging with increasing clarity. Like his predecessors as far back as the eighteenth century, Spock devoted a large part of his book to dealing with misbehavior in children—anger, jealousy, whining, tantrums and disobedience—which even the best "firm and friendly" parenting skills have difficulty solving in the malnourished child on a blood-sugar rollercoaster.

Knowledge about nutrition has increased exponentially since Spock wrote *Baby and Child Care*, and most modern books on the subject give lip service to the importance of vitamins and minerals, and fats and oils, not only for physical health, but for brain development, behavior and emotional development. But the information in modern baby books is conflicting, with much of it obviously wrong. And this brings us to the burning question: when it comes to children (and their parents), what constitutes a healthy diet?

THE ENDURING
OBSERVATIONS OF WESTON A. PRICE

One year before *Baby and Child Care* appeared in print, a dentist named Weston A. Price published a book called *Nutrition and Physical Degeneration* (1945). Price was well known and well respected in his field—he had published a textbook on dentistry and was head of research for the National Dental Association. *Nutrition and Physical Degeneration* contained a number of Price's articles, which had appeared separately over the years in dental journals, and included several new chapters in which Price summarized his findings.

Nutrition and Physical Degeneration describes a series of unique investigations, which engaged the author's attention and energies for over ten years. Price was disturbed by what he found when he looked into the mouths of his patients. Rarely did an examination of an adult client reveal anything but rampant decay, often accompanied by serious problems elsewhere in the body such as arthritis, osteoporosis, diabetes, intestinal complaints and fatigue.

But it was the dentition of younger patients that gave him the most cause for concern. He observed that crowded, crooked teeth were becoming more and more common, along with what Price called "facial deformities"—overbites, narrowed faces, underdevelopment of the nose, lack of well-defined cheekbones and pinched nostrils. Such children invariably suffered from one or more complaints that sound all too familiar to today's parents—frequent infections, allergies, anemia, asthma, poor vision, lack of coordination, fatigue, learning disorders and behavioral problems—not to mention the fact that as they reached maturity, their lack of physical attractiveness made them unhappy.

Price did not believe that such "physical degeneration" was mankind's natural state. He was rather inclined to believe that Nature intended physical

perfection for all human beings, and that children should grow up free of ailments.

Price's bewilderment gave way to a unique idea. He would travel to various isolated parts of the world, where the inhabitants had no contact with "civilization," to study their health and physical development. His investigations took him to isolated Swiss villages and a windswept island off the coast of Scotland. He studied traditional Eskimos, Indian tribes in Canada and the Florida Everglades, South Sea islanders, Aborigines in Australia, Maoris in New Zealand, Peruvian and Amazonian Indians and tribesmen in Africa.

These investigations occurred at a time when remote pockets of humanity, untouched by modern inventions, still existed, yet when one modern invention, the camera, allowed Price to make a permanent record of the people he studied. The photographs Price took, the descriptions of what he found and his startling conclusions are preserved in *Nutrition and Physical Degeneration*. Yet this compendium of ancestral wisdom did not enjoy the popularity that greeted Spock's child rearing manual; in fact, even today, Price's book is relatively unknown, although it has remained in print since 1945.

Nutrition and Physical Degeneration is the kind of book that changes the way people view the world. No one can look at the handsome photographs of

PARADISE LOST

"As a child I had an experience similar to that of Weston Price. My family spent six weeks each summer traveling to different parts of the world. Our favorite was the Pacific Islands, so I was there four times, from 1958 to 1968. In that space of time, we noticed dramatic changes in the children on the islands. My father was a gynecologist (infertility specialist) and my mother was an anthropologist/sociologist, so we noticed these things! On our last voyage, when our cruise ship arrived, the crew told us we had to wait to disembark because the Sara Lee coffee cakes got off first. They told us they would be sold out of the stores within twenty-four hours.

"On our first visit, the children we saw were round-faced, with wide beautiful smiles and gleaming even teeth. They always smiled, laughed and ran around playing. By the last visit, they looked like poor Americans, with pinched faces, darkened uneven teeth and sullen expressions. There was more picking on one another than playing. The South Pacific was no longer paradise. During that time, the French completely transformed Papeete, Tahiti for their nuclear program and American Samoa was likewise changed. Even in Hawaii the same thing was evident."

Letter to *Wise Traditions*, Winter 2000

so-called primitive people—faces that are broad, well-formed and noble—without realizing that there is something very wrong with the development of modern children. In every isolated region he visited, Price found tribes or villages where virtually every individual exhibited genuine physical perfection. In such groups, tooth decay was rare and dental crowding and occlusions—the kind of problems that keep American orthodontists in yachts and vacation homes—nonexistent. Price took photograph after photograph of beautiful smiles, and noted that the natives were invariably cheerful and optimistic. Such people were characterized by "splendid physical development" and an almost complete absence of disease, even those living in physical environments that were extremely harsh.

Price described babies and children who were robust, healthy, alert and curious. He noted that primitive village life was rarely interrupted by the sound of a child crying. The cheerful optimism of young and old especially impressed the peripatetic dentist—parents in these cultures did not need advice on dealing with anger, tantrums, whining and destructive conduct because these types of behavior did not exist. And when every individual in a society was attractive, well-formed and healthy, jealousy was rarely an issue. Price came to the conclusion that what his contemporaries referred to as "defects in moral character" were not the result of poor parenting skills or bad genetics but poor nutrition.

The fact that "primitives" often exhibited a high degree of physical perfection and beautiful straight white teeth was not unknown to other investigators of the era. The accepted explanation was that these people were "racially pure" and that unfortunate changes in facial structure were due to "race mixing." Today dentists insist that crowded teeth, narrow faces and other deformities are inherited, or are the result of eating "soft foods."

Price found the racial mixing theory unacceptable. Very often the groups he studied lived close to racially similar groups that had come in contact with traders or missionaries, and had abandoned their traditional diet for foodstuffs available in the newly established stores—sugar, refined grains, canned foods, condensed and pasteurized milk and devitalized fats and oils—what Price called the "displacing foods of modern commerce." In these peoples,

he found rampant tooth decay, infectious illness and degenerative conditions. Children born to parents who had adopted the so-called civilized diet had crowded and crooked teeth, narrowed faces, deformities of bone structure and reduced immunity to disease.

Price concluded that race mixing had nothing to do with these changes. He noted that physical degeneration occurred in children of native parents who had adopted the white man's diet while mixed race children whose parents had consumed traditional foods were born with wide handsome faces and straight teeth. "Individual beauty is a matter of both design of the face and regularity and perfection of the teeth," wrote Dr. Price. "Nature always builds harmoniously if conditions are sufficiently favorable, regardless of race, color or location."

The notion that facial narrowing is due to genetics does not hold up to simple logic: the parents and grandparents of children with facial deformities did not have crooked teeth and facial deformities. Genetic changes do not take place in one generation. And the facial structure of an individual is apparent from the day of birth; it continues to manifest during infancy when the only food is a soft food—milk.

The diets of the healthy "primitives" Price studied were all very different: In the Swiss village where Price began his investigations, the inhabitants lived on rich dairy products—unpasteurized milk, butter, cream and cheese—dense rye bread, occasional meat and organ meats, bone broth soups and the few vegetables they could cultivate during the short summer months. The village was known for the beauty of its women and the strength and athletic prowess of the men; during athletic contests the men drank bowls of pure cream.

The children never brushed their teeth—in fact their teeth were often covered with green slime—but Price found that only about one percent of the teeth had any decay at all. The children went barefoot in frigid streams during weather that forced Dr. Price and his wife to wear heavy wool coats; nevertheless, childhood illnesses were virtually nonexistent, and the village had never known a single case of tuberculosis.

A key finding—one that amazed Dr. Price—was

the emphasis primitive peoples put on special, nutrient-dense foods for parents before conception, for pregnant and nursing mothers, and for children during their growing years, when the body is formed and the connections in the brain are made—for these so-called primitive peoples, childhood was indeed a separate and distinct stage of life. Without the help of scientists or doctors, they instinctively knew that formation and growth require extra nutrition, and that parents needed to prepare themselves in advance so that good nutrition was available from the moment of conception.

For the Swiss villagers, this nutrient-dense food was a special kind of butter—the deep orange butter that came from their cows when they first went to pasture in the spring. They believed that when the cows were eating rapidly growing, bright green grass, the butter they produced was especially nutritious. In fact, the spring butter was a sacred food to the isolated mountaineers, honored with a special ceremony in their churches, in which they placed a bowl of spring butter on the altar and lighted a wick in it to acknowledge its life-giving properties.

Hearty Gallic fishermen living off the coast of Scotland consumed no dairy products. Seafood formed the mainstay of the diet, along with oats made into porridge and oatcakes. The special food for pregnant women and children was fish heads stuffed with oats and chopped fish liver—children consumed stuffed fish heads, not Cheerios and skim milk, every morning for breakfast.

The Eskimo diet, composed largely of fish, fish roe and marine animals, including seal oil and blubber, allowed Eskimo mothers to produce one sturdy baby after another without suffering any health problems or tooth decay. Their sacred food was salmon roe, preserved in the spring and consumed frequently, they told Dr. Price, so they could have healthy babies.

Well-muscled hunter-gatherers in Canada, the Everglades, the Amazon, Australia and Africa consumed game animals, particularly the parts that civilized folk tend to avoid—organ meats, glands, blood, marrow and fat—along with a variety of grains, tubers, vegetables and fruits that were available. Native Americans prepared a kind of milk out of bone marrow for growing children.

African cattle-keeping tribes like the Maasai consumed virtually no plant foods—just meat, blood and milk. Marriage was preceded by a period of special feeding. Many African tribes considered liver a sacred food.

South Sea islanders and the Maori of New Zealand ate seafood of every sort—fish, shark, octopus, shellfish, sea worms—along with pork meat and fat, and a variety of plant foods including coconut, manioc, yams and fruit. They exposed themselves to considerable danger by hunting the shark, because they considered the shark's liver a sacred food, necessary for healthy babies. In addition, the men ate the male reproductive organs of the shark and the women ate the female reproductive organs, to prepare for conception and pregnancy.

Whenever these isolated peoples could obtain sea foods they did so—even Indian tribes living high in the Andes. Andean Indians put a high value on fish roe, which was available in dried form even in the most remote villages. Like the Eskimos thousands of miles to the north, they consumed fish roe in order to have healthy babies.

Insects were another common food in all regions except the Arctic, but especially in Africa. We do not eat insects in the West, but a look through a microscope at stored grains that have not been fumigated is enough to clinch the argument that until recently, most of humankind inadvertently consumed insects.

The foods that allow people of every race and every climate to be healthy are nutrient-dense natural foods—meat with its fat and especially organ meats, whole unprocessed milk products from grass-fed animals, fish, shellfish, insects, whole grains, tubers, vegetables and fruit—not newfangled concoctions made with white sugar, refined flour, processed milk and rancid, chemically altered vegetable oils—not puddings, fruit juice, sugar water and condensed milk.

Price took samples of native foods back to his laboratory in Cleveland and subjected them to analysis. He found that the diets of healthy peoples contained at least four times more minerals and water-soluble vitamins—vitmin C and B complex—than the diet of modernized peoples. Price would undoubtedly find a greater discrepancy today, as we enter the twenty-first century, due to continual depletion of our soil fertility through industrial farming practices, and the wholesale acceptance of processed foods. What's more, among traditional populations, grains, legumes and tubers were prepared in ways that increased vitamin content and made minerals more available—soaking, fermenting, sprouting and sour leavening.

It was when Price analyzed the native foods for fat-soluble vitamins that he got a real surprise. The diets of healthy native groups contained at least ten times more vitamin A and vitamin D than the diet of modernized peoples! These vitamins are found only in animal fats—butter, lard, egg yolks, fish liver oils—and foods with fat-rich cellular membranes like liver and other organ meats, fish eggs and shellfish.

Price referred to the fat-soluble vitamins as "catalysts" or "activators" upon which the assimilation of all the other nutrients depend—protein, minerals and vitamins. In other words, without the dietary factors found in animal fats, all the other nutrients largely go to waste.

Price discovered another fat-soluble vitamin that was a more powerful catalyst for nutrient absorption than vitamins A and D. He called it "Activator X." All the healthy groups Price studied consumed foods rich in Activator X. In fact, these were the very foods they considered so important for fertility and growth—fish liver oil, fish eggs, organ meats and the deep yellow spring and fall butter from cows eating rapidly growing green grass.

The therapeutic value of foods rich in the vitamins A, D and the X Factor was recognized during the years before the Second World War. Price found that the action of "high-vitamin" spring and fall butter was nothing short of magical, especially when small doses of cod liver oil were also part of the diet. He used the combination of cod liver oil and high-vitamin butter oil, made by extracting the unsaturated oils in butter from the harder fats through a slow centrifuge process, with great success to treat osteoporosis, tooth decay, arthritis, rickets and failure to thrive in children.

The identification of Activator X remained a mystery until recently; we now know that Activator X is vitamin K_2, the animal form of vitamin K.[2] Research on vitamin K_2 dovetails perfectly with Dr. Price's findings. Price's lab tests identified Activator X in butterfat, fish eggs, organ meats and animal fats; modern research confirms the presence of vitamin K_2 in butterfat, organ meats and animal fats.

Vitamin K_2 is synthesized by animal tissues, including the mammary glands, from vitamin K_1, which is found in association with the chlorophyll of green plants in proportion to their photosynthetic activity—thus the presence of vitamin K_2 in the spring butter so prized by the Swiss villagers. When cows eat rapidly growing green grass, rich in vitamin K_1, they transform this precursor into vitamin K_2, which is then carried in the butterfat.

Modern science has discovered that vitamin K_2 activates cells to produce proteins after signaling by vitamins A and D—hence the synergy of cod liver oil, rich in vitamins A and D, with high-vitamin butter or high-vitamin butter oil, rich in vitamin K_2.

Price's research indicated that Activator X plays an important role in reproduction, infant growth, facial structure, mineral utilization, bone density, protection from cavities, and protection from fatigue; it supports mental development and neurological health. Price even cured a boy of seizures with a combination of cod liver oil and high-vitamin butter oil.

Modern research has revealed that sperm possess a vitamin K_2-dependent protein; thus the vitamin plays an important role in reproduction. Vitamin K_2 activates proteins responsible for the deposition of calcium and phosphorus in the bones and teeth; the presence of vitamin K_2 in the saliva prevents cavities. And while vitamin K_2 contributes to the development of strong, dense bones, it also protects against the calcification and inflammation of blood vessels and the accumulation of atherosclerotic plaque.

Vitamin K_2 supports energy production in the body—deficiency induces fatigue in laboratory animals.

The brain contains one of the highest concentrations of vitamin K_2, where it is involved in the synthesis of the myelin sheath of nerve cells, thus contributing to learning capacity; and vitamin K_2 is involved in the synthesis of lipids called sulfatides in the brain, the absence of which induces seizures.

Most significantly, vitamin K_2 contributes to infant and childhood growth by preventing the premature calcification of the cartilaginous growth zones of the bones, including the bones of the face. Thus vitamin K_2 supports the development of a wide facial structure, capacious sinus cavities, long nose and attractive high cheekbones. A specific sign of vitamin K_2 deficiency is a "sunken in" structure of cheeks and nose, what Dr. Price referred to as "the underdevelopment of the middle third of the face."

Other dietary practices among healthy primitive peoples included the use of bones, usually as a nourishing bone broth; careful preparation techniques for grains, legumes and nuts; and the use of fermented foods, all of which increase nutrient content and improve digestibility of these foods.

Those groups that consumed milk were characterized by tall stature; milk from cows, goats, sheep, reindeer, camels or water buffalo was always consumed raw and often fermented.

MODERN ADVICE

Unfortunately, the modern world has largely ignored—or even ridiculed—the findings of Dr. Weston Price. Instead, formula feeding and canned baby food have become the foods of choice for infants, and lowfat diets for children are enshrined as national policy.

Most books on infant feeding warn that vitamin A is toxic and that vitamin D must be obtained through a supplement. Vitamin K_2, so necessary for growth, bone density and mental development, is rarely mentioned.

The American Academy of Pediatrics recommends no special foods for pregnancy other than a prena-

---

BAD ADVICE IN BABY BOOKS

"Your body's need for fat [during pregnancy] is minimal, reduce your intake by trimming fat off meat, using less butter, drinking low-fat milk, boiling or steaming foods. . . "
> *The Complete Book of Pregnancy and Childbirth* by Sheila Kitzinger, Knopf, 2003

"Limit total fat intake to 25 to 30 percent of total calories by cutting back on saturated fats in fatty meats and dairy products. . . . You can't eat butter because its high saturated fat content increases the risk for heart disease. . . "
> *Nutrition for a Healthy Pregnancy* by Elizabeth Somer, MA, RD, Owl Books, 2002

"Choose lean meats and trim fat from meat before cooking. With poultry, remove skin."
> *The Everything Pregnancy Nutrition Book* by Kimberly A. Tessmer, RD, LD,
> Adams Media Corporation, 2005

"Saturated fats are the least healthy (fat) and are best used in small amounts. Go easy on butter, fat found in meats, coconut, coconut oils and palm oil."
> *Mothering Magazine's Having a Baby, Naturally* by Peggy O'Mara
> (editor of *Parenting* magazine) and others, Atria 2003

"Babies don't need any oil. . . Children do not need whole milk. They do not need that for the developing brain. That myth is old, was never true and has been discredited."
> *Listening to Your Baby* by Jay Gordon, MD, Perigee Books, 2002

"Your milk has every vitamin, mineral and other nutritional element that your baby's body needs. . . . There's no need to worry about the quality of your milk. Eating more won't make more milk and not eating enough won't make less milk."
> *The Womanly Art of Breastfeeding*, Eighth Edition, La Leche League, 2010

tal vitamin pill and an extra three hundred calories per day; for babies, they suggest cereals as the first food, starting at four months.

The Baby Book, the best-selling tome by William and Martha Sears, contains no dietary recommendations whatsoever for pregnant mothers and warns against saturated fats in foods like eggs and butter for children older than two years. Both the American Academy of Pediatrics and William and Martha Sears specifically follow USDA dietary recommendations, calling for lowfat milk after the age of two.

Not surprisingly, *The Baby Book* devotes a large portion of its pages to dealing with behavior problems, digestive disorders, rashes and respiratory problems like asthma and bronchitis, considering such unfortunate conditions as normal in the course of the childhood years.

Modern books on baby and child care largely warn against the foods formerly considered important for growing children: raw whole milk, butter, liver and other organ meats, bone broths and egg yolks. Cautionary statements against seafood are common, due to misplaced concerns about mercury, and cod liver oil is roundly condemned as a source of "toxic" vitamin A. Fat-phobia now reaches its bony pointed finger down to those who need it most, the very young.

The day is not far off when we will view these puritanical and unscientific restrictions as a severe form of child abuse, worse than corporal punishment, over-strict parenting, child labor or the Victorian suppression of natural instincts.

Even more serious is the medical establishment's wholesale acceptance of soy foods—known to be toxic—starting with soy-based formula for the vulnerable infant and progressing to soy milk, soy protein and tofu for the toddler. Pregnancy and childcare magazines in particular have heavily promoted soy foods as "natural" or "alternative" health foods for growing children, putting the soy-fed generation at risk for nutrient deficiencies, growth problems, digestive disorders, learning disorders, hormonal disturbances and infertility.

Another obsession shared by modern child rearing "experts" is germs. While sterile conditions are necessary in the operating room and in the treatment of open wounds, the rampage against germs in baby's day-to-day environment is not only futile, but counterproductive.

During the last twenty years, the old paradigm—that the intestinal tract should be sterile and that germs attack us and make us sick—has given way to the discovery of beneficial bacteria and the many ways in which they support good health. The new paradigm recognizes the necessity of up to six pounds of beneficial bacteria lining the intestinal tract. These microorganisms play many important roles: they help digest our food, they prevent the absorption of toxins and heavy metals like mercury, they keep the few species of harmful bacteria at bay, they support the immune system, they produce vital nutrients and they even play a role in the production of feel-good chemicals.

Thus a key goal for today's parents lies in creating the conditions necessary for the proliferation of beneficial bacteria in the intestinal tract and, through good nutrition, the creation of a healthy symbiotic relationship between the infant and the multitudes of "germs" with which he comes in contact.

As lowfat diets, soy foods and sterile environments will soon be relegated to the dust heap of discarded medical ideas, so too will the practice of vaccinations. A child vaccinated according to the official schedule today receives over three dozen shots before entering school, starting with day one after birth. Profit and influence have prevented physicians from admitting the harm done by so many vaccines (or even any vaccines), all carrying a load of neurotoxins, all interfering with the development of natural immunity.

Modern baby books tend to gloss over the consequences of bad advice about nutrition and dangerous interventions like vaccination; unfortunately, without the tools of good nutrition and a recognition of the body's innate wisdom, there is not much useful advice these books can give to a parent whose child has severe asthma, allergies, frequent infections, cancer, so-called "genetic" disorders, disruptive behavior, growth problems and learning disorders—not to mention the living hell of autism, now afflicting as many as one child in seventy.

These conditions burden not only the child, but the child's whole circle of relatives; they disrupt family life, drain finances and create devastating emotional conflicts. Modern baby books do not prepare parents for the tragedy of serious disease; and when disease occurs, they insist that nothing can be done, that the cause is "genes" or "germs," against which we are helpless.

In spite of—or perhaps because of—the advice of well meaning "experts" and health officials, modern parents in fact tend to be anxious, hesitant and distrustful of the natural world; clearing baby's path with antibacterial wipes; slathering on sunscreen before dressing their children (just in case they might be exposed to the sun); clamoring for strong drugs including antibiotics at the first sign of a sniffle; vaccinating against every possible illness, trundling their youngsters off to lessons, sports and preschool. In short, they focus on everything but what children need most from their parents: good nutrition provided in an atmosphere of freedom to develop, balanced with careful discipline and unconditional love.

RUDOLF STEINER ON THE DEVELOPMENT OF THE CHILD

It was the Austrian philosopher, social thinker and esotericist Rudolf Steiner (1861-1925) who first discussed childhood as a separate stage of existence.

According to Steiner, the human being is actually composed of four bodies: a physical body, which is the material body that we perceive with our senses; the etheric or life body, which comprises the plant-like, liquid and electronic forces in the body; the astral or emotional body, often referred to as the soul, which houses our instinctive and subconscious life and which we share with the animal kingdom; and the ego, mental or thinking body, which houses the spirit and is unique to the human being.

Each seven years of human development corresponds to the development of one of these four bodies.

It is during the first seven years of existence, from birth to the change of teeth, says Steiner, that the forces of development are focused most intently on the physical body—a concept echoed in the practices of so-called primitive peoples with their emphasis on special nutrient-dense foods during the period of pregnancy and early growth.

During the second seven-year period, the etheric or life body unfolds; during this state, children are subject to the various illnesses of childhood, such as measles and mumps.

The emotional body reaches maturity during the sometimes stormy adolescent years, from the onset of puberty at age fourteen to the age twenty-one.

The ego body, the forces of clear thinking and individualism, emerge only during the fourth stage, from age twenty-one until age twenty-eight.

Steiner describes the child up to the age of seven as "one big sensory organ," with which most parents—observing their toddlers putting objects into their mouths or making a beeline for an electrical socket or dish of cat food—would agree.

During this age, the child learns by imitating, and his most important activity is play. The modern tendency to force intellectual learning on young children, and to structure their lives with classes, lessons and team sports, deprives children of the vital development that accrues from unstructured, imaginative play, and can have serious consequences on the child's emotional and intellectual development. A child deprived of time and freedom for play during the early years may tend to engage in escapist, childish activities for the rest of his life. And well nourished children will learn to read, write, study and think when the time is appropriate; we do children no service by forcing them into these activities before the seventh year.

In agreement with many other philosophers of his day, Steiner believed that within every human being was an "ideal human being," a complete and harmonious ego capable of giving love in perfect freedom; and that only such human beings could give rise to a harmonious, just and free human community.

Thus, the role of the parent is important indeed, and we would agree with the early writers of child rearing books that the way we bring up our children determines the character of human society in the years to come. But we do not say this to instill hesitancy or anxiety, only to provide inspiration, along with practical guidelines.

Steiner warned against extremes. The life fully lived, he said, was a life consciously and precisely guided between opposing tendencies—between materialism and mysticism, between discipline and relaxation, between structure and laissez-faire. This is good advice for parents torn between strict "parentist" and relaxed "childist" philosophies of child rearing, between "helicopter" and hands-off parenting. Parents do well when they avoid extremes, providing gentle discipline but also freedom to play within the structure of family life, good nutrition through delicious meals, and an example of relaxed self-discipline, above all avoiding the extremes of constant disapproval and smothering affection.

And while your child is engaged in the very serious business of growth and play, you as parent can observe and enjoy. For the universe holds no greater wonder than the developing child, especially the very healthy developing child; and if parents know how to provide the foods for optimal physical growth, and the environment for optimal emotional and spiritual growth, they can sit back, relax and let Nature do the rest.

FOR MORE INFORMATION

Nutrition and Physical Degeneration by Weston A. Price, DDS, published by the Price-Pottenger Nutrition Foundation, www.ppnf.org.

Raising America: Experts, Parents and a Century of Advice About Children by Ann Hulbert.

Chapter 1
Preparing for Your Baby

This book puts a primary emphasis on nutritional preparation before and during pregnancy—more than any other book on this subject and more than on any other subject in this book. The diet of both mother and father before conception, and the diet of the mother during pregnancy, will determine to a very large extent the appearance, intelligence and physical health of their baby, and in addition will contribute to their child's emotional and mental well-being.

No other society is as careless about preparation for pregnancy and birth as our own; our haphazard approach stands in sharp contrast to the wisdom and dedication that Dr. Weston A. Price observed in traditional cultures, which often practiced a period of special feeding for men and women before conception, and always provided special nutrient-dense foods during pregnancy, lactation and growth. Even worse is the modern corpus of appalling advice—a society that advocates lowfat or vegetarian diets, or endorses processed foods for pregnant women and growing children, is a society that has lost its way, has sacrificed the health of its young people to convenience, dogma and financial gain.

When things go wrong, when baby is born too early, or with a birth defect, or exhibits some abnormality in growth and behavior, genetics often gets the blame. By blaming genetics, we absolve ourselves of responsibility. But modern research has shown us that nutrition in fact affects the expression of the genes, and poor nutrition can so adversely affect genetic expression that "defects" persist for several generations.

The production of healthy babies indeed constitutes a partnership between ourselves and the Creator; God provides the blueprint, the genetic code, while we, the parents, provide the building materials. Together we can build magnificent body temples to house the souls of future generations, the souls who will make the planet a better place, the souls who will ensure that peace and justice reign on the Earth.

We write these words not to discourage you or to frighten you, but to *inspire* you to adopt the best dietary practices you can, because the rewards, both to yourselves and to your offspring, are very great.

WHAT IS A HEALTHY BABY?

A healthy baby is robust, well formed, energetic and free of birth defects; a healthy baby has a broad face, strong bones and a wide palate, allowing the teeth to grow in straight; a healthy baby has clear skin, good eyesight and keen hearing; a healthy baby has a good immune system, rarely catches a cold or gets sick; a healthy baby has a good digestive system, nurses well, does not spit up food and has normal

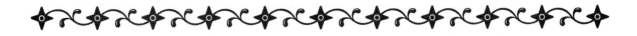

bowel movements; a healthy baby is free of allergies, rashes and asthma; a healthy baby has a good disposition, rarely cries, is cheerful and outgoing, smiles frequently and sleeps well; a healthy baby is alert and curious, babbles and takes directions early; a healthy baby passes her milestones, such as sitting up, crawling, standing and speaking, on schedule; a healthy baby responds to affection but can also amuse herself and play alone without needing attention. Healthy babies grow up into healthy, intelligent, attractive, self-disciplined and high-functioning adults.

Good nutrition for ensuring a truly healthy baby needs to start before baby is conceived. If you have been following a nutrient-dense diet according to the principles outlined in this chapter for some time, then your period of preparation need only be about six months. But if you have been consuming a standard American diet, full of junk food, or alternatively if you have been following a so-called "healthy" lowfat, vegetarian or vegan diet, you should count on two to three years of preparation before conception. This may seem a long time for those eager to have a family, but we would urge you not to rush. A malnourished or depleted body needs time to recover, and that recovery needs to take place before, not during, your pregnancy.

See the sidebar, opposite, for a list of foods to consume in preparation for a healthy pregnancy, as well as a list of foods to avoid. Many of the recommended foods may be unfamiliar to you; you may even have been told that our recommended foods are bad for a pregnant woman and her developing baby. You may even find some of these foods difficult to eat. Let's discuss the importance of each of these dietary elements one at a time. (For sample recipes, see Recipes.)

COD LIVER OIL

Until the end of the Second World War, cod liver oil served as the number one supplement for pregnant women and growing children—doctors, nurses, health officials, teachers, ministers, Sunday school teachers and government agencies, all urged the population to take cod liver oil in order to protect themselves from infectious disease and ensure strong bones and teeth.

Books on infant feeding recommended cod liver oil starting in the third month of life, even cod liver oil drops as early as the third week.

With the advent of antibiotics, the campaign for cod liver oil waned; today government agencies discourage cod liver oil, especially for pregnant women, claiming that the vitamin A in cod liver oil can contribute to birth defects (see Sidebar, page 17).

Actually, the vitamin A content of cod liver oil is the most important reason for taking this old-fashioned supplement. Vitamin A is critical for the optimal expression of the genetic potential, for strong bones, healthy skin, keen eyesight, mineral metabolism, hormone production, mental stability and even the ability to plan for the future and stick to tasks.[1]

It is vitamin A that gives the undifferentiated fetal stem cells (sometimes called germ cells) their sig-

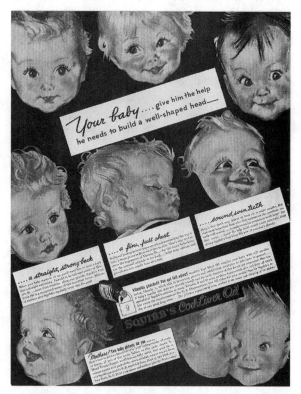

A 1930s ad for Squibbs cod liver oil. "Your baby . . . give him the help he needs to build a well-shaped head. . . a straight, strong back. . . a fine full chest . . . sound even teeth. . . Daily use is important." Cod liver oil taken before conception and during pregnancy gives your baby the benefits of vitamins A and D before he is even born.

THE DIET FOR HEALTHY BABIES

The diet for producing a healthy baby—and for keeping baby's parents healthy during pregnancy, throughout baby's growing years and beyond—should start before conception and includes the following:

- Cod liver oil to supply about 20,000 IU vitamin A and at least 2000 IU vitamin D per day.
- 4 cups whole raw milk daily and/or 5-6 ounces aged raw cheese.
- At least one egg daily, preferably from pastured chickens, with as many additional yolks as possible added to smoothies, salad dressings, scrambled eggs, custards, homemade ice cream, etc.
- 4 tablespoons butter or ghee daily, preferably from pasture-fed cows; 1/4-1/2 teaspoon high-vitamin butter oil daily is optional.
- 2-4 ounces fresh liver (beef, lamb, chicken, duck, turkey, goose) at least two times per week
- Fresh seafood, two to four times per week, particularly fish eggs, shellfish, oily fish like sardines, and wild salmon.
- Fresh beef, pork or lamb daily, always consumed with the fat.
- Oily fish or lard daily, for vitamin D; duck fat or goose fat occasionally for vitamin K_2.
- 2 tablespoons coconut oil daily, used in cooking, smoothies, or melted in hot water.
- Lacto-fermented condiments and beverages.
- Bone broths used in soups, stews and sauces.
- Properly prepared whole grains, legumes and nuts.
- Fresh vegetables and fruits, preferably organic and in season.
- Unrefined salt.

It is also important to avoid all processed foods, fast foods and junk foods containing:

- *Trans* fatty acids (partially hydrogenated oils).
- Liquid commercial vegetable oils.
- Refined sweeteners such as sugar, high fructose corn syrup, yacon syrup, agave "nectar."
- Artificial sweeteners such as Equal, Nutrasweet and Splenda.
- White flour, boxed breakfast cereals and improperly prepared grains.
- Modern soy products.
- Caffeine and caffeine-like substances (coffee, tea and chocolate).
- Microwaved and irradiated food.

In addition, avoid:

- Tap water containing fluoride, chlorine and other chemicals.
- Exposure to pesticides, herbicides and industrial chemicals.
- Cigarettes.
- Alcohol.
- Vaccinations.
- Synthetic vitamins.
- Drugs, even prescription drugs.

nals to differentiate into the various organs, such as heart, liver and lungs. If a women with low vitamin A status becomes pregnant, the heart in the fetus cannot form properly, and the newly pregnant woman may suffer a miscarriage; or, the heart may form incorrectly, resulting in a serious birth defect.

Each organ system begins development during a specific window of time. Vitamin A regulates the differentiation of the primitive cells into cells specific to each organ system, in essence signaling to the genes their marching orders so they "know" where to locate themselves and what kind of tissues to become. If vitamin A is lacking during any of these brief periods, the organs develop abnormally or not at all.[2]

According to recent research, even partial vitamin A deficiency affects the sensitive developing central nervous system; vitamin A plays a key role in the development of the visual system, the retina of the eye, the inner ear, the spinal cord, the craniofacial area including the sinus passages and dental arches, and the thymus, thyroid and parathyroid glands.[3]

During mid-gestation, vitamin A is required for fetal lung development. In vitamin A-deficient animals, congenital malformations in the urogential system occur.

Most interesting is new research on the effect of vitamin A on kidney development. Vitamin A deficiency results in a reduced number of nephrons (kidney cells) in the kidney. Lower numbers of nephrons mean the kidneys will not work at optimal levels and may doom the individual to dialysis later in life.[4]

Another fascinating avenue of research has shown that vitamin A holds the key to what scientists call the "holy grail" puzzle of developmental biology: the existence of a mechanism that ensures the exterior of our bodies develop symmetrically while the inner organs are arranged asymmetrically. Vitamin A provides the signal that buffers the influences of asymmetric cues in the early stages of development, and allows the body to develop symmetrically. In the absence of vitamin A, the exterior of our bodies develops asymmetrically, resulting in the right side shorter than the left side.[5] A shorter right foot or smaller right eye is a sign of mild vitamin A deficiency in utero.

After the formation of all the organ systems, vitamin A supports their growth. Chronic vitamin A deficiency during pregnancy compromises the liver, heart and kidneys and impairs lung growth and development during the last weeks of gestation.[6]

A key role of vitamin A is to provide protection against environmental chemicals, such as dioxins, and estrogenic substances in pesticides, plastics and the lining of tin cans. These substances can cause birth defects, so in a toxic world, the protective role of vitamin A is critical.[7]

Many books for expectant parents insist that pregnant women can get adequate vitamin A from leafy green plant foods and orange and yellow vegetables and fruits. These foods contain carotenes, the precursors to vitamin A. Humans are able to convert a small portion of carotenes into true vitamin A, but not enough to meet the high requirements for reproduction and pregnancy. In fact, too much dietary carotene carries a certain amount of risk. In addition to conversion to vitamin A, carotenes can also be converted into a number of potentially harmful products within the cell, compounds that may cause cancer and even interfere with vitamin A activity.[8]

Unfortunately, the U.S. Food and Drug Administration (FDA) and other government agencies warn pregnant women to avoid foods like liver and cod liver oil, claiming that too much vitamin A from these foods can cause birth defects. A review of the scientific literature (see Sidebar, opposite) shows that these concerns are unwarranted.

However, vitamin A consumed without vitamin D can be problematic. Studies in Scandinavia have correlated high vitamin A intake with osteoporosis and increased hip fractures. But these harmful effects occur only when vitamin D intake is low—in Scandinavia, where vitamin D is lacking due to the long winters, vitamin A added to breakfast cereals and other processed foods leads to vitamin A overdose. Vitamin A taken alone will result in a deficiency of vitamin D, and it is this deficiency that leads to bone problems. Vitamins A and D work together, and when there is adequate intake of vitamin D, vitamin A is toxic only at extremely high levels.[9]

The beauty of cod liver oil is that it can provide vitamins A and D together—two vitamins that are difficult to obtain in adequate amounts in the Western diet but that traditional cultures consumed in large amounts. Vitamin D works hand in hand with vitamin A to ensure optimal development of the fetus. Vitamin D consumed before pregnancy will prepare the mother's bones, teeth, organs and brain for the additional stresses of pregnancy.

Fathers should also take cod liver oil—vitamin A is needed for sperm production in men and vitamin A protects the sperm against damage from environmental chemicals such as dioxins and bisphenol A.[10]

VITAMIN A AND FETAL DEVELOPMENT

The U.S. Food and Drug Administration (FDA) and other government agencies warn pregnant women to avoid foods like liver and cod liver oil, claiming that too much vitamin A from these foods can cause birth defects.

The claim that intakes of vitamin A over 10,000 IU per day can increase the risk of birth defects can be traced back to a 1995 paper published by a group of researchers at Boston University.[11]

The researchers followed almost twenty-three thousand women over the course of their pregnancies and found that women who consumed more than 10,000 IU vitamin A during the first trimester gave birth to offspring with a greater risk of certain types of birth defects.

However, the study had some serious flaws. Most of the vitamin A came from multivitamins. The authors did not distinguish between various food sources—and most "food" vitamin A comes from fortified breakfast cereals—so the cause of the birth defects may well have been something else in the multivitamins or in the cereals. Three groups of experts wrote to the journal questioning the authors' classification of the types of defects.[12]

Most importantly, the authors may have underestimated the rate of certain types of birth defects in the group with low vitamin A intake. The rate of total birth defects among the twenty thousand women consuming less than 10,000 IU was only 1.5 percent; by contrast, the generally accepted background rate is 3-4 percent. The rate of defects among the three thousand women consuming more than 10,000 IU of vitamin A was 3 percent—on the lower end of normal.[13]

The most serious objection to this study is the fact that it conflicts with all the other evidence. For example, a 1990 study conducted in Spain found that among twenty-five thousand births, doses of vitamin A over 40,000 IU per day carried a 2.7-fold higher risk of birth defects, but doses of vitamin A up to 20,000 IU or between 20,000 and 40,000 IU both carried a 50 percent *lower* risk of birth defects compared to no supplementation.[14]

A 1996 study of over five hundred thousand births found that the children of women supplementing with at least 10,000 IU of vitamin A in addition to a multivitamin had a lower risk of birth defects than those of women who did not supplement, although the association could not be distinguished from the effects of chance.[15]

A 1997 study of fifteen hundred births found no relationship between birth defects and use of vitamin A supplements, fortified breakfast cereals, organ meats or liver.[16]

A 1999 prospective study of three hundred eleven mothers who consumed between 10,000 and 300,000 IU of vitamin A in the first trimester and a similarly sized group that did not supplement with vitamin A found no evidence of an increased risk of major malformations with increasing dose. The median dose was 50,000 IU.

The supplemented group as a whole had a 50 percent *lower* risk of major malformations than those who did not supplement, and there were no major malformations in offspring born to mothers consuming more than 50,000 IU.[17]

The preponderance of the evidence clearly favors the view that 20,000 IU of supplemental vitamin A per day during pregnancy is safe and may even reduce the risk of birth defects.

The best source of vitamins A and D is high-vitamin fermented cod liver oil (see Sources). Cod liver oil also provides an important omega-3 fatty acid called DHA, docosahexaenoic acid, needed for brain development.

The Weston A. Price Foundation recommends 20,000 IU of vitamin A and 2,000 IU of vitamin D from cod liver oil during pregnancy. This can be obtained from just under two teaspoons high-vitamin cod liver oil, an amount that also supplies about two grams of omega-3 fatty acids—the same amount shown in one study to prevent premature delivery.[18]

We hope that this lengthy discussion has convinced you of the importance of taking cod liver oil. Still, for many, the idea of taking this oily, smelly substance can be daunting. Here is yet another reason to begin a special nutrient-dense diet long before you conceive—you may need time to get used to new and unusual foods like cod liver oil.

The best way to take cod liver oil is to mix it with a small amount of warm water, whole raw milk or fresh juice, stir and gulp down quickly. Alternately, you can take cod liver oil in capsules, but this will be more expensive—because many capsules are needed to get an adequate dose of vitamins A and D—and possibly not as effective. If you find that cod liver oil makes you burp, or that you experience the taste of cod liver oil long after taking it, try taking it immediately before eating. It may help to divide your dose into three, taking a smaller dose before each meal. A teaspoon of Swedish bitters mixed with water taken with the same meal may also help (during pregnancy, use the special formulation for pregnant women--see Sources).

It is important that the cod liver oil you take provide the right ratio of vitamin A to vitamin D. Some commercial brands of cod liver oil contain very little vitamin D. The ratio of vitamin A to D should be ten units or fewer of vitamin A to one unit of vitamin D.

The fermented high-vitamin cod liver oil we recommend is sold under several brand names. It is made according to old-world processing techniques and filtered at low temperature to remove impurities. It is never heated and contains all the original vitamins, with nothing synthetic added. The ratio of A to D is about eight to one. Slightly less than two teaspoons per day will supply, in addition to 20,000 IU vitamin A, about 2500 IU vitamin D. For brands of lower potency, you will need about four teaspoons

THE DOCUMENTED BENEFITS OF COD LIVER OIL

A number of studies have demonstrated the benefits of using cod liver oil during pregnancy.

- Rats fed cod liver oil during pregnancy give birth to offspring that have higher cognitive performance than controls at six months. If rats are fed a protein-deficient diet during pregnancy, their offspring have disturbed glucose metabolism; if they are also fed cod liver oil along with the protein-deficient diet, however, the glucose metabolism of their offspring is normal.[19]

- In Norway, use of cod liver oil during pregnancy was associated with a 70 percent reduced risk of type 1 diabetes.[20]

- A study of over ten thousand infants in Finland conducted between 1966 and 1997 showed that direct supplementation of 2,000 IU vitamin D from cod liver oil per day to infants in the first year of life virtually eradicated the risk of type 1 diabetes over the next thirty years.[21]

- Women who used liquid cod liver oil in early pregnancy gave birth to heavier babies, even after adjusting for the length of gestation and other confounding factors. Thus cod liver oil protects against the dangers of low birth weight and ensures that the infant starts life at a good, robust weight.[22]

- Children born to mothers who took cod liver oil during pregnancy and lactation scored higher on intelligence tests at age four compared with children whose mothers took corn oil.[23] Vitamins A and D are necessary for the optimal formation and function of the brain; in addition, cod liver oil supplies a special fat called DHA, also very necessary for brain function.

per day to obtain 20,000 IU vitamin A and 2000 vitamin D. (For recommended brands of cod liver oil, see Sources.)

Skate liver oil is another good choice, as is halibut liver oil, but not ordinary fish oils. These are made using a highly industrial process, tend to be rancid, and are not good sources of vitamins A and D. Use of fish oils during pregnancy may be associated with excessive bleeding at birth (see page 85).

EGGS AND EGG YOLKS

Egg whites provide perfect protein and egg yolks contain a powerhouse of nutrients, chief among them being choline, which is critical for the development of the brain. Choline is especially important for the formation of cholinergic neurons (neurons that use the neurotransmitter acetylcholine), which takes place from day fifty-six of pregnancy through three months after birth; and for the formation of the connections between these neurons, called synapses, which occur at a high rate through the fourth year of life.[24]

When choline is lacking, these connections cannot take place; adding choline to the diet in later years will not compensate for missing choline during growth—the window of opportunity, when the body is programmed to make these connections, will have closed.

The mother's intake of choline—lots of choline—can have a beneficial effect for the entire life of her offspring. Rats fed three times the normal choline requirement during pregnancy give birth to offspring with remarkably resilient nervous systems. These offspring have a lifelong thirty percent increase in visuospatial and auditory memory; they grow old without developing any age-related senility; they are protected against the assaults of neurotoxins; and they have an enhanced ability to focus on several things at once.[25]

The RDA for non-pregnant women is 425 mg choline per day. The RDA for pregnant women is 450 mg per day, only 25 mg more. However, rat studies suggest that an amount two to three times more may provide your baby with lasting benefits.

Egg yolks are the richest source of choline, containing about 680 mg per 100 grams, or 115 mg per yolk. It is not necessary to eat more than one egg white per day in preparation for conception and during pregnancy, but you cannot eat too many yolks! You need four yolks to satisfy even the modest government recommendations. Choline also occurs in liver and dairy foods, and to a lesser extent in meats (especially pork), nuts and legumes, but to ensure an adequate supply you should consume at least two egg yolks per day—and more is better. Add extra egg yolks to scrambled eggs and omelets, consume raw egg yolks in smoothies, eat them in custards, soufflés and homemade ice cream, or mix them with hot rice or oatmeal.

Egg yolks are also a wonderful source of cholesterol, yet another important nutrient that our government officials have demonized. Prospective parents should in no way limit cholesterol intake—all sex hormones are made from cholesterol as are the hormones the body makes to deal with stress. Mothers need extra cholesterol to help the fetus develop the brain and nervous system, as well as the intestinal tract, and a cholesterol-rich diet should continue throughout the period of growth—and indeed throughout life.

Egg yolks also provide vitamins A, D, K_2 and E as well as folate, biotin and important minerals like iron, zinc and selenium; the levels of vitamins and minerals will be higher if the eggs come from hens allowed to roam on green pasture in the sunlight. In a study conducted by *Mother Earth News*, folate levels were over two hundred times higher in pastured eggs than in eggs from chickens raised in confinement.[26] Organic eggs are a second best choice with supermarket eggs coming in third. But even if conventional supermarket eggs are your only choice, don't be afraid to eat liberally of the yolks. The future intellectual ability of your child may depend on it.

BUTTER

Butter is the queen of fats, especially when it comes from grass-fed cows. Grass-fed butter will be a rich source of vitamins A, D, K_2 and E—needed for the development of body and brain—as well as selenium, copper, zinc and chromium. Butter provides iodine—critical for thyroid function. It is rich in cholesterol and also contains lecithin, needed for the proper utilization of cholesterol. And butter contains DHA, vital for brain development and function.

All these nutrients are fairly heat stable, so will survive pasteurization. But raw butter contains an anti-stiffness compound called the Wulzen factor, which is destroyed by heat.

Most importantly, butter provides arachidonic acid (AA), an under-appreciated type of fat that is essential for healthy skin, intestinal integrity and brain function. The many roles of AA include promotion of sustained, goal-oriented behavior by supporting dopamine production in the central nervous system; prevention of excito-toxicity and epilepsy; formation of the cell-to-cell junctions essential to skin and intestinal health; and support of the immune response and the resolution of inflammation. It is essential to fertility and to blood clotting.[27] The principal sign of AA deficiency is dry, scaly skin (the water evaporates due to lack of cell-to-cell junctions).

It's not hard to get the recommended four tablespoons of butter into your daily diet. Use butter liberally on sourdough bread or crackers, put it on oatmeal, sauté your vegetables and meats in butter or

RAW MILK SAFETY

According to the FDA, raw milk is "inherently dangerous" and should not be consumed, especially by pregnant women. Actually, the government's own statistics show that raw milk is a very safe food. Data gleaned from U.S. government websites and government-sanctioned reports on foodborne illnesses show that the risk of contracting foodborne illness by consuming raw milk is much smaller than the risk of becoming ill from other foods.

The key figure that permits a calculation of raw milk illnesses on a per-person basis comes from a 2007 Centers for Disease Control (CDC) FoodNet survey, which found that 3.04 percent of the population consumes raw milk, or about 9.4 million people, based on the 2010 census.[28] This number may in fact be larger as raw milk is growing in popularity. For example, sales of raw milk increased 25 percent in California in 2010, while sales of pasteurized milk declined 3 percent.

A compilation of published reports of illness attributed to raw milk from 1999 to 2010 shows that during the eleven-year period, illnesses attributed to raw milk averaged forty-two per year.[29] Many of these cases are unconfirmed, but using these numbers, we find that the rate of illness from raw milk is about .00044 percent, hardly a basis for calling milk "inherently dangerous." There are an estimated 48,000,000 cases of foodborne infections per year in the U.S. in a population of about 300,000,000. The rate of illness from all foods can be calculated at 16 percent. Thus, one is at least 35,000 times more likely to contract illness from other foods than from raw milk.

Another way of looking at the data is as follows: Between 1998 and 2005, there were over 10,000 documented outbreaks that contributed to 199,263 documented cases of foodborne illness. Raw milk was associated with 0.4 percent of these cases, a number that is probably exaggerated due to extreme government bias. There is no way to quantify whether any one of these foods is safer than another from this data, but it is clear from the data that there is no basis for singling out raw milk as "inherently dangerous."

It is important to note that there have been no deaths attributed to raw milk for many years. Pasteurized milk killed dozens of people during the 1980s and three people in Massachusetts in 2007; pasteurized mother's milk killed four infants in 2003; and pasteurized cheese killed seven people in Europe in 2009. Recently we have had deaths from cantaloupe, spinach, luncheon meat, red peppers and peanuts. Raw oysters kill about fifteen people per year, but the FDA has no plans to ban the sale of raw oysters.[30]

It is irresponsible for government officials to oppose raw milk, claiming that it is inherently hazardous. *Rather, government data show that raw milk is inherently safe.*

ghee, add it to vegetables and sauces. And remember that cream is mostly butterfat, so use cream liberally in soups and sauces, on hot oatmeal, in homemade ice cream and as whipped cream on fruit.

For those with a very low tolerance to dairy protein, use ghee (which is butter with the milk proteins removed) instead of butter.

WHOLE RAW MILK
AND/OR RAW MILK CHEESE

Our recommendation to consume raw milk during pregnancy runs completely counter to U.S. government recommendations. According to the Food and Drug Administration, "drinking raw milk is like playing Russian roulette with your health," and is especially dangerous for pregnant women.

What these government agencies don't tell you is that the dangers of raw milk are greatly exaggerated, and reports associating raw milk with illness are highly biased.[31] Furthermore, any food that is not handled properly can cause illness—including pasteurized milk—and raw milk is unique among the foods we consume in that it contains numerous factors that actually kill pathogens while strengthening the immune system.

Raw whole milk from pasture-fed cows provides a complete source of nutrition that is easy to digest and assimilate. While there are not many published studies comparing raw with pasteurized milk, the few that we do have indicate that raw milk is vastly superior to pasteurized for building strong bones and teeth, for protecting against infection, allergies and asthma and for building immunity. In addition, many consumers of pasteurized milk diagnosed as lactose intolerant can consume raw milk without difficulty.[32]

The milk pregnant women consume should be not only raw, but full fat from grass-fed cows.

As described in *Nutrition and Physical Degeneration* by Weston Price, the Maasai tribes of Africa allowed men and women to marry only after spending several months consuming milk from the wet season when the grass was especially lush and the milk much denser in nutrients. Maasai milk is higher in fat and cholesterol and lower in sugar than commercial American milk. The highest quality Maasai milk, used for preconception diets, is even richer: compared to commercial American milk, it has over twice the cholesterol, nearly three times the fat, and over five times the quantity of choline than the milk available in grocery stores.[33]

RAW MILK AND *LISTERIA*

The FDA often cites raw milk as causing infection with *Listeria monocytogenes*, a deadly food-borne pathogen that can result in severe illness and fetal death, premature birth or neonatal illness and death.

Yet a 2003 USDA/FDA report found that compared to raw milk, there were over five hundred more illnesses from *Listeria monocytogenes* due to deli meats and twenty-nine times more illness from *Listeria monocytogenes* due to pasteurized milk. On a per-serving basis, deli meats were *ten* times more likely to cause illness from *Listeria monocytogenes* than was raw milk.[34] Yet FDA does not issue public warnings for pregnant women to avoid pasteurized milk and deli meats—a clear double standard.

In a response to a Freedom of Information Act request, the Centers for Disease Control provided data on raw milk outbreaks 1993-2005—a thirteen-year period. In this report, CDC listed *no* cases of food-borne illness from raw milk caused by *Listeria* during the period.[35]

What *can* cause severe illness from *Listeria* infection is soft, unaged cheese, both raw and pasteurized. In 2009, there were four deaths in Europe from pasteurized soft cheese;[36] and there have been numerous illnesses and miscarriages from soft, unaged "Mexican style" cheese made from raw milk. Pregnant women would do well to avoid soft unaged cheese of every type; but fluid raw milk and aged cheeses made from raw milk are safe and healthy foods for pregnant women.

Compared to grain-fed milk, grass-fed milk (and cheese from grass-fed milk) is much higher in fat-soluble vitamins, pigments, conjugated linoleic acid (CLA) and omega-3 fatty acids. Weston Price showed that the content of vitamin A and vitamin K_2 increased markedly in butterfat during the rainy lush season.[37] As the quality of grass increases, we can presume that the content of other grass-related nutrients—such as pigments, vitamin E and CLA—will also markedly increase in the milk.

As with any new food, raw milk may take some getting used to. Some people report slight constipation or runny stools on first consuming raw milk—this is why future mothers need to get used to this wonderful food before becoming pregnant. And of course, it is important to obtain your milk from a clean source. In some states you can purchase carefully regulated raw milk in stores; in states where raw milk is available only from farms, be sure to visit the farm and talk with the farmer. The milk should come from cows fed mostly green grass or hay with only a small amount of grain, be milked under clean conditions and chilled quickly after milking. In addition, it is important for the farmer to have the milk tested regularly to ensure low bacteria counts and an absence of pathogens.

For additional benefits, raw milk can be cultured to make butermilk, kefir or yogurt. Fermented milk products are even easier to digest than sweet milk, and they provide beneficial bacteria for the digestive tract.

If you cannot obtain raw milk where you live, then consume raw cheese, which is legal and available in

RAW MILK VERSUS PASTEURIZED

Studies carried out in the early part of the 1900s showed that raw milk was vastly superior to pasteurized milk for growth, for building strong bones and teeth, for protecting against illness, and even for behavior.[38] New studies indicate that raw milk is highly protective against asthma and allergies.[39] Reseach shows that many of the vitamins and minerals in raw milk are lost during pasteurization or are poorly absorbed after heat treatment:

VITAMIN C: Raw milk but not pasteurized can resolve scurvy. ". . . Without doubt. . . the explosive increase in infantile scurvy during the latter part of the 19th century coincided with the advent of use of heated milks. . ."[40]

CALCIUM: Animal studies show the formation of longer and denser bones on raw milk compared to pasteurized. The calcium levels in raw and pasteurized milk are the same, but the body uses the calcium from raw milk more effectively.[41]

FOLATE: The carrier protein for folate is inactivated during pasteurization.[42]

VITAMIN B_{12}: Raw milk contais a binding protein for vitamin B_{12} that results in complete assimilation; the activity of this enzyme is diminished by pasteurization.[43]

VITAMIN B_6: Animal studies indicate B_6 is poorly absorbed from pasteurized milk.[44]

VITAMIN A: Beta-lactoglobulin, a heat-sensitive protein in milk, increases intestinal absorption of vitamin A. Heat degrades vitamin A.[45]

VITAMIN D: Vitamin D in raw milk is bound to lactoglobulins; pasteurization cuts assimilation in half.[46]

IRON: Lactoferrin, which contributes to iron assimilation, is inactivated during pasteurization.[47]

IODINE: Levels of iodine are lower in pasteurized milk.[48]

MINERALS: Minerals in milk are bound to proteins that assure assimilation; these proteins are inactivated by pasteurization; Lactobacilli, destroyed by pasteurization, enhance mineral absorption.[49]

all states; raw cheese is also available through the Internet (see Sources).

The goal is to consume 1500 mg calcium per day, which is provided by five cups of whole milk or seven to eight ounces of cheese. You will obtain some calcium from other foods, so four cups of whole raw milk or five to six ounces of raw cheese—or some combination of milk and cheese—should be adequate for your calcium needs.

In addition to calcium and fat-soluble vitamins, raw dairy foods also provide phosphorus, B vitamins including B_6 and B_{12}, vitamin C, cholesterol and CLA, all in a form that is easy for the body to absorb—thus raw milk is particularly important for those who suffer from malabsorption and other digestive problems.

If you are intolerant of all dairy products, even raw and fermented dairy products, you will need to pay extra attention to other sources of calcium, such as bone broths, anchovies and sardines.

LIVER

Liver was considered a sacred food in almost all traditional cultures, necessary for strength, stamina and for the production of beautiful, healthy babies. There is good reason for the reverence accorded to liver, because of all the foods in the human diet, liver is the most nutrient-dense. For example, beef liver contains over 50,000 IU vitamin A per 100 grams—chicken, duck and goose liver about 30,000 IU per 100 grams—and about 110 mg vitamin B_{12} per 100 grams, over sixty times more than the amount found in beef.

In addition, liver is an excellent source of phosphorus, iron, zinc, copper, vitamin B_2, vitamin B_6, choline, biotin and folate. Liver actually contains more vitamin C per gram than apples or carrots.[50] In addition, chicken, duck and goose liver are among our best sources of vitamin K_2.[51]

Vitamin K_2 is critical for the development of your baby's bone structure, teeth, blood and brain. In conjunction with vitamins A and D, liberal amounts of vitamin K_2 in the diet ensure wide, attractive facial development, with plenty of space for the teeth to come in straight. Vitamin K_2 is also found in the fats of grass-fed animals, such as meat fats, butter and cheese, but poultry liver is the best source of vitamin K_2 in western diets.[52]

Unfortunately, for many people, eating liver represents a real challenge. A large portion of young people today have never eaten liver even once in their lives, and they find the taste and texture objectionable.

But there are many palatable ways to eat liver: fried in bacon fat with bacon and onions, puréed with bread crumbs and made into dumplings, enjoyed as paté, Braunschweiger or liverwurst. (See Recipes and Sources.)

By the way, cooking lamb or beef liver, rich in vitamin A, in lard or bacon fat, rich in vitamin D, provides a synergistic combination of these two key vitamins.

For those who can't stand even these gourmet versions, you can take desiccated liver capsules (see Sources). Some even swallow raw frozen liver cut into pea-sized pieces. Liver and other nutritious organ meats can also be grated raw or ground and mixed with ground beef or lamb in meat loaf, chile and casseroles.

The important thing is that you prepare for conception by eating liver in one form or another at least twice a week, and then continue the practice during pregnancy. Not only will liver help ensure a healthy child, but it will give you strength, stamina and a healthy outlook throughout your pregnancy.

SEAFOOD

A real battle rages among U.S. government agencies about whether or not to recommend seafood for pregnant women. Those who object cite higher levels of mercury in fish, as well as PCBs and other toxins. But defenders of seafood for pregnant women point out that although women who have higher levels of mercury in their blood tend to have children with lower intelligence, those who eat two or more servings of fish per week have babies of higher intelligence. The beneficial effects are credited to the omega-3 fatty acids in fish, but fish is also a good source of iodine and other trace minerals that support neurological function.

The findings of the Avon Longitudinal Study of Parents and Children (ALSPAC), a UK study involving about fourteen thousand women and their children, show that the benefits of eating most types of seafood during pregnancy far outweigh any risks.[53] The most important finding: women who eat twelve ounces or less of seafood per week were almost 50 percent more likely to have children with low verbal IQ scores compared with women who exceeded this amount. At age three, children whose mothers ate less seafood during pregnancy were more likely to have social and communication problems with their peers and by ages seven and eight, they tended to have more behavioral problems and trouble with fine motor skills.

Part of the confusion about whether fish consumption contributes to the mental development of the next generation comes from the fact that our exposure to mercury is not limited to the mercury in the fish we eat. Mercury can be in the air, in processed foods (such as high fructose corn syrup) and, most troubling, in amalgam fillings, which outgas mercury fumes directly into the mouth and brain.[54] And the absorption rate of mercury from fish depends on a number of factors, including the health of our gut flora. Healthy bacteria in the intestinal tract will actually trap food-borne mercury and prevent its absorption.[55] Adequate selenium and glutathione levels in the body also protect against mercury. The best source of glutathione is raw milk.[56]

In the context of the healthy diet that we recommend, fish consumption before and during pregnancy is both safe and beneficial, although we would caution against overconsumption of large fish like swordfish and tuna (which tend to concentrate mercury), and commercial freshwater fish like catfish (which can be very high in pollutants like PCBs).

And don't neglect the more nutrient-dense types of seafood, including the skin on fish fillets, the vitamin A-rich heads (for making fish soup, see Recipes), shellfish such as shrimp, crab, lobster, mussels and oysters, and above all, fish eggs (also called fish roe).

Caviar—salted fish roe—is associated with wealth and luxury, but Weston Price discovered that fish eggs were prized as a fertility food among cultures as diverse as the Alaskan Eskimo and the South American Incas. In China, fish eggs are said to bestow intelligence—especially skill in arithmetic—on growing children, and the Europeans honor caviar as an aphrodisiac.

Science completely validates these traditions; we now know that fish eggs are rich in vitamins B_{12}, vitamin K_2, cholesterol, choline, selenium, calcium, magnesium, vitamin A, zinc, iodine, trace minerals and DHA—all necessary for healthy reproduction and the development of the endocrine system, the nervous system and the brain. Caviar is also extremely rich in vitamin D—containing over 10,000 IU per tablespoon according to an independent analysis carried out by the Weston A. Price Foundation.

Not all caviar is hugely expensive—American paddlefish caviar, pale blond caviar and salmon roe can be had for a reasonable price, and a single ounce (two tablespoons) will stretch for two or three meals. (See Sources for well-priced caviar and Recipes for delicious ways of serving this quintessentially healthy food.)

MEAT

Fresh meat can and should be included in the diet every day—this includes lamb, beef, pork, goat, poultry and game. Whenever possible, this meat should come from naturally raised, grass-fed animals.

Meat should always be consumed with the fat—or in the case of poultry, with the skin. If the meat is lean, cook it in a fat like lard or butter, or eat it with butter or a cream-based sauce. The fat provides valuable nutrients and makes it easier for you to digest the meat.

Meat is a rich source of complete protein, iron and zinc, all needed for building baby's body, blood and brain; meat fats provide important minerals, fatty acids and the anti-cancer substance CLA. And, like butter, meat fats provide arachidonic acid (AA), so important for neurological development (11 percent of the brain is arachidonic acid), gut integrity and beautiful rash-resistant skin.

OILY FISH OR LARD

The large amount of vitamin A you will be consuming from liver needs to be balanced by additional vitamin D, found in foods like oily fish or lard. Don't be afraid to cook in lard—pasture-fed lard is stable and healthy, and it provides a particularly rich source of vitamin D (see Sources). Oily fish like anchovies and sardines are another source of vitamin D: they make a great snack. The bones are also a good source of calcium.

COCONUT OIL

This wonderful fat will strengthen your immune system and protect you against infection, will give you plenty of energy without causing unwanted weight gain, will nourish healthy bacteria in the colon, and may even contribute to the optimal development of your baby's brain and nervous system. You can use coconut oil for gentle sautéing or add it to smoothies, but the best way to take it is to melt one or two tablespoons in hot water or herb tea. As a natural pick-me-up, coconut oil is a great substitute for coffee or tea.

BONE BROTHS

Homemade broth made from the bones of chicken, duck, beef, lamb or fish is a magic gelatin-rich food that will help you digest your food, will contribute to strong bones, tendons and connective tissue in both yourself and your developing baby, and will protect the integrity of your digestive tract. For those who have trouble digesting meats, adding a gelatin-rich sauce often solves the problem.

Homemade broth is rich in the amino acid glycine, which is conditionally essential during pregnancy. Usually our bodies are able to make enough glycine to meet our basic survival needs; during pregnancy, however, additional glycine must be obtained from food. Glycine is the limiting factor for protein synthesis in the fetus, and thus almost certainly a limiting factor for fetal growth. Glycine is also needed for the synthesis of the placenta and protection of both mother and baby from toxins and stress.[57]

The fetus can obtain glycine from two sources: the placenta transports glycine from the mother's blood, or it uses folate to manufacture it from an-

---

THE GAPS DIET

The Gut and Psychology Syndrome (GAPS) diet, formulated by UK physician Natasha Campbell-McBride, MD, is designed to heal the intestinal tract and help the body detoxify. The diet eliminates all grains, sugars and starches, which all contain large amounts of complex sugars called disaccharides. These are digested by disaccharidases, enzymes produced by the lining of the small intestine. When the intestine is damaged or inflamed, production of disaccharidases all but ceases, and these undigested starches then feed yeasts and other undesirable microorganisms in the gut; they also wreak havoc on the immune system and even cause changes in behavior. Eliminating these carbohydrate foods for a period allows the intestine to heal and disaccharidase production to resume. The diet includes copious amounts of homemade bone broth to heal the digestive tract as well as lacto-fermented foods, animal protein and good fats.

The GAPS diet can be highly beneficial for a myriad of conditions, including leaky gut syndrome, digestive disorders, chemical sensitivities and psychological disorders such as ADD, ADHD, depression and autism. Details of the diet, which we recommend for children with digestive and learning disorders, are found in Appendix II.

However, the diet is not appropriate or safe for pregnant and breastfeeding women as it is a diet that encourages detoxification, and dislodged toxins may threaten the fetus or infant.

If you suffer from digestive disorders, the GAPS diet may be highly effective in curing them; but it should be undertaken *before* pregnancy, with a six-month interval between ending the diet and the beginning of pregnancy. The same can be said for any detoxifying or unusual diet—pregnancy is not the time to participate in dietary extremes or experiments.

other amino acid called serine. The mother's best source of glycine is collagen-rich foods such as skin and cartilage, or bone broths. When she consumes these foods, there will be plenty of glycine on hand for her baby.

Glycine balances methionine, an amino acid found in eggs and meat. When we consume large amounts of methionine from muscle meats, we need glycine to safely dispose of it; otherwise it can disrupt cellular communication, leading to a variety of problems, such as mental disorders or cancer.[58] It is therefore best to always consume muscle meats with sources of extra glycine such as bones and skin.

Folate from liver, legumes and green vegetables works together with glycine to help the body clear excess methionine.[59] It is important, therefore, for the expectant mother to liberally match her egg and muscle meat consumption not only with glycine-rich skin and bones but also with folate-rich liver, legumes and greens.

LACTO-FERMENTED CONDIMENTS AND BEVERAGES

Lacto-fermentation is a process that preserves foods, including vegetables, fruits, milk, meat and fish. The process involves bacteria working primarily on sugars and starches to produce lactic acid, a natural preservative. (Alcoholic fermentation involves yeasts working on sugars to produce alcohol, also a preservative.) Lacto-fermented foods are rich in enzymes, lactic acid and good bacteria, which together help digestion.

Good bacteria in the gut are critical to good health. In addition to their role in digestion, they keep potentially harmful microorganisms like Candida in balance and parasites at bay, they strengthen the immune system, they produce important nutrients, and they even produce feel-good chemicals. Most importantly, good bacteria coat the intestinal tract with a biofilm that serves as our first line of defense against environmental toxins. Good bacteria lining the gut will latch on to mercury and take it out of the body; ditto for toxins like dioxins. Scientists are beginning to realize that the good bacteria lining our intestinal tract provide an important component of our immune system.[60]

Good bacteria in mom's gut will also flourish in her birth canal and even in her milk ducts. Baby's environment in the womb is thought to be sterile, but the bacteria that baby encounters during birth are the bacteria that will populate his own intestinal tract. Thus it is critical that pregnant women encourage the growth of beneficial bacteria in the gut; and since these good bacteria prevent the absorption of environmental chemicals that can harm the developing fetus, mothers need to encourage the growth of good gut bacteria well before baby is conceived. The vehicle for inoculating the intestinal tract with good bacteria, and for keeping them there, is lacto-fermented foods.

The most familiar lacto-fermented food is traditional sauerkraut—raw sauerkraut preserved by lacto-fermentation, not by using sugar or vinegar, nor by canning or pasteurizing. Many other plant foods besides cabbage can be preserved in this way—cucumbers, carrots, beets, turnips, onions, herbs, fruits like apples and berries, even pineapple (see Recipes).

Buttermilk, yogurt and kefir are also lacto-fermented foods and will be especially beneficial if they are made at home from raw milk rather than in a factory (see Recipes). Other lacto-fermented foods include traditionally made salami and *gravlax* (Scandinavian lacto-fermented salmon).

The principle of lacto-fermentation can also be applied to beverages and used to produce healthy versions of ginger ale and fruit sodas (see Recipes). A popular lacto-fermented beverage called kombucha is available in most health food stores. Fermented grain drinks, including kvass from Russia, are excellent sources of good bacteria. A medicinal beverage called beet kvass can be especially helpful for treating Candida overgrowth and reestablishing healthy gut flora after antibiotic use (see Recipes).

If you are new to lacto-fermented foods, you should introduce them slowly. As with any new food, they can cause temporary changes, such as loose stools or even detoxification reactions like hives. Kombucha and beet kvass are especially useful for detoxification—something that needs to happen well before conception and not during pregnancy.

WHOLE GRAINS, LEGUMES AND NUTS

Whole grains, legumes and nuts can provide excellent nutrition—in particular magnesium to balance the calcium in dairy products—but only if prepared carefully. While rich in nutrients, these foods also contain anti-nutrients that can block assimilation, interfere with digestion and irritate the intestinal tract—none of which should occur while you are pregnant or preparing for a pregnancy.

Proper preparation involves soaking whole grains or freshly ground whole grain flour in a warm, slightly acidic medium, such as water with a small amount of lemon juice, vinegar, buttermilk, yogurt, kefir or whey added; or soaking them in full-strength buttermilk, yogurt or kefir.

The combination of warmth, moisture and slight acidity over time breaks down the anti-nutrients, neutralizes irritants like tannins, increases vitamin content, liberates minerals and makes the grains much more digestible (see Recipes). Genuine sourdough techniques for making bread accomplish the same thing, as well as "digest" gluten.

Legumes provide choline, folate, phosphorus and many important minerals, including magnesium. But legumes contain high levels of enzyme inhibitors, which can block digestion; phytic acid, which can block mineral uptake; as well as difficult-to-digest carbohydrates. Legumes need to be well soaked and then well cooked.

Nuts are a nutritional powerhouse, our best source of magnesium; but they are high in phytic acid, which can block mineral assimilation; in enzyme inhibitors, which can cause irritation and indigestion; and in oxalic acid, which can block calcium assimilation and lead to kidney stones. Nuts like almonds, pecans, walnuts, macadamia and cashews should be soaked in salt water for six to eight hours, then drained and dehydrated in a warm oven or dehydrator (see Recipes). They can then be used in desserts, stuffings and sauces, or eaten in moderate quantities as a nutritious snack food.

FRESH VEGETABLES AND FRUITS

While most books on pregnancy put vegetables and fruits first on the list, we put them near the end.

Vegetables and fruits lend variety and interest to the diet, but they are not nearly as nutrient-dense as animal foods—the emphasis for a healthy pregnancy and optimal fetal development should be on meat and organ meats, dairy foods, eggs and seafood.

Vegetables and fruits contain only a fraction of the nutrients per gram found in meats, dairy foods and organ meats. However, they are good sources of vitamin C, folate and minerals like magnesium. Most importantly, fruits and vegetables make great vehicles for good fats like butter and cream; in fact, the nutrients in fruits and vegetables are more easily assimilated when they are served with these healthy fats.

Leafy green vegetables are a good source of folate, a critical nutrient for the growing fetus. But they also contain oxalic acid, which can block calcium uptake and form painful deposits in the joints, kidneys and other organs. Foods like spinach, chard, mustard greens and kale should be well cooked and served with liberal amounts of butter, lard or fatback.

Cruciferous vegetables like cabbage, broccoli and Brussels sprouts contain goitrogens that can block thyroid function and use up valuable iodine; they are fine if cooked or fermented and eaten in moderation.

In fact, you will get a lot more out of most fibrous vegetables if they *are* cooked. The human digestive tract is not designed to deal with a lot of raw fiber. If you have trouble with digestion or suffer from acid reflux (GERD), even salads should be avoided. (Tender lettuce and salad greens tend to be low in fiber so most people can eat them raw.)

Potatoes, sweet potatoes and similar starchy vegetables are rich in disaccharides. If you have suffered from intestinal damage, such foods may be extremely difficult to digest until the gut heals. If you have no trouble digesting such starchy foods, they can be included in the diet—always with plenty of butter, of course.

High-pectin fruits like apples, pears, peaches and nectarines may be more digestible if cooked—and delicious served with whipped cream or homemade ice cream. But many fruits can be eaten raw—

MAKING THE TRANSITION

The desire for a normal pregnancy and healthy offspring is a great motivator for making improvements in diet and lifestyle. Fortunately, the foods that you can and should be eating are delicious and satisfying. They provide good substitutes for nearly every type of processed food. Consult the Weston A. Price Foundation Shopping Guide for brand names and sources of healthy food products.

INSTEAD OF. . .	CONSUME WITH CONFIDENCE
Pasteurized, homogenized, reduced-fat commercial dairy products	Whole raw milk and cheese from pasture-fed cows
Commercial yogurt	Homemade yogurt and kefir made from raw, whole milk
Commercial luncheon meats containing many additives	Additive-free artisan preserved meats, such as salami, sausage, bacon, ham, liver paté and liverwurst
Lean commercial meats and skinless chicken	Grass-fed meats, consumed with the fat; grass-fed poultry consumed with the skin
Fast food hamburgers	Homemade hamburgers using full fat, grass-fed meat
Farmed fish; skinless fish fillets	Wild seafood including fish skin, shellfish and fish eggs
Bottled sauces filled with MSG and other additives	Gravies and sauces made with homemade bone broths
Margarines and spreads	Butter
Cooking oils	Cook in grass-fed lard, butter, ghee, duck fat and goose fat; or coconut oil or olive oil
Commercial salad oils	Cold-pressed or extra virgin olive oil
Commercial salad dressing	Make your own with cold-pressed or extra virgin olive oil and other natural ingredients
Fast food French fries	Potatoes sautéed in lard, butter or olive oil; baked or mashed potatoes with plenty of butter
Egg substitutes; egg whites	Real eggs from pastured hens, mostly the yolks
Fish oils	Cod liver oil
Artificial flavors, MSG	Natural herbs and spices; sauces made from bone broth
Commercial pickles	Lacto-fermented pickles and sauerkraut

MAKING THE TRANSITION

Soft drinks	Lacto-fermented sodas such as ginger ale, kvass and kombucha
Extruded breakfast cereals	Oatmeal, soaked overnight and cooked, served with butter or cream, a natural sweetener and chopped crispy nuts
Potato chips, corn chips and other snack foods	Plain pork cracklings, crispy nuts
Commercial bread	Genuine sourdough bread
Commercial refined salt	Unrefined salt
Commercial ice cream	Homemade ice cream made with egg yolks from grass-fed chickens, heavy cream (not ultrapasteurized) and natural sweeteners
Commercial cookies, sweets, highly sweetened desserts	Homemade cookies, custards and desserts using natural sweeteners, egg yolks, crispy nuts and other healthy ingredients
Caffeine (coffee, tea, chocolate, soft drinks, energy drinks)	Lacto-fermented sodas, coconut oil melted in hot water, coffee substitutes such as Dandy Blend and Cafix

berries, tropical fruits (which supply helpful enzymes for digesting protein) and citrus fruits (which are a good source of vitamin C).

Do your best to purchase organic vegetables—remember that most pesticides are estrogenic and could adversely affect the development of the fetus. Pesticides also tend to be high in cadmium, a toxic metal. There will be a lot more nutrition in vegetables and fruits that are raised without pesticides, produced locally, vine ripened and consumed in season.

SALT

Your body needs salt—without salt you can digest neither carbohydrates nor protein. Cellular metabolism depends on the sodium from salt, and salt supports adrenal function.

Salt also plays a critical role in your child's neurological development because sodium activates an enzyme needed for the production of glial cells in the brain—these are the cells that support logical and creative thinking.[61]

Formula makers discovered the role of salt in a very tragic way when they came out with a low-sodium formula; children who consumed this formula suffered permanent neurological damage.[62] Mothers need to maintain a good sodium status throughout pregnancy and breastfeeding.

The best salt for a healthy pregnancy is unrefined salt (see Sources), which provides not only sodium chloride but also magnesium and many trace minerals. Refined salt is devoid of these nutrients and also contains an aluminum compound that prevents the salt from clumping, so that it "pours when it rains."

THE DANGERS OF PROCESSED FOODS

Avoid processed foods. Period. The ingredients in processed food spell nothing but trouble for prospective parents, pregnant and nursing mothers, and growing children.

First and foremost are the *trans* fats found in partially hydrogenated oils, margarines and shortenings, and hidden in processed foods like cookies, crackers, bread, pastries, chips and other snack foods. Commercial fried foods are another source of *trans* fats. *Trans* fats interfere with growth and neurological development; consumption of *trans* fats is associated with low-birth-weight babies—and low birth weight is associated with a myriad of problems in the infant, even chronic illness like heart disease later in life. *Trans* fats impair growth and interfere with learning ability. Even a tiny amount of *trans* fats in the diet of the pregnant and nursing mother can result in reduced visual acuity.

When *trans* fats are incorporated into the cell membrane they inhibit receptors and enzymes. *Trans* fats are the chief cause of type 2 diabetes, a condition in which the cell membrane receptors for insulin do not work. They also interfere with hormone production, disrupting sexual development and causing the infant to be less resistant to stress.[63]

Do not be fooled by labels stating that a product contains zero *trans* fats; that simply means that the serving sizes have been made ridiculously small so the total per serving contains less than one-half gram of *trans*. And *trans* fats in mono- and diglycerides do not require labeling and are not counted in the totals; likewise for *trans* fats formed during the deodorizing of liquid vegetables oils.

As the dangers of *trans* fats have become widely known, the industry has returned to using more liquid oils in processed food products. But these have their own dangers. Vegetable oils from corn, soy, cottonseed, canola, safflower and sunflower seeds contain fragile polyunsaturated fatty acids that are heavily damaged by high-temperature processing. The result is a product loaded with free radicals, the toxic breakdown products of processed oils, which can cause cancer, depress the immune system and impair growth.

In addition to cooking oils, products like ready-made dressings, toppings, dips and spreads all contain these harmful oils. Use butter and cream instead, and make your own salad dressing using pure olive oil.

Refined sweeteners in processed food should also be avoided as much as possible. The metabolism of sugar uses up large amounts of vitamins, minerals and enzymes and creates a roller-coaster of high and then low blood sugar levels. The list of conditions caused by consumption of sugar is a long one, and includes diabetes, hypoglycemia, more frequent infectious illness, heart disease, cancer, digestive problems, endocrine problems, infertility, skin problems, obesity, increased desire for alcohol, coffee and tobacco, Candida overgrowth, bone loss, dental decay, hyperactivity, violent tendencies and depression. Clearly it's best to kick the sugar habit before you get pregnant as a prelude to strictly limiting sugar in your growing family.

High fructose corn syrup and its cousins agave "nectar" and yacon "syrup" are even worse than sugar, especially for the period of growth. Currently the preferred sweetener in soft drinks and many food products aimed at children, high fructose sweeteners cause serious abnormalities in test animals, particularly growing animals. Fructose has a detrimental effect on the liver and in conjunction with copper deficiency (widespread in the U.S.) interferes with the production of collagen.[64] If you want a child who is sturdy and strong, who doesn't injure easily, and whose liver is capable of dealing with environmental toxins, do your best to avoid high fructose corn syrup. Agave "nectar" or "syrup" and yacon "syrup" contain even more free fructose than high fructose corn syrup.

Artificial sweeteners, such as Equal, Nutrasweet and Splenda, are not good alternatives. Sold as Equal, Nutrasweet and AminoSweet, aspartame can cause severe neurological reactions including headaches, seizures and a dangerous sudden drop in blood pressure. Linked to brain cancer and damage to the retina of the eye, aspartame stimulates the release of insulin and plays havoc with neurotransmitters. And there is no evidence that aspartame as a substitute for more caloric sugar leads to weight loss; on the contrary, many people show increased food consumption on a diet containing aspartame.[65]

The other main artificial sweetener, sucralose (sold as Splenda) is equally problematic. Test animals fed sucralose developed a shrunken thymus gland (hence reduced immunity), enlarged liver and kidneys, a decrease in red blood cells and a tendency to diarrhea. Most serious for those wishing a normal pregnancy and healthy children, sucralose caused prolonged or aborted pregnancy, low birth weight in offspring and reduced growth rate.[66]

Clearly these toxins should have no place in the diet of pregnant women, or those hoping to conceive. Fortunately there are many natural sweeteners that parents can use in moderation to satisfy their sweet tooth—such as raw honey, maple syrup, Rapadura (dehydrated cane sugar juice) and maple sugar—without posing a threat to their offspring. Lacto-fermented beverages like kombucha, which are available commercially and also easy to make, provide an excellent and healthy replacement for soft drinks (see Recipes and Sources).

Next we come to the plethora of grain products on the market, starting with white flour, depleted of nutrients and spiked with bleaching agents. White flour is the main ingredient of pasta, crackers, pastries, cookies and most commercial bread, food products that also contain industrial oils, refined sweeteners and, in the case of bread, dozens of additives.

GENETICALLY MODIFIED FOODS

The evidence that genetically modified (GM) foods—plants with foreign genes inserted into the DNA—cause health problems, especially to the fetus and to growing chidlren, continues to mount:

- Scientists at the Russian Academy of Sciences reported between 2005 and 2006 that female rats fed Roundup Ready-tolerant GM soy produced excessive numbers of severely stunted pups with more than half of the litter dying within three weeks, and the surviving pups completely sterile.[67]

- In 2005, scientists at the Commonwealth Scientific and Industrial Research Organization in Canberra, Australia reported that a harmless protein in beans (alpha-amylase inhibitor 1) transferred to peas caused inflammation in the lungs of mice and provoked sensitivities to other proteins in the diet.[68]

- From 2002 to 2005, scientists at the Universities of Urbino, Perugia and Pavia in Italy published reports indicating that GM soy affected cells in the pancreas, liver and testes of young mice.[69]

- In 2004, Monsanto's secret research dossier showed that rats fed MON863 GM corn developed serious kidney and blood abnormalities.[70]

- In 1998, Dr. Arpad Pusztai and colleagues formerly of the Rowett Institute in Scotland reported damage in every organ system of young rats fed GM potatoes containing snowdrop lectin, including a stomach lining twice as thick as controls.[71]

- Also in 1998, scientists in Egypt found similar effects in the guts of mice fed Bt potato.[72]

- The U.S. Food and Drug Administration had data dating back to early 1990s showing that rats fed GM tomatoes with antisense gene to delay ripening had developed small holes in their stomachs.[73]

- In 2002, Aventis company (later Bayer Cropscience) submitted data to UK regulators showing that chickens fed glufosinate-tolerant GM corn Chardon LL were twice as likely to die compared with controls.[73]

- In 2012, researchers found that female rats fed Roundup Ready-tolerant GM corn developed large tumors and dysfunction of the pituitary gland; males also developed tumors and exhibited pathologies of the liver and kidney.[74]

Obviously, GM foods should not be fed to children and should be completely avoided by pregnant women. Fortunately, this is fairly easy to do when following our diet, which necessarily excludes processed foods. The three main GM food crops are corn, soy and canola oil, with GM sugar beets now entering the marketplace. Some papayas and crooked neck squash are genetically engineered, with more fruits and vegetables in the pipeline. GM ingredients are not allowed in organic foods, so the best defense is to eat only organic versions of any crop that has GM varieties, and to avoid products that contain corn, soy, canola oil and refined sugar.

Whole grain breads can be equally problematic, as the grains are ground at high temperatures (hence rancid) and are not subject to the careful preparation techniques that make them digestible. Many so-called healthy breads contain added gluten, which is extremely hard to digest and can even cause toxic shock in some people. And most breads today contain soy flour, to be avoided at all costs.

Cold breakfast cereals are made by a high-pressure, high-temperature process called extrusion, which distorts the delicate proteins in grains—similar to the distortion of delicate milk proteins that occurs during pasteurization—and renders them toxic to the nervous system.[75] That can translate into problems with concentration and behavior, as well as digestive problems (there are as many nerve endings in the gut, the second brain, as there are in the brain). These cereals may even be somewhat addictive, so the difficult adjustment to life without them needs to take place well before you conceive.

Soy products should be strictly avoided—they are loaded with phytoestrogens that can cause hormonal imbalances and thyroid problems, and oxalates and enzyme inhibitors that can cause extreme digestive distress. In addition, they contain high levels of phytic acid that can block the uptake of important nutrients like zinc, calcium, iron and magnesium.[76]

Phytoestrogens are strong anti-fertility agents that may prevent you from becoming pregnant; and if you consume soy foods while pregnant, these endocrine disruptors can cross the placenta and have an adverse effect on the infant. Even at very low levels, exposure to genistein, the main phytoestrogen in soy, caused behavior changes in rodents, including increased signs of stress, decreased social contact and altered sexual expression.[77]

Another concern is additives in our food. The average American consumes nine pounds of additives per year, including preservatives, dyes, bleaches, emulsifiers, antioxidants, artificial and "natural" flavors, conditioners, extenders, anti-caking agents and thickeners.

The most dangerous additive is the neurotoxic free glutamic acid, also known as monosodium glutamate (MSG), often disguised as hydrolyzed vegetable protein, yeast extract or "natural" flavors. Any-

thing hydrolyzed, autolyzed or extracted is likely to contain free glutamic acid. Citric acid and sodium and calcium caseinates contain free glutamic acid, as does powdered milk added to reduced-fat dairy products. Modern soy products contain free glutamic acid (MSG), which is formed during processing. In addition MSG may be added to mask the soybean's bitter taste.[78]

Next comes caffeine and caffeine-like substances, in all their guises—coffee, tea, soft drinks, energy drinks and chocolate. Caffeine gives you a lift by stimulating the secretion of adrenaline, and then the adrenal cortex needs to work very hard to produce the corticoid hormones that bring the body back to homeostasis. The result over time is nutrient depletion and adrenal exhaustion.

An interesting theory holds that a woman with depleted adrenal function can "steal" adrenal hormones from her developing fetus, condemning the newly born child to compromised adrenal function from the moment of birth.[79] The corticoid hormones produced by the adrenal glands regulate almost every aspect of our metabolism, including blood sugar levels, blood pressure, mineral metabolism, healing and stress responses. They are also involved in the production of sex hormones.

One of the most important gifts you can give to your child is strong, well functioning adrenal glands, and that means kicking the caffeine habit well before you conceive.

Finally, a word on microwaved and irradiated foods. These processes destroy nutrients and render the delicate fatty acids rancid.[80] Stick to old fashioned cooking methods and avoid microwaved and irradiated food. A good substitute for the microwave is a countertop convection toaster oven. This cooks food rapidly and evenly using old fashioned heat.

ADJUSTING TO A NUTRIENT-DENSE DIET

If you are already familiar with the principles of healthy traditional diets, and have been putting them into practice for some time, your pre-pregnancy diet need only involve increasing your intake of cod liver oil and nutrient-dense foods—like egg yolks, raw dairy products, liver and fish eggs—for a period of about six months before conception.

MENUS FOR NUTRIENT-DENSE MEALS

Here are some suggestions for nutrient-dense meals (for recipes, see Appendix III). As you can see, eating a healthy diet does not mean depriving yourself in any way.

BREAKFAST: High-fat and nourishing, to get your day off to a good start

- Pastured eggs, any style, with good quality bacon, optional sourdough toast and butter, fresh fruit, glass of raw milk
- Soaked oatmeal with pastured butter, cream and/or egg yolks mixed in, natural sweetener, glass of whole raw milk
- Smoothie made with homemade kefir and/or yogurt, fresh fruit, natural sweetener, egg yolks and coconut oil
- Homemade pancakes with butter, natural sweetener, and MSG-free sausage or bacon, glass of raw milk
- Oyster fritters, fresh or stewed fruit with cream
- Raw cheese, additive–free ham with sourdough bread and butter
- Paté with sourdough bread or crispy pancakes, stewed or fresh fruit with cream
- Smoked salmon and cream cheese on sourdough bread or crispy pancakes

LUNCH: Keep it simple! Lunch is the perfect opportunity to consume nutrient-dense sacred foods.

- Homemade soup with sourdough bread, butter and raw cheese
- Caviar or salmon roe with sour cream on crispy pancakes
- Chicken liver paté on crispy pancakes, sourdough bread or endive leaves
- Salad of lettuce or baby greens, with chopped meat, bacon, anchovies, raw cheese, tomatoes and croutons fried in butter, lard or duck fat.
- Omelet containing extra egg yolks
- Leftovers from previous dinner
- Tacos or taco salad using organ meat mixture (see Recipes), tortillas fried in lard
- Salmon Salad (Salade Niçoise)
- Chicken or salmon salad

DINNER:
Start with homemade soup or salad

Main course of
- Meat, organ meat, fish or poultry with broth-based sauce
- Fresh vegetables with plenty of butter
- Potato, sweet potato, brown rice or other whole grain (optional)

Dessert of
- Fresh or stewed fruit
- Homemade ice cream
- Raw cheese with sourdough bread or crackers
- Cookie, homemade with natural ingredients

BEVERAGES: Whole raw milk, kombucha, lacto-fermented soft drinks, sparkling water with squeeze of lemon and a pinch of salt.

NOTE: If you are gaining too much weight, eliminate the starch (potato, sweet potato, brown rice or other whole grain) and forgo the dessert.

But if all this is new to you, if your diet has consisted largely of junk food and fast food, if you have been practicing a vegetarian, vegan or lowfat diet, or if you are suffering from a serious health problem, then you will need to make a lot of changes and stick to your new diet for two or even three years before conception. It helps to keep the goal in mind: a healthy, robust, beautiful, intelligent child.

An excellent resource for those embarking on a healthy traditional diet is the Weston A. Price Foundation, especially your nearest local chapter, which can help you find raw milk and pastured animal products.[81] Some prospective parents have even changed jobs and moved to a new location to have better access to healthy food—remember, you will need these foods not only before and during pregnancy, but for your family as it grows. Local chapters of the Weston A. Price Foundation often put on classes to help you learn basic cooking methods for grains, fermented foods, broth and organ meats.

The Foundation also publishes a yearly Shopping Guide that provides sources of healthy foods availably nationally. The Foundation's realmilk.com website lists sources of raw milk by state.

If you have been on a lowfat diet for any length of time, or if you suffer from low cholesterol, you may have trouble digesting all the recommended fatty foods. (Bile salts, needed for fat digestion, are made out of cholesterol.) If this is the case, start slowly with small amounts of fats, and build up gradually. Swedish bitters, one teaspoon in water taken morning and evening, will help your liver produce bile for fat digestion; another helpful product is ox bile, one tablet taken with meals (see Sources). Ox bile can be taken throughout pregnancy, but not Swedish bitters as it contains angelica root, which is not recommended for pregnant women.

If you have had your gall bladder removed, you can still consume a diet containing plenty of healthy fats. Your liver can still make bile, but since you lack a gall bladder to store the bile, it is important to adhere to a consistent eating schedule so your body gets used to secreting bile at mealtimes. Again, it may be helpful in this situation to take an ox bile tablet with meals.

Some people have trouble digesting meat, in which case it is helpful to consume meat with bone broth—either cut up in a bone broth soup or consumed with a broth-based sauce. Hydrochloric acid (see Sources) taken with meals can also be helpful. This product may also be taken through pregnancy. And remember that meat is much more digestible when consumed with fat.

Often when individuals learn that they need not fear fats, and then give themselves the go-ahead to consume them, they find that they want to gorge themselves on fats—as if finally given permission to provide their depleted bodies with the nutrients lacking for so long. Do not worry if you "overindulge" in healthy fats like butter, lard and coconut oil or rich foods like paté and bacon—you are simply making up for lost time. You may even gain weight, in which case you should cut back on carbohydrate foods. As soon as the body's nutritional requirements are satisfied, your appetite for fats will decline somewhat, and you will probably easily lose the weight you gained. You may also find that your cravings for sweets and carbohydrates go away.

For those who have a sweet tooth, a switch to a high-fat, nutrient-dense diet will often cure cravings. In any event, you need not give up sweet foods—just switch to homemade desserts sweetened with natural sweeteners like honey, maple syrup, maple sugar, Rapadura (dehydrated cane sugar juice) or molasses. Homemade treats such as custards and ice cream are a wonderful way to increase your egg yolk intake. The same goes for high-carbohydrate refined foods like bread and pasta—slather them with plenty of butter or cream sauce and you will find that you end up eating far less of these carbohydrate-rich foods. Likewise, addictions to stimulating foods like coffee, tea, sodas and chocolate often evaporate with the implementation of a healthy diet; lacto-fermented beverages, coffee substitutes consumed with plenty of real cream, and coconut oil in hot herb tea are all great replacements and take the sting out of giving up the caffeine habit.

OUR TOXIC WORLD

Unfortunately, prospective parents have more to be vigilant about than just food. Modern men and women are living in a sea of chemicals—many of them estrogenic, hormone-disrupting chemicals—from pesticides, herbicides, plastics bottles and tin can linings, air pollution, flame retardants, air fresheners, household cleaning products, perfumes and industrial toxins. It goes without saying that you should reduce your exposure as much as possible, starting with your own home. Don't use pesticides, air fresheners and harsh chemicals in your house or apartment, and don't use pesticides and herbicides on your own lawn or garden. Minimizing exposure is important not just before and during your pregnancy, but also while your children grow.

If you cannot avoid exposure to chemicals due to your work or proximity to factories or conventional farms, you should increase your cod liver oil intake—vitamin A provides the number one protection against toxic chemicals.[82] It is also wise to increase your intake of fermented foods—good bacteria lining the gut will prevent the absorption of many of these chemicals.

It's best to avoid doing any decorating or renovations in your house or apartment immediately before or during your pregnancy—there are lots of toxic chemicals that outgas from building materials, fresh paint, new carpets and new fabrics.

Tap water is a concern, as it usually contains fluoride, chlorine and other chemicals—all toxic—as well as pharmaceutical drugs from antibiotics, birth control pills and cholesterol-lowering medications. The solution is bottled water—in glass bottles—delivered to your home, or a filter on your tap water (see Sources).

By the way, it is not necessary to consume large amounts of water before and during pregnancy; water in large amounts actually upsets the body's homeostasis and can be depleting—not to mention send you running to the bathroom frequently. Much better to hydrate your body with lacto-fermented beverages and bone broths. The best way to hydrate your body is to consume plenty of healthy fats, because fats provide the most energy on the cellular level—much more than carbohydrates and proteins, and the by product of this energy is water.[83] If you do like to consume a lot of water, try sparkling water with a squeeze of lemon and a pinch of salt—a kind of instant healthy soft drink.

It goes without saying that you should not smoke before, during or after your pregnancy, and alcohol consumption should be curtailed to a very strict minimum. Recreational drugs pose a very grave danger to your offspring.

As with cravings for sweets and carbohydrates, you may find that your new high-fat, nutrient-dense diet will help more serious addictions go away. When the body is well nourished with the right fats and plenty of cholesterol, it can make its own endogenous feel-good chemicals so that the temporary feel-good effects of sugars, drugs, alcohol and cigarettes are no longer needed.

ELECTROMAGNETIC FIELDS

As if prospective parents didn't have enough to worry about, the new generation is threatened by the invisible pollution of electromagnetic fields. All objects produce an electromagnetic signature but scientists estimate that the electromagnetic radiation from cell phones, cell towers, Wi-Fi and similar technologies is 3000 percent greater than that found in the natural world. Strong electromagnetic fields near high-tension power lines can also have very negative effects. Since the brain, heart and every cell operate electronically, interference is a given, especially for the fetus and the growing child. It is well known that high levels of electromagnetic radiation can cause breaks and splits in DNA that can lead to birth defects, growth problems and health problems like allergies and asthma. There is growing evidence of a link between strong electromagnetic fields and leukemia.[84]

If you live close to high-tension power lines or a cell tower, you will want to move to a safer location long before you become pregnant. If you can, install DSL or cable rather than Wi-Fi in your home or apartment. If you must use a cell phone, use an earpiece and avoid conversations longer than two minutes. Even portable phones emit a strong electromagnetic signal, so use an old fashioned landline telephone connected with a cord. Men should know that cell phones operating on their belts or in a pocket can lower sperm count and cause the production of abnormal sperm.[85]

Conventional electrical equipment can also emit strong electromagnetic fields that can be damaging when close to the body. The worst offenders are electric blankets and alarm clocks next to your bed—so use warm comforters and a battery-powered alarm clock instead. Fluorescent light bulbs, including the new screw-in "energy saving" light bulbs, emit "dirty electricity" so stick to old-fashioned incandescent bulbs or the new LED bulbs.

Smart Meters, for remote reading of electricity use, emit very strong radiation and have made many sensitive individuals very ill; fortunately legislation in some states is allowing people to opt out and retain their old fashioned analog meters.[86]

We know of no research on whether diet can protect us to a certain extent from the damages of electromagnetic fields, but it makes sense that a diet that strengthens the brain, heart and cell membranes will provide considerable immunity. That means plenty of stable saturated fats from animal products, as well as the full complement of nutrients contained in the diet outlined above. Choline from egg yolks and liver may also be highly protective.

PHARMACEUTICAL DRUGS

Following the thalidomide tragedy in the 1950s, when thousands of children were born with gross deformities after their mothers took the drug to prevent morning sickness and miscarriage, the medical profession adopted a wisely conservative stance. For several decades, pregnant women heard stern warnings against taking *any* prescription or over-the-counter drug during pregnancy. Now that the thalidomide scandal has faded from memory, the warnings have become less stern. With the more laissez-faire attitude, women are again taking various drugs while they are trying to conceive or during pregnancy, drugs whose effects on the unborn are unknown. The best policy is to just say no to any and all pharmaceutical compounds.

Especially dangerous are cholesterol-lowering drugs, sometimes promoted to women of child-bearing age. These drugs—called statins—are a Class X teratogenic, meaning that they can cause serious birth defects. If you become pregnant while taking a statin, the damage may be done before you even know you have conceived.

Birth control pills can deplete the very nutrients your baby needs for neurological development.[87]

They are not a good idea under any circumstances (for safe methods of birth control, see Chapter 11), but if you have been taking them, you should wait at least two years after discontinuing them before you get pregnant. Many women report that the pill also significantly disrupts intestinal flora.

Another problematic pharmaceutical: antibiotics. Antibiotics wipe out gut flora and can lead to serious digestive problems, problems that can be passed on to your baby because she will also lack beneficial organisms in the digestive tract. Dr. Natasha Campbell-McBride, author of *Gut and Psychology Syndrome*, argues convincingly that lack of beneficial gut flora, often initiated with the mother's use of antibiotics, is a major factor in autism. Antibiotics can lead to an overgrowth of candida and other harmful yeasts, which produce chemicals that can severely affect the brain. All antibiotics should be strictly avoided for at least two years before conception and during pregnancy, and every effort should be made to rebuild a healthy gut flora if you have taken these drugs.

Vaccines are drugs injected directly into the bloodstream; vaccines can contain up to four neurotoxins—mercury, aluminum, formaldehyde and free glutamic acid—and represent a shock to the immune system. (Vaccines that are "mercury-free" tend to be high in aluminum.) Vaccines pose a very real risk of miscarriage as well; they should be strictly avoided at all times but especially during pregnancy (see Chapter 6).

PRENATAL VITAMINS

Conventional books on pregnancy and childbirth put a big emphasis on prenatal vitamins, and no wonder; the recommended pregnancy diets are so obviously lacking in nutrients that the only solution is supplementation with synthetic vitamins. And that's just the problem—the vitamins in prenatal formulations are synthetic. That means the body may have trouble absorbing and using them, or even that these drug-like compounds may have negative effects. The healthy pre-industrialized peoples that Dr. Weston Price described did not take prenatal vitamins; they got the vitamins and minerals they needed from nutrient-dense foods.

In recent times we have seen a big push for pregnant

women to take folic acid. But the synthetic folic acid in prenatal vitamins and added to processed foods is a chemical that is not normally found in foods or the human body. It can be converted into usable forms of folate, but this conversion is limited to about 200 mcg per single dose in healthy volunteers;[88] it may be even more limited during long-term exposure or in certain people.

Unlike natural folate from food, synthetic folic acid does not cross the placenta.[87] While the synthetic supplements do seem to prevent neural tube defects, how much better to consume a folate-rich diet. Folate-rich foods include liver, egg yolks, legumes and greens.

An interesting study from India points out the need for balancing folate with vitamin B_{12}. The study looked at vegetarian women who got plenty of folate from legumes and green vegetables; however 60 percent were deficient in vitamin B_{12}. Those who had the highest levels of folate but were also deficient in B_{12} tended to have babies who were small and who became overweight and insulin resistant at six years—a recipe for diabetes in adulthood.[88] Most prenatal vitamins do contain B_{12}; but folic acid is added to many foods these days, especially grain foods favored by vegetarains.

HERBS AND NATURAL REMEDIES

Gentle herb teas such as echinacea for colds, chamomile for sleep, slippery elm for digestion and constipation, ginger for upset stomach and pregnangy-formulated Swedish bitters for digestion are safe for pregnancy, but remember that all herbs can have a mild drug-like effect, and some herbs should be completely avoided by pregnant women. These include red clover and alfalfa (which have estrogenic effects) and numerous herbs including black cohosh, blue cohosh, angelica, arnica, black walnut, blue flag, castor oil, catnip, chicory, comfrey, dong quai, ephedra, elder, feverfew, henbane, licorice, lobelia, ma huang, poke root, uva ursi and wormwood, which all can cause miscarriage. (For a complete list of herbs to avoid during pregnancy, see www.92024.com/herbsnpregnancy.htm.) Remember that with herbs, as with all pharmaceutical drugs, the motto should be "when in doubt, go without."

DETOXIFICATION

For those with serious health problems or with a history of exposure to pesticides, industrial chemicals and environmental pollution, the period of dietary preparation should also be a period of detoxification. Nutritionist Kaayla T. Daniel, PhD, CCN, warns parents that if they are toxic, their babies will be toxic. She sees many babies born with high levels of one or more of the following: aluminum, mercury, cadium and lead, as well as toxic levels of the needed minerals manganese and copper. She notes that these toxic babies are more likely to have allergies, and even be allergic to breast milk. Asthma, attention deficit disorder, behavioral problems, crankiness and excessive crying characterize the offspring of toxic parents.

Daniel notes that the high-fat, nutrient-dense diet described in these pages often helps women struggling with fertility problems become pregnant (and helps dad make her pregnant)—but these women become pregnant before they have adequately prepared themselves for pregnancy. Even though the biological clock is ticking, women who have struggled with fertility need to take the extra time to detoxify before allowing themselves to become pregnant.

The detoxification regime should be a gentle one that includes foods like gelatin-rich bone broths, lacto-fermented foods and beverages (including a medicinal lacto-fermented beverage called beet kvass, see Recipes) and plenty of saturated fat (which supports the detoxification process). Hot baths with Epsom salts and magnesium-rich clays can be helpful for relaxation and detoxification. Baking soda and salt baths (one pound of each) weekly can help clear the body of radiation damage, and are a good policy after any x-rays or airplane trips.

Dr. Daniel recommends a diatomaceous earth product (see Sources), taken one tablespoon per hundred pounds of weight per day in water, to help pull toxic metals from the digestive tract.

For anyone who is extremely toxic, or wants to speed up this process, consultation with an alternative or naturopathic physician who uses lab assessment and has experience helping people eliminate toxic metals is warranted.

If you have amalgam fillings in your mouth, it would be wise to have them replaced by composites that have been tested and found to be non-toxic and compatible for your body. Be sure that your dentist is a biological dentist experienced in methods developed by the IAOMT (International Academy for Oral Medicine and Toxicology) and who can instruct you on gentle detoxification during the course of the removals. Mercury filling removal may take a year or more depending upon the number of fillings and the overall health of the individual. Incorrect procedures can result in worsened mercury toxicity and heightened exposure to the unborn child, so prospective mothers should be willing to travel to the right dentist if one is not available locally. To find a holistic dentist, check with the your local chapter of the Weston A. Price Foundation.

NOT FOR MOTHERS ONLY

While this chapter has focused on pre-conceptual and pregnancy diets for mothers, the dietary principles outlined here are important for the whole family. Diet affects not only fertility in women and proper development of the fetus, but also hormone levels and sperm quality in men.

Most importantly, the right diet will support good health and peaceful family life throughout the years. Nutrient-dense foods not only prevent illness, they provide sustained energy and support the kind of patient, relaxed, goal-oriented behavior that translates into a happy family life. When both mom and dad follow a nutrient-dense diet and avoid junk foods, their children will naturally do the same, especially during the critical early years.

THE DIET FOR DADS: JUST AS IMPORTANT[89]

New discoveries in biology continue to validate the practices of traditional peoples, who fed special nutrient-dense foods not only to prospective mothers but also to fathers-to-be.

Scientists have known for years that smoking, drinking and recreational drugs can lower the quality of sperm. Recent discoveries indicate that what men eat, the toxins they are exposed to, the traumas they endure and their age at the time of conception can leave biological traces on their children, and even their grandchildren.

For example, male rats that are starved before mating produce offspring with lower blood sugar, altered levels of corticosterone (which protects them against stress) and insulin-like growth factor 1 (which helps babies develop).

Southeast Asian men who chew betel nuts, a food that contains an alkaloid affecting metabolic functions, are more likely to have children with weight problems and heart disease, and these effects may extend to the grandchildren.

When male rats mate after traumatizing exposure to larger, aggressive rats, their offspring tend to be anxious and depressed, overreacting to social stress.

And a large body of research indicates that the children of older men are more likely to suffer from autism and schizophrenia.

None of these studies looked at whether a nutrient-dense diet given before mating could mitigate the problems of malnutrition, exposure to toxins and stress, and even the decline in sperm quality that comes with age, but it makes sense that it would. Fathers as well as mothers need to consume plentiful amounts of the sacred foods, so rich in fat-soluble activators, to built up reserves, clear toxins, help the body recover from stress, and support the production of strong and viable sperm. Truly, both sexes need to prepare for a healthy baby!

FOR MORE INFORMATION

Nourishing Traditions by Sally Fallon, with Mary G. Enig, PhD, NewTrends Publishing.

The Whole Soy Story by Kaayla Daniel, PhD, CCN, NewTrends Publishing.

The Untold Story of Milk by Ron Schmid, ND, NewTrends Publishing.

"Mad as a Hatter: How to Avoid Toxic Metals and Clear Them From the Body," by Kaayla T. Daniel, PhD, CCN and Galen D. Knight, PhD, www.westonaprice.org/environmental-toxins/mad-as-a-hatter.

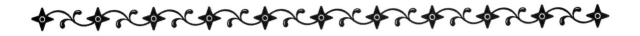

Chapter 2
Nutrition for Fetal Development

Biological human life begins at conception, the moment when the male sperm enters the female ovum. At this instant, the new organism possesses its own unique combination of some twenty thousand genes and becomes capable of growth and cell division. After that, things happen very fast. By day twenty-three, often before the expectant mother even knows she is pregnant, the heart has formed; by day forty, brainwaves can be recorded.

Growth and development of the fetus during these early weeks depends on the nutritional stores that the expectant mother has built up during the preconceptual period; and the development that occurs during the ensuing months will draw on the expectant mother's pregnancy diet and the nutritional environment of the womb. The quality of nutrition before and during these nine months produces lifelong effects on the structure of the body, the shape of the face, the placement of the teeth, and the function of the brain, kidneys, lungs and cardiovascular system. The nutritional environment of the womb determines the risk of degenerative disease later in life, the resistance to infection, range of intellect and even the quality of emotions from childhood to old age.

THE FIRST TRIMESTER

During ovulation, an egg is released from the ovary and moves into a tube called the oviduct. At conception, the sperm and egg combine within the oviduct to form a zygote. The genes from each parent combine into pairs and the zygote possesses a new, unique genome that every cell into which it divides will inherit.

The embryonic state of fetal development, which takes place from conception to approximately the eighth week of pregnancy, constitutes the most critical stage, when all systems are undergoing important foundational development. The period of tissue differentiation during the first two months is the period when the growing fetus is most susceptible to damage from drugs and chemicals (called teratogens), viral infections, x-rays, electromagnetic radiation and poor nutrition. Much critical development takes place before a woman even knows she is pregnant, so nutritional and environmental preparation for pregnancy must begin well before conception.

Certain developmental problems often occur together. For example, kidney problems and hearing problems are often found together because the kidneys and the inner ears develop at the same time.

Over the course of the first seven days, the zygote divides into a hollow ball of cells as it moves through the oviduct toward the uterus. By the seventh day, it becomes embedded in the uterine wall. At this point

it is called an embryo. The primary yolk sac begins to form, along with the amniotic sac and tissues that give rise to the placenta and umbilical cord.

The embryo then becomes multilayered through the process of gastrulation, during which the morphology of the embryo is dramatically restructured by cell migration. After the second week, the development of the embryo is in full swing. In the third week the heart is formed outside the body, and development of the brain, spinal cord and gastrointestinal tract begin. Teratogens introduced during this period, or lack of nutrients, may cause severe birth defects, such as the absence of one or more limbs or a heart that is outside the chest cavity at birth.

At four weeks, cellular division continues, with the cells separating into those that will make up the placenta and those that will make up the baby.

By the fifth week of the pregnancy the embryo has an outer layer consisting of the brain, nerves and skin. The middle layer becomes the bones, muscles, blood vessels, heart and sex organs. The inner layer holds the stomach, liver, intestines, lungs and urinary tract.

Through the process of neurulation, the embryo develops a spinal cord. The vertebral column is formed, and by the end of the sixth week of pregnancy the embryo has a head and trunk of the body. The eyes, limb buds, and other features begin to form, along with the lower jaw, the larynx and rudiments of the ear and eye. The heart, which is still outside the body, now beats at a regular rhythm. Teratogens or lack of nutrients at this period may cause problems involving the esophagus, vertebrae, eyes, face, hands and feet.

By the sixth week of pregnancy, the embryo is approximately one-half inch long and weighs a fraction of an ounce. In week six, the nose, jaw, palate and lung buds form. The fingers and toes form, but may still be webbed. The "tail" recedes; the heart is almost fully developed. Teratogens or lack of nutrients at this point may leave the baby with heart problems or a cleft lip.

During week seven, the eyes move forward on the face and the eyelids and tongue begin to form. Teratogens or lack of nutrients at this point may cause

heart and lung problems, a cleft palate and ambiguous genitalia.

At eight weeks, the embryo resembles a human being. The intestines begin to form and teeth start growing under the gums. The facial features continue to develop and the external ears appear. External genitalia become visible. The long bones begin to form and the muscles are able to contract. Teratogens at this period may still cause heart problems and stunting of the fingers and toes.

After eight weeks, the growing organism is called a fetus. At this point, all organ systems are present and functioning; out of forty-five hundred body structures present in the adult, four thousand are present at the eight-week point.

By the end of the third month of pregnancy, the fetus is completely formed. The head is large, fingers and toes are distinct, external genitalia are clearly male or female. The fetus may have begun moving its arms, legs and head. Beating at up to one hundred sixty beats per minute, the heart of the fetus now has four chambers. Kidneys are becoming functional, and intestines have begun to develop. The umbilical cord is now fully formed. By the end of the first trimester, the fetus is about three inches long and weighs just over one ounce.

THE SECOND TRIMESTER

During the first month of the second trimester, the baby undergoes a rapid growth spurt. The fetus develops a firm grip, begins to somersault, hiccups and sucks its thumb. Through sucking, the fetus swallows some of the amniotic fluid, and a thin dark substance called meconium is made in the intestinal tract. The skin of the fetus is almost transparent, so much so that blood vessels can be seen. He begins to develop fat under his thin skin. Fine hair called lunago develops on the head. Nostrils by this time are almost formed and the eyes move from the sides to the front of the head. The kidneys begin to process bodily fluids, and the liver begins to function as it should. Bones also begin to harden at this time. The heart beats one hundred twenty to one hundred fifty times per minute, processing twenty-five quarts of blood every day. Brain waves are detectable.

During the fifth month, eyebrows and lashes appear and nails appear on fingers and toes. This is an exciting time for the parents as the mother can feel the fetus moving and the fetal heartbeat can be heard with a stethoscope. Internally, a five-month-old fetus has functional sebaceous glands and the pituitary gland is mature enough to release thyroid-stimulating hormone. Myelination of the spinal cord commences, and the testes in a male fetus begin to descend.

In the beginning of the sixth month, the fetus nestles into position to sleep, stretches upon waking, has a startle reflex and can hear. All the eye components are developed, footprints and fingerprints are forming and the entire body is covered in a cream cheese-like substance called *vernix caseosa*. By the end of the second trimester, fetal skin is now red and wrinkled and lanugo hairs have darkened. The spinal cord continues development and the lungs begin to secrete surfactant, a substance that allows gas exchange necessary for breathing.

THE THIRD TRIMESTER

Once into the third trimester, babies have a chance of survival if born prematurely. In the last half of this trimester, rapid growth takes place, especially in the skeletal system. Infants born six weeks prematurely have only half the calcium and phosphorus laid down in the bones as infants carried to term.

By the twenty-fourth week, the baby will weigh approximately 1.3 pounds (0.6 kilograms). During the period of time from the twenty-fifth to the twenty-eighth week, lung development is marked, as the baby prepares to breathe air at birth. By the twenty-eighth week, 90 percent of babies born will survive, although breathing may be an issue. Ligaments form, nostrils open and brain development proceeds at a fast rate. The baby's retinas begin to form, and she can completely open her eyes at this point.

From the twenty-ninth to the fortieth week, fetal development is focused on the development of the lungs. For the most part, all of the major systems and organs are complete. The baby's job is to fatten up to face the environment outside of the protective womb. In the eighth month, myelination of the brain begins. The baby begins to develop immunities needed to survive. At thirty-seven weeks, the baby will continue to add approximately one ounce

per day to his body weight. This week marks a pregnancy as full term, when the baby can be delivered without any fear of complications, although a pregnancy may span as many as forty-two weeks.

None of this growth and development can take place without nutrients. Fats and carbohydrates fuel the growth. Fats and cholesterol form cell membranes. Amino acids form structural proteins and enzymes. Vitamins and minerals act as cofactors for those enzymes or as regulators of the entire process of growth. These nutrients are uniquely supplied by the mother's diet.

SEXUAL DIFFERENTIATION

Modern people live in a sea of estrogens—from pesticides, household products, cosmetics, plastics, the lining of tin cans and isoflavones in soy foods. The dangers of these estrogenic substances, especially coupled with a poor diet, are apparent when we focus on the fetal development of the sexual organs.

At the inception of the embryo, as sperm meets egg, sex chromosomes from the mother (X) and from the father (either X or Y) are combined to provide the potential of gender—but not the key to sexual differentiation. Sexual differences are determined by a gene on the Y chromosome called the SRY gene, which suppresses the female program of development—the female sex in humans is the default position for sexual development—and which allows for the growth of the testes. In the absence of the SRY gene, a gonad develops into an ovary even if the genetic makeup of the embryo is XY.

Through the actions of the SRY gene, cells of the normal gonad differentiate to produce the hormones and factors that allow for masculinization. In the testis, testosterone becomes the predominantly produced hormone. The presence of testosterone has the effect of turning the female gonads into the male gonads.

In females, however, the absence of the SRY gene causes the gonads to continue developing into ovaries. The ovary does produce testosterone, but most of that testosterone is quickly converted into estrogens, none of which can be converted back into androgens (male hormones). The lack of significant androgen levels and the presence of estrogens together allow the formation of the female reproductive organs and the female organization of the urinary tract.

Significant deviations in the levels of the appropriate sex hormones can cause severe consequences in reproductive and urogenital development, especially at the time of fetal growth and the period before puberty. In humans, the process of masculinization or feminization is not a black-and-white proposition but a process that takes place on a continuum over the years.

The Prader scale measures a person's development on that continuum by looking at the development and location of the urethral opening and the location of the testicles or labia compared to the glans or clitoris, respectively. The development of the male body plan, and hence the process of defeminization, depends on the presence of androgens along with the absence of estrogens, while the development of the female body plan depends on the presence of estrogens along with the lack of androgens.

This complicated process depends on good nutrition, especially vitamin A and saturated fats, to support hormone production; and a careful avoidance of estrogenic chemicals starting well before pregnancy. Above all, avoidance of soy products, loaded with estrogenic compounds, both before and during pregnancy, is critical for ensuring normal sexual differentiation.

NUTRITION FOR FETAL DEVELOPMENT . . . AND FOR LIFE

The scientific community is showing increasing interest in what is called the "developmental origins theory." This theory postulates that the nutritional environment in the womb affects not only the risk of defects immediately apparent at birth, but also the lifelong risk of degenerative disease.

Weston Price supported an early version of this theory in the 1930s and 1940s. In *Nutrition and Physical Degeneration*, for example, he proposed that an increased risk of tuberculosis was largely deter-

HYPOSPADIAS

Hypospadias is a birth defect in which the opening of the urethra appears on the underside of the shaft of the penis. The opening can be anywhere from the tip to the scrotum or even the perineum, although it usually occurs an inch or so from the usual end site. In some cases, it appears so far back as to create doubt about the gender of the child. The condition can usually be repaired surgically so that it will not interfere with urination and sex. Undescended testicles and inguinal hernia are the most common associated anomalies found in boys with hypospadias.

Hypospadias is one of the most common congenital birth defects. It now occurs in one out of one hundred twenty-five live male births. Since the 1960s, seven European countries and the United States have published independent reports on increasing rates of hypospadias. Severe cases have seen the largest increase. This is not a worldwide trend, for hypospadias is rarely found in less affluent and less industrialized nations.

Hypospadias results when hormonal disturbances result in incomplete virilization around the eighth week of gestation. Exposure to pesticides, plastics and industrial chemicals is a likely culprit, but so is exposure to estrogenic soy.

In a longitudinal study of pregnancy and childhood, researchers found that vegetarian mothers were five times more likely to give birth to a boy with hypospadias than a mother on an omnivorous diet. Lesser risk factors included taking iron supplements or catching the flu during the first trimester of pregnancy. There were no significant differences pertaining to maternal smoking, drinking, age or having twins. The researchers concluded: "It is important to note that there is biological evidence that vegetarians have a greater exposure to phytoestrogens and thus a causal link is biologically feasible. . . . As vegetarians have a greater exposure to phytoestrogens than do omnivores, these results support the possibility that phytoestrogens have a deleterious effect on the developing male reproductive system."[1] Soy is the likeliest culprit as no other commonly eaten food is high in phytoestrogens.

mined by a deformation of the chest cavity that began taking shape in the womb and paralleled the deformation of the dental arch that results in crowded teeth. He also demonstrated an association between delinquent behavior and deformities of the dental arch and found the same association with nondelinquent but mentally retarded children as well.

The modern developmental origins theory observes that birth weight is determined in part by embryonic and fetal nutrition; and low birth weight is in turn associated with an increased risk of heart disease, stroke, high blood pressure, diabetes and kidney disease. To explain these observations, the theory proposes that poor nutrition during pregnancy causes changes in the growth and development of the internal organs, which in turn affects the lifelong risk of degenerative disease.

The British researcher David J. Barker first proposed the developmental origins theory in the 1980s to explain a puzzling paradox: as British prosperity increased, so did heart disease; yet geographically, the most heart disease was found in the poorest places in Britain. Barker found geographical associations of heart disease with infant mortality, but not with smoking or dietary fat.

Yet even infant mortality had declined over the course of the century, just as prosperity had gone up. When he accounted for a time lag between cause and effect of more than fifty years, however, the paradox was resolved—something was determining the risk of disease at or near birth, not late in life when the disease develops.[2]

Barker and his team of researchers then studied the birth weight of individuals born between 1911 and 1930 in Hertfordshire. This allowed them to study the association at the level of individuals rather than local districts. Infants carried to term with birth weights between 8.5 and 9.5 pounds had a 45 percent lower risk of heart disease than infants carried to term weighing less than 5.5 pounds; they had a similarly lower risk of stroke, a nearly 70 percent lower risk of insulin resistance, and a slightly lower blood pressure in the seventh decade of life. The risk declined steadily and evenly between 5.5 and 9.5 pounds and began increasing thereafter. Later, other researchers found similar trends in the United States and southern India.[3]

Data from the three-month Dutch famine that occurred during World War II suggests that specific types of diseases are associated with specific windows of development during pregnancy. Women who were exposed to this famine during their first trimester gave birth to offspring with an increased risk of cardiovascular disease; women exposed during their second trimester gave birth to offspring with an increased risk of kidney disease; women exposed during their third trimester gave birth to offspring with an increased risk of insulin disorders.[4]

Developmental origins theorists have offered several explanations for these associations: poor nutrition could alter the development of the pancreas, which secretes insulin, and the liver, which secretes cholesterol and blood clotting proteins; muscle tissue could program itself for insulin resistance in order to spare glucose and amino acids for the brain when the supply of these materials is limited; overgrowth of the left ventricle of the heart—which itself is independently associated with cardiovascular disease—could be a response to the need to supply a greater volume of blood to the brain at the expense of the other tissues.[5]

Just as Weston Price had associated the skeletal defects that occur because of poor prenatal nutrition with the risk of disease in childhood and adolescence, researchers are now associating the defects of the internal organs that occur due to poor nourishment with the risk of disease in adulthood and old age.

The ideal birth weight according to these studies appears to be between 8.5 and 9.5 pounds. These figures exclude infants whose birth weights are low because of premature delivery; it is the rate of fetal growth, not the birth weight itself, that counts. The theory does not suggest that the risk of disease is affected only by the rate of growth within the womb—simply that the nutritional environment during this period makes an incomplete yet permanent contribution to that risk.

Genetics has little if anything to do with birth weight. A 1995 study examined sixty-two cases of egg donor pregnancies. The birth weight of the baby was not correlated with the donor's weight, the donor's birth weight, or the birth weights of the donor's other children; it was, however, correlated with the recipient's weight.[6] This study shows that birth weight is determined by the environment that the womb provides rather than the genome present at conception.

An intake of meat protein below 25 grams per day during late pregnancy and an intake of carbohydrate above 265 grams per day during early pregnancy are associated with a decrease in birth weight. A low intake of animal protein relative to carbohydrate is also associated with an increase of blood pressure at forty years of age.[7] In order to obtain adequate glycine for growth, meat and egg protein should be balanced with the liberal use of liver, skin, bone broths, legumes and green vegetables.

The use of cod liver oil is independently associated with birth weight: that is, use of cod liver oil results in bigger babies, regardless of other factors.[8] Seven out of twelve trials have shown that folic acid supplementation increases birth weight.[9] Iron deficiency compromises fetal growth[10] and a major deficiency in any vitamin or mineral is likely to do the same.

Modern science continues to confirm what primitive peoples knew instinctively: that optimal fetal development depends on a nutrient-dense diet. A generous intake of all nutrients—especially the fat-soluble vitamins, essential fatty acids, biotin, folate, choline and glycine—will supply the developing fetus with everything it needs for robust and vigorous growth and a long, healthy life to come.

The following is a review of the key nutrients needed to support this development—nutrients that need to be in good supply at the moment of conception and continued throughout the period of pregnancy and birth.

VITAMIN A

In *Nutrition and Physical Degeneration*, Price described the early work on vitamin A deficiency during pregnancy and the preconception period. In diverse species of laboratory animals, this deficiency produced spontaneous abortion; prolonged labor and death of the mother and her offspring during labor; eye defects including the complete absence of eyes; defects of the snout, dental arches and lips; displacement of internal organs including the kid-

neys, ovaries and testes; and deafness due to degeneration of the nervous system.[11]

We now know that vitamin A is necessary for the differentiation and patterning of all of the cells, tissues and organs within the developing body. It is especially important for the development of the communication systems between the sense organs and the brain—these systems are highly compromised in tragic conditions like autism.

Even mild vitamin A deficiency compromises the number of functional units called nephrons in the kidneys, which could predispose a person to poor kidney function later in life. The number of cells in the kidneys is highly dependent on vitamin A status during embryonic and fetal development.

Vitamin A is also necessary during fetal development and through adult life to maintain the presence of cells lining the lungs, which are covered in hair-like projections called cilia.[12] These hairs sweep away debris and foreign material, protecting the lungs from pollutants and infectious diseases. During and after the formation of all these systems, vitamin A is necessary for their continued growth.

The RDA of vitamin A for pregnant women is only 2,600 IU—just 300 IU more than the RDA for women who are not pregnant. To obtain this figure, the scientists at the Institute of Medicine (IOM) made the following calculation: first, they ascertained from previous reports the amount of vitamin A stored in the livers of fetuses that were spontaneously or voluntarily aborted between thirty-seven and forty weeks; second, they doubled this figure, assuming that half of the fetal vitamin A stores exist in the liver; and third, they divided this amount over the number of days in the last trimester, during which they presumed this vitamin A would accumulate.[13]

There are several problems with this calculation. Since the fetuses were aborted, we have no idea what their future health would have been like—their visual acuity, their hearing, their intelligence, their facial and dental features, their reproductive health, or their length of life.

And the function of vitamin A, of course, is not to be stored but to be used. The fetus does not simply hold on to vitamin A to use it after birth, but rapidly uses and metabolizes it to regulate the entirety of its growth and development.

We do not have exact figures for the vitamin A content of the preconception and pregnancy diets used by the groups that Price studied, but they were certainly higher than 2,600 IU per day. These groups prized organ meats, especially liver, and used them on a regular basis—there are over 50,000 IU vitamin A in one serving of liver. Preconception and pregnancy diets added additional foods rich in fat-soluble vitamins.

Considering the ubiquitous role of vitamin A in the development of every organ system of the body, and considering how tightly the body regulates the level of the activated form, we should expect a generous helping of vitamin A-rich organs, cod liver oil and animal fats to support perfect fetal development, not to throw it off course. The preponderance of the evidence suggests that this is the case.

VITAMIN D

In the late third trimester, the fetal skeleton enters a period of rapid growth that requires calcium, phosphorus and vitamin D. An infant born six weeks prematurely has laid down only half the calcium into its bones as an infant carried to term.

There is evidence that vitamin D plays a role in lung development,[14] and it probably plays a much larger role in fetal development in general due to vitamin D's interaction with vitamin A.

At birth, the infant's blood level of vitamin D is closely correlated to that of the mother.[15] Adequate levels of vitamin D protect the newborn from tetany, convulsions and heart failure.[16]

The rapid skeletal growth that occurs in late pregnancy taxes the vitamin D supply of the mother and her blood levels drop over the course of the third trimester. One study conducted in Britain showed that 36 percent of new mothers and 32 percent of newborn infants had no detectable vitamin D in their blood at all; another showed that 60 percent of infants born to white mothers in the spring and summer had levels under 8 nanograms per milliliter (ng/mL), a level that is overtly deficient.[17]

In spite of these findings, government agencies and the American Academy of Pediatrics continue to advocate a mere 400 IU vitamin D for pregnant women. Moreover, the Academy directs mothers to keep their infants out of the sun, dress them in protective clothing, and liberally cover them in sun block. The Academy admits that breast milk is deficient in vitamin D—due, of , to the low intake of vitamin D during pregnancy and lactation that it advocates.

We recommend a healthy 2,000 IU per day of vitamin D from cod liver oil, and additional amounts from fatty fish, fish eggs, shellfish and grass-fed butter, egg yolks and lard. Although no studies have directly assessed the use of this dose during pregnancy, a study of over ten thousand infants in Finland conducted between 1966 and 1997 showed that direct supplementation of 2,000 IU per day to infants in the first year of life virtually eradicated the risk of type 1 diabetes over the next thirty years.[18]

VITAMIN E

Vitamin E was originally named "Fertility Factor X" in 1922 because rats could not reproduce without it. Two years later, researchers dubbed it "tocopherol" from the Greek *tokos*, meaning "childbirth," and *ferein*, meaning "to bring forth." Its precise role in rat fertility remains unclear and scientists have yet to conclusively demonstrate that it is essential to human reproduction.

Mice lacking the gene for the protein that transports vitamin E across the placenta conceive offspring that die within eleven to fifteen days. The nutritional transport system of the placenta is observably malformed by the ninth day. The human placenta makes the same protein, so the role of vitamin E in constructing the nutritional transport system of the human placenta is probably similar. Vitamin E, then—despite the lack of published proof—is almost certainly essential to human reproduction.[19]

Unrefined vegetable oils are high in vitamin E, but they are also high in polyunsaturated fatty acids (PUFA), which deplete the body of this nutrient. Commercial refined vegetable oils have been stripped of vitamin E to begin with, so consumption of these products greatly increases the body's vitamin E requirements. The vitamin E content of grass-fed animal fats is four times higher than that of grain-fed animal fats. Butter can be an especially rich source if it comes from grass-fed animals. Nuts, seeds, fresh fruits and vegetables and freshly ground grains also contain vitamin E.

VITAMIN K

Compared to vitamins A and D, very little is known about the role of vitamin K in embryonic and fetal development. The enzyme that uses vitamin K to activate vitamin K-dependent proteins first shows up in the skeletal and nervous tissue of the embryo.[20] Two vitamin K-dependent proteins are present in the first trimester.[21] These proteins help lay down calcium salts in bone tissue and keep calcium out of the soft tissues where it does not belong.

In 1997, an infant was born to a mother who took Warfarin during pregnancy. This drug interferes with the normal clotting mechanism of the blood by creating an effective vitamin K deficiency. During the early development of the middle third of the infant's face, the cartilage of her septum calcified; at birth, her nose was a stub. Since only twenty percent of the septum protrudes from the face, a mere ten percent reduction in its length can cut the length of the nose in half. She also had cavities and plaques in her spinal cord; she required oxygen due to respiratory distress at birth; and she was quadriplegic by twenty months.[22]

This tragic case of severe deficiency illustrates the essential role of K vitamins in the development of proper facial proportions and the much more important and fundamental development of the nervous system. This case also demonstrates the wisdom in avoiding all drugs during pregnancy.

Vitamin K_2 has a higher rate of transport across the placenta than vitamin K_1.[23] When mothers receive injections of vitamin K_2, the placenta rapidly accumulates it and then releases it slowly to the fetus over time.[24] Vitamin K_1 is found in leafy greens, while vitamin K_2 is found in fermented foods such as natto and sauerkraut and grass-fed animal fats—goose and duck fat and liver, aged cheese, and to a lesser extent butter, egg yolks and fatty meats.

DHA

The fetus, infant and adult can all convert the omega-3 fatty acid found in plant oils, alpha-linolenic acid (ALA), into the elongated docosohexaenoic acid (DHA)—but the rate of this conversion is no more than one percent at all ages and stages of development. DHA may be necessary for the formation of neurons and for the synthesis of the important brain lipid phosphatidylserine; it is also the precursor to an important compound that protects neurons when they are assaulted by oxidative stress.

The fetus hoards DHA from the mother and incorporates it into its brain at ten times the rate at which it can synthesize it.[25] (Maternal loss of DHA may be a contributing factor to postpartum depression.) DHA can be obtained primarily from cod liver oil and fatty fish and in small amounts from grass-fed animal fats.

BIOTIN

Biotin is a B vitamin but has also been called "vitamin H." Researchers have studied its role in pregnancy for decades but only recently have discovered that marginal biotin deficiency during this critical period is the norm.

In pregnant rats, a diet containing 5 percent egg white produced a marginal biotin deficiency. The activity of biotin-dependent enzymes declined 10 percent in the mother. Yet in the fetus, the activity of these enzymes decreased a full 50 percent. Although the mother had no obvious symptoms herself, her offspring suffered an increased risk of limb and palate defects. These effects were all reversed when biotin was added to the diet in addition to egg whites.[26]

Whether marginal biotin deficiency causes birth defects in humans is an open question, but the results of the rat studies merit attention to increasing one's intake during pregnancy. Most foods contain some of this vitamin, but it is primarily found in liver and egg yolks.[27]

Egg whites contain a glycoprotein called avidin that strongly binds to biotin and prevents its absorption. Cooking neutralizes avidin, but not completely. Frying destroys 67 percent, boiling the egg white directly for two minutes destroys 60 percent, and poaching only destroys 29 percent.[28] Raw egg whites, then, should be strictly avoided, and cooked egg whites should be consumed in moderation— and never without the yolk. The addition of pure egg yolks to scrambled eggs, smoothies and ice cream will help boost biotin status.

FOLATE

Folate is the vitamin whose essential role in pregnancy is most widely known. It is necessary for the production of new DNA, and new DNA is needed for new cells. The growing life within the womb engages in constant cell division, and the mother must expand her blood supply with the production of new red blood cells as well—these activities demand a generous supply of folate.[29]

Adequate folate intake prevents neural tube defects (defects of the brain and spinal cord) and increases birth weight. It may also prevent spontaneous abortion, mental retardation and deformations of the mouth, face and heart.[30]

The pregnancy RDA for folate is 600 micrograms (mcg) per day. This figure is based on the amount needed to prevent the folate concentration of the mother's red blood cells from dropping during pregnancy and on urinary markers indicating the amount of folate being used. It assumes that only half of the vitamin is absorbed from food, although this figure is just an average; the rate of folate absorption is dependent on zinc status—one good reason for consuming red meat and shellfish, the best sources of zinc, throughout pregnancy.

Synthetic folic acid is a chemical that is not normally found in foods or the human body. It can be converted into usable forms of folate, but this conversion is limited to about 200 mcg per single dose in healthy volunteers;[31] it may be even more limited during long-term exposure or in certain people.

Synthetic folic acid, the kind added to processed foods, does not cross the placenta; folate crosses the placenta only in the form of the naturally occurring isomer. Since the synthetic supplements do prevent neural tube defects, pregnant women should use them if they are not going to eat folate-rich diets; whenever possible, however, it is best to meet the folate requirement from foods. Folate-rich foods include liver, legumes and dark green vegetables.

CHOLINE

Choline is related to folate because the body can turn it into a compound called betaine, which can be substituted for folate in certain chemical reactions. Perhaps for this reason, a low intake of choline is associated with a four-fold increased risk of neural tube defects.[32]

Choline has a much more direct role, however, in the development of the brain. It is especially important for the formation of cholinergic neurons (neurons that use the neurotransmitter acetylcholine). This process takes place from day fifty-six of pregnancy through three months postpartum; and choline is needed for the formation of the connections between these neurons, called synapses, which occurs at a high rate through the fourth year of life.[33]

It bears repeating that rats fed three times the normal choline requirement during pregnancy give birth to offspring with very resilient nervous systems. These offspring have a lifelong 30 percent increase in visuospatial and auditory memory; they grow old without developing any age-related senility; they are protected against the assaults of neurotoxins; they have an enhanced ability to focus on several things at once; and they have a much lower rate of interference memory. Interference memory occurs when a past memory interferes with an immediate memory—for example, when a past memory of where you parked your car on a previous day interferes with your ability to find it when you exit the store.[34]

In addition, choline protects the fetus from chronic stress-related illness later in life. When mom is under stress during pregnancy, the levels of stress hormones in baby also rise, leading to reduced ability to deal with stress after birth.[35] Extra choline during the third trimester protects against this unfortunate outcome.[36]

The RDA for non-pregnant women is 425 milligrams (mg) per day. The RDA for pregnant women is 450 mg per day, only 25 mg more. The increase is based on the typical transfer of choline to the fetus and accumulation in the fetus. Rat studies, however, suggest that an amount two to three times this may provide the offspring with lasting benefits. Choline can be obtained from liver, egg yolks, and high-quality grass-fed dairy foods; it can be obtained to a lesser extent from meats, cruciferous vegetables, nuts, and legumes.

GLYCINE

The amino acid glycine is conditionally essential during pregnancy. Usually, we are able to make enough of it ourselves to meet our basic survival needs; during pregnancy, however, it must be obtained from food. It is the limiting factor for protein synthesis in the fetus, and thus almost certainly a limiting factor for fetal growth.[37]

As detailed in Chapter 1, the fetus can obtain glycine from two sources: the placenta transports glycine from the mother's blood, and it uses folate to manufacture it from another amino acid called serine. The mother can obtain glycine primarily from collagen-rich foods such as skin and bones or bone broths.

Glycine is depleted in the clearing of excess methionine, another amino acid. Eggs and meat are the main sources of methionine—it not only constitutes a greater percentage of their total protein but these foods are also higher in total protein than plant foods. It is important, therefore, for the expectant mother to liberally match her egg and muscle meat consumption with glycine-rich skin and bone broths and folate-rich liver, legumes and greens.

SULFUR

It is essential that a woman consume abundant sulfur-containing foods during pregnancy. Of particular concern is taurine, the only sulfonic amino acid, which is found exclusively in animal-based foods. Taurine is the most common free amino acid in the body, and it is present in the newborn child at three times the adult level. Taurine plays an important role in the neural development of the fetus.[38] While our physiology is capable of synthesizing taurine, this will deplete supplies of sulfur-containing amino acids for other important needs—for protein building and for protection from oxidative damage.

Another crucial role sulfur plays in the fetus involves the safe transport of cholesterol, sex hormones and neurotransmitters to all the fetal tissues, particularly the brain. This is achieved by attaching sulfate to these molecules, making them both temporarily inactive and water-soluble. In fact, the levels of cholesterol sulfate skyrocket in the placental villi during the last trimester of pregnancy.[39] It is believed that cholesterol itself is unable to penetrate the placental barrier (because it is not water soluble), so sulfation is what allows the mother to deliver cholesterol to the developing fetus.

Cholesterol plays a crucial role in the developing brain. It is unclear whether the fetus is capable of synthesizing cholesterol, but if not, then the mother must supply it. Serum sulfate deficiency is characteristic of autism, and so insufficient cholesterol sulfate delivery to the fetal brain due to insufficient

SEROTONIN AND THE INFANT BRAIN

Serotonin, the body's natural feel-good chemical, is critical for the developing fetus. In addition to supporting brain development, serotonin may be involved in the development of the heart and pancreas. In the infant and in adults, serotonin supports a feeling of well-being.

Synthesis of serotonin begins in the hind brain and then gradually moves to the forebrain. New findings indicate that before the forebrain can produce serotonin, the placenta produces it and provides this vital substance to the developing fetus.

Disruption of serotonin development in the fetus can leave permanent alterations in brain function and behavior, such as autism and Down Syndrome.

Serotonin is manufactured from the amino acid tryptophan. Best sources are animal sources such as egg white, turkey, pork and hard cheeses like Parmesan and Cheddar. Nuts and seeds also provide tryptophan.[41]

sulfate supply from the mother may be a significant factor in autism.[40]

Sulfur is found in highest concentration in our two favorites, egg yolks and liver, along with cholesterol for which it has such an affinity. These should be the premier foods during pregnancy, along with a good source of calcium such as raw milk or cheese. Other good sources of sulfur include onions and molasses.

SATURATED FAT

The relentless attack on saturated fats by the medical establishment and in the press has not spared pregnant women. Studies purporting to show that saturated fat is bad for the pregnant woman and her developing baby have vectored many an expectant mother to a nutrient-poor diet based on polyunsaturated vegetable oils, or to one in which all fats are severely lacking.

Yet, nearly half the fatty acids in human breast milk are saturated, suggesting that dietary saturated fats are critical to the development of infants and young children.[42] Saturated fats are so important during these critical stages of development that their abundant presence in breast milk is universal among mammals. The biochemical reason is clear: saturated fats make up nearly half of our cell membranes, where they anchor proteins to specific locations, participate in signaling activities, and transport cellular components. They also form an important source of energy and, of course, carry the all-important fat-soluble vitamins.

It would therefore seem illogical to insist that saturated fats in the expectant mother's diet are harmful to either the mother or her unborn child, yet many studies in recent years have claimed to show just that. One recent study, for example, claimed that a "high-saturated-fat diet" fed to pregnant and lactating rat dams caused obesity and brain inflammation in the dams and their pups.[43] What media reports never mention, however, is that the fat used in these diets is only about one-third saturated. Another third is monounsaturated and the remaining third polyunsaturated, meaning these diets are much lower in saturated fat and six times richer in polyunsaturated fat than breast milk. The fat, moreover, is provided in the context of purified sugar, starch and milk protein, with added supplements of vitamins and minerals. In short, these diets contain purified ingredients rather than whole foods. Negative effects likely result from their refined ingredients rather than from their modest content of saturated fat.

Several human studies have attempted to blame problems that occur in pregnancy on saturated fat. A retrospective study found that mothers who gave birth to children with congenital heart defects ate more saturated fat than other mothers, but the difference was only one gram per day, which amounts to less than a half-teaspoon of butter.[44] These same mothers also had lower intakes of niacin and riboflavin, and the authors provided no compelling reason to blame the extra gram of saturated fat in their diets.

One randomized trial examined the effect of advising pregnant and breastfeeding mothers to eat a diet that "targeted excessive saturated fat and low fiber consumption." The aim was to reduce the blood levels of an unusual form of insulin in their infants, one that predicts the risk of future metabolic disorders. The diet was successful, but unfortunately the authors did not describe the diet in detail.[45]

A final study was a randomized trial testing the effect of a "low-cholesterol, low-saturated fat diet" on pregnancy complications. The diet reduced the risk of premature delivery by ten-fold[46] and improved indices of blood vessel function in the umbilical artery.[47] The diet, however, was not simply low in cholesterol and saturated fat. It restricted coffee and was high in fatty fish, whole grains, fruits, vegetables, legumes, olive oil, nuts, olives, seeds, vitamin C, vitamin E, vitamin D and magnesium. With these many changes, why should we blame saturated fat or cholesterol, compounds we know to be essential to a developing human being because they are so abundant in breast milk?

Ultimately, the totality of the evidence provided by these studies suggests that pregnant and breastfeeding mothers should eat a diet based on nutrient-dense whole foods. Such a diet inevitably provides a healthy amount of saturated fat and cholesterol along with plenty of vitamins and minerals needed to keep a mother strong and produce a healthy baby.

OTHER NUTRIENTS

It is safe to assume that the requirements for all vitamins and minerals are increased during pregnancy—calcium, zinc, iodine, magnesium, iron, cholesterol, protein, saturated and unsaturated fatty acids, B vitamins, vitamin C and many other nutrients are needed for the growth and optimal development of the fetus, as well as the nourishment of the mother. These will be provided by raw dairy products and the many nutrient-dense foods that ccontain the nutrients listed above.

We cannot stress enough the importance of obtaining these nutrients from high-quality natural foods, prepared in the home, starting months before pregnancy begins and continued through pregnancy, lactation and beyond.

FOR MORE INFORMATION

"Vitamins for Fetal Development," by Chris Masterjohn, www.westonaprice.org/childrens-health/vitamins-for-fetal-development-conception-to-birth.

"Effects of Antenatal Exposure to Phytoestrogens on Human Male Reproductive and Urogenital Development," by Bernard Poggi, www.westonaprice.org/soy-alert/phytoestrogens-and-male-reproductive-development.

The Whole Soy Story by Kaayla Daniel, PhD, CCN, NewTrends Publishing.

EFFECTS OF SATURATED FAT ON PREGNANT WOMEN

Human studies purporting to show the perils of consuming saturated fat during pregnancy have focused on weight gain, high blood sugar and diabetes. Many are based on dietary recall questionnaires, which are notoriously inaccurate.

Among retrospective studies, one found women who developed blood sugar problems during pregnancy ate more saturated fat than those who did not,[48] while another found no relationship.[49] Two prospective studies found that pregnant women who developed blood sugar problems consumed no more saturated fat than other women.[50] One prospective study reported conflicting findings: pregnant women who developed blood sugar issues consumed less saturated fat than other women, but after making statistical adjustments for other risk factors their saturated fat intake appeared higher.[51] Even so, intake of baked goods, ice cream, chips, candy, and soda had a much stronger relationship with blood sugar levels in this study than intake of saturated fat.

A final prospective study found that women who ate more saturated fat and processed foods gained more weight during pregnancy than other women, but concluded that this was simply because they ate more calories.[52] Randomized trials have shown that cutting saturated fat during pregnancy decreases weight gain if calories are also cut,[53] but not if calorie intake remains the same.[54] The only randomized trial that examined the effect of saturated fat on blood sugar in pregnant women compared the effects of two different meals in ten women with gestational diabetes. Blood sugar and insulin were lower after the meal rich in saturated fat than after the meal rich in monounsaturated fat. The authors concluded that "saturated fat may be useful in controlling postprandial glucose."[55]

Chapter 3
A Healthy Pregnancy

I'm pregnant! For most women, this is a joyful moment, especially joyful if you have prepared for pregnancy with good nutrition.

The most obvious sign of pregnancy is a missed menstrual period. If you want to know for sure whether or not you are pregnant, you can do a pregnancy test. These work by detecting a hormone called human chorionic gonadotropin (HCG) in the blood or urine. The embryo begins to produce HCG on implantation in the uterus; this helps maintain progesterone production, which is critical for a pregnancy in humans.

HCG production usually begins about six days after the merger of egg and sperm. But studies show that in up to 10 percent of women, implantation does not occur until later, after the first day of the missed period. The amount of HCG then rapidly builds up with each day of pregnancy.

At-home pregnancy tests measure HCG in the urine; to measure HCG in the blood requires a doctor's visit. Home pregnancy tests are accurate if used correctly and at the right time—no earlier than one week after a missed period—and have the advantage of providing a private and inexpensive confirmation of pregnancy.

FATIGUE

A common early sign of pregnancy, especially the first pregnancy, is fatigue or, more specifically, the need for sleep. This usually passes after a few days, or at most a few weeks, but while it lasts, don't fight it! Get as much sleep as your body tells you it needs! That may mean frequent naps, even a cat nap at work.

The key point is not to be tempted by caffeinated drinks to keep yourself awake. A glass of raw milk or a mug of broth is a much better pick-me-up; molasses and coconut oil in hot water also work well (see Recipes). The important thing is to get the sleep you need during the early weeks of your pregnancy.

PREGNANCY DIET

If you have prepared for pregnancy with the diet outlined in Chapter 1, you will not need to make any fundamental changes to the way you eat. The one caveat is foods likely to carry *Listeria monocytogenes*. Infection with *L. mono* during pregnancy can cause miscarriage.

Contrary to government pronouncements, raw milk is not a likely source of *L. mono* (see page 21).

However soft unaged cheeses—both raw and pasteurized—can carry the organism and should be avoided during pregnancy. Another common source is deli and luncheon meats. In any event, for those who have taken care to build up healthy gut flora prior to pregnancy, the risk of serious infection from *L. mono* is low.

What if you have discovered these dietary guidelines only after becoming pregnant? All the more important to implement them right away, eliminating refined carbohydrates and processed foods, while incorporating as many nutrient-dense foods into your diet as you can. However, foods that may cause an allergic or die-off reaction, such as kombucha, should be introduced very slowly if you have not consumed them before your pregnancy. If you are new to raw milk, start with just one-fourth cup per day, sipped at room temperature, and build up gradually to the recommended one quart per day.

Likewise, with animal fats, if you are not used to including butter and other healthy fats in your diet, start slowly and build up gradually. (For strategies on digesting fats, see page 34.)

Food cravings—the subject of so many jokes about pregnant women—tend to focus on fatty foods like ice cream and sour foods like pickles, foods that supply critical nutrients for pregnant women—the fat-soluble vitamins in animal fats and vitamin C and beneficial bacteria in properly made pickles. The pre-conceptual diet described in Chapter 1 provides these components in abundance, thus making food cravings unlikely. However, if you do crave fatty and sour foods, be sure to satisfy your cravings with foods of the best possible quality—butter, cream and egg yolks from grass-fed animals and true lacto-fermented condiments.

MORNING SICKNESS

In contrast to cravings, morning sickness can rob you of an appetite during the critical early weeks of pregnancy. Morning sickness, also called *nausea gravidarum* or vomiting of pregnancy, is a condition that affects more than half of all pregnant women, to a greater or lesser extent. The nausea can be mild or so severe that it leads to actual vomiting. It is usually present in the early morning, but can occur at any time of day, often triggered by sensitivity to odors. The nausea usually tapers off at the end of the first trimester. However sick you may feel, be reassured by the fact that having morning sickness is not associated with any increase in adverse outcomes in your developing child. But the specter of morning sickness, when you may pass several weeks with little food, makes pre-conceptional dietary preparation with nutrient-dense foods to build up nutritional stores all the more necessary.

There are many theories on what causes morning sickness. One involves increased hormone levels. Estrogen levels may increase by up to one hundredfold during pregnancy. This theory has fallen from favor because studies find no consistent evidence of differences in estrogen levels between women who experience sickness and those who don't. However, it may be that women who experience morning sickness lack the enzymatic mechanisms for clearing the hormone. Likewise, increased progesterone in pregnancy relaxes the muscles in the uterus, which, according to the theory, also relaxes the stomach and intestines, leading to excess stomach acid and acid reflux.

The current theory on morning sickness holds that it is an evolved trait that protects the fetus from toxins ingested by the mother. Proponents of this theory note that many plants contain chemical toxins that serve as a deterrent to human consumption. Adult humans, like other animals, have defenses against plant toxins, including extensive arrays of detoxification enzymes manufactured by the liver and the surface tissues of various other organs. In the fetus, these defenses are not yet fully developed, and even small doses of plant toxins, which have negligible effects on the adult, could be harmful or lethal to the embryo.

According to this theory, pregnancy sickness causes women to experience nausea when exposed to the smell or taste of foods that are likely to contain toxins injurious to the fetus, even though they may be harmless to the mother.

This line of reasoning has led to the view that morning sickness is a functional adaptation and not a pathology. Studies have found that women who have no morning sickness are more likely to miscarry or bear children with birth defects, presumably because they are more likely to ingest substances that

CELIAC DISEASE AND PREGNANCY

Celiac disease is the inability to digest gluten-containing grains, such as wheat, barley and rye. As with related conditions, such as irritable bowel syndrome (IBS), Crohn's disease and colitis, poor cell-to-cell junctures in the gut lining result in poor assimilation of nutrients leading to malnutrition and absorption of allergenic protein fragments. The best time to address these problems is before you get pregnant; indeed celiac disease and related conditions often result in infertility or miscarriage. Miscarriage occurs 31 percent more in undiagnosed celiac patients than in the normal population.[1]

Malnourishment certainly plays a large role in causing infertility and miscarriage, but in addition, a recent study has shown that the anti-TTG antibody produced in response to gluten exposure in celiac disease actually binds to the placenta.[2] This may compromise placental function, putting patients at higher risk for miscarriage and problems with the fetus.

The good news is that that once the diagnosis of celiac disease is made, and a gluten-free diet is initiated, the majority of women have a resolution of their symptoms and their fertility rates return to whatever is normal for their age.

Celiac disease often manifests initially as anemia, due to poor absorption of iron and possibly also vitamin A—vitamin A is needed for iron assimilation as well as for gut integrity. If celiac disease is suspected, you will want to test for serum iron levels in addition to folate and B_{12}, vitamin D and zinc. Our diet for pre-pregnancy, pregnancy and lactation, outlined in Chapter 1, should be followed strictly, leaving out all gluten-containing grains, for at least six months and up to two years before getting pregnant. Gelatin-rich bone broth should be a regular part of the diet for its gut-healing properties.

What if you have celiac disease and find yourself pregnant? Again, the first line of defense is our nutrient-dense diet, strictly avoiding all gluten-containing grains. Eat plenty of iron-rich foods like liver, red meat and egg yolks, butter and meat fats for arachadonic acid (needed for tight cell-to-cell junctures in the gut) and cod liver oil every day without fail for vitamins A and D. It's a good idea to check serum iron levels several times during pregnancy and to follow the suggestions for anemia during pregnancy and lactation (page 58).

One word of caution: the many gluten-free foods now available in the grocery stores tend to be highly processed and contain soy as a major ingredient. Many suffering from celiac disease never get better until they cut out the soy as well as the wheat.

are toxic to the fetus. But the hormonal theory is an equally good explanation for the observation that women who do not experience morning sickness are more likely to miscarry. Lack of sufficient amounts of estrogen, progesterone and other hormones could easily lead to miscarriage, as well as birth defects.

A glaring inconsistency in the "toxin" theory is the fact that the foods most likely to trigger nausea are fatty animal foods, not plant foods. This has led to revisions in the original premise: morning sickness protects the pregnant woman from bad meat, likely to carry pathogenic organisms, in addition toxins from plant foods.

In any event, long-term nausea that makes eating difficult should not be considered normal. While morning sickness occurs throughout the developed world, it seems to be rare or nonexistent among truly primitive peoples, so we can only assume that morning sickness is not a natural reaction to pregnancy, but a situation that occurs due to insufficient clearing of hormones, a detoxification effect or some kind of deficiency that is common in civilized diets.

One logical explanation for pregnancy nausea is a lack of bile. The body makes sex hormones out of cholesterol, and the body makes bile, needed to digest fats, from cholesterol as well. If not enough cholesterol is available to handle the excess requirements of pregnancy, then most available cholesterol will be sequestered to the production of estrogen and progesterone, with not enough available for the production of bile. In this situation, ingestion of fatty foods could indeed cause nausea.

Whatever the cause of morning sickness, pregnant women should never take anti-nausea medications such as Zofran or promethazine, which in addition to unknown effects on your developing baby, can have some severe side effects for pregnant moms, including dizziness, drowsiness, dry mouth, nausea, vomiting and weakness.

A now discredited drug for morning sickness is thalidomide. The thalidomide tragedy, in which thousands of babies were born with gross deformities of the arms and legs, originated in West Germany, where the drug was first developed and prescribed. In the U.S., Frances Oldham Kelsey, MD, of the FDA refused to approve thalidomide for use as a treatment for morning sickness. However, millions of tablets were distributed to physicians during a clinical testing program, leading to the same tragic outcome in the U.S.

Thalidomide was withdrawn in 1961; the following year Congress enacted laws requiring tests for safety during pregnancy before a drug can receive approval for sale in the U.S. But no woman should risk her unborn baby's health based on confidence in "safety tests during pregnancy" administered by the drug companies and subsequently rubber-stamped by FDA. The days when physicians cautioned women to avoid all drugs during pregnancy have passed, but it is still the only safe policy for pregnant women to follow. (That means avoiding all antibiotics, and over-the-counter drugs like aspirin and Advil as well.)

An important dietary therapy for morning sickness is to avoid low blood sugar. That means consuming plenty of fats and eating frequently enough to avoid having an empty stomach.

If fats are causing nausea, take Swedish bitters formulated for pregnancy (one-half teaspoon in water) or an ox bile tablet with each meal (see Sources). Be sure to eat fatty foods with sour lacto-fermented foods, which help digest the fats. If lacto-fermented foods cause nausea, try squeezing fresh lemon juice on your food to provide a sour taste.

The most common alternative treatments for morning sickness are ginger, acupuncture and supplements of vitamin B_6. Vitamin B_6 status tends to be marginal or low in women suffering severe morning sickness. Pyridoxal-5-phospate (a form of vitamin B_6) in sublingual tablets may help, but you should

HOLISTIC TREATMENTS FOR MORNING SICKNESS

- Raw milk or bone broth with added coconut milk, sipped throughout the day.

- Acupuncture.

- Ginger tea or ginger capsules, 1 capsule three times per day, plus plenty of ginger in your food.

- Sublingual tablets of pyridoxal-5-phosphate (a form of vitamin B_6) or Max Stress B from Premier Research (see Sources), 1 teaspoon in water twice per day. These B vitamins are made using natural fermentation and in many cases have at least taken the edge off the morning sickness. Another choice is Thorne B Complex #12 which contains both forms of the vitamin together (see Sources).

- Ox bile tablet with meals and/or Swedish bitters formulated for pregnancy (see Sources).

- Lacto-fermented condiments, such as sauerkraut, with rich and fatty foods.

- Plenty of fat with each meal to keep blood sugar stable.

- Magnesium salts baths (see Sources).

- Homeopathic remedies recommended for morning sickness include Sepia, Pulsatilla and Nux Vomica.

first try obtaining the vitamin from food. Two good sources of vitamin B_6 are liver and bananas—bananas might be more palatable than liver in cases of severe morning sickness, but a nicely seasoned liver paté, consumed in the evening when you are feeling fine, could be just the ticket for avoiding nausea the next morning.

Prolonged and severe morning sickness might be a sign of pyroluria, a condition requiring abnormally high levels of vitamin B_6 and zinc. Self tests for pyroluria are available on the Internet.[3]

By all means try acupuncture if nausea persists and prevents you from eating a healthy diet. In one study, use of acupuncture for morning sickness helped patients feel better without any adverse effects.[4] An earlier study found that acupuncture was "clinically useful" for treating the condition.[5] Many have found relief with acupressure wrist bands.

Raw milk is an excellent treatment for morning sickness. We know of severe cases of nausea that were relieved only by sipping whole raw milk throughout the day. Raw milk provides complete nourishment, including very usable vitamin B_6, along with unadulterated fats that can stabilize blood sugar. For increased effectiveness, add some powdered ginger and a little molasses to the milk, set the glass in simmering water and heat gently.

In addition to raw milk, or if raw milk is not available, bone broths with added coconut milk or cream can be sipped between meals to avoid nausea. Fresh ginger can be added to bone broths or simply to hot water, making a ginger tea.

Some women have reported relief wth magnesium salts baths (see Sources). Magnesium-rich foods include nuts and legumes.

Finally, if you have been vomiting or unable to eat, it is critical to avoid dehydration. Sparkling water with a squeeze of lemon juice plus a generous pinch of salt is your best bet for quenching thirst—and the lemon juice and salt may also help cut down on the nausea. Bone broths also work as good hydrators.

WEIGHT GAIN

According to the official view, a woman of average weight before pregnancy should gain twenty-five to thirty-five pounds during pregnancy, and up to forty-five pounds if carrying twins. Underweight women should gain twenty-eight to forty pounds while overweight women may need to gain only fifteen to twenty-five pounds during pregnancy.

As a general rule, you should gain about five pounds during your first three months of pregnancy and one pound per week during the remainder.

Why so much weight gain when the baby is born weighing only about eight pounds? Here's where the extra pounds go:

Baby	8 pounds
Placenta	2-3 pounds
Amniotic fluid	2-3 pounds
Breast tissue	2-3 pounds
Increased blood supply	4 pounds
Extra fat stores	5-9 pounds
Uterus increase	2-5 pounds
Total	25-35 pounds

It's helpful to have guidelines, but the last thing you should do during pregnancy is worry excessively about your weight—strict attention to limiting weight gain often leads pregnant women to restrict their intake of nutritious food. If you gain fifty pounds, but still feel well, don't worry about it. It's better for your baby for you to gain a little too much weight than not enough.

If you feel you are gaining more than a little too much, cut back on carbohydrate foods like potatoes and bread, but not on nutritious animal foods like raw milk, butter, seafood and meat.

EXERCISE DURING PREGNANCY

It's important to exercise during pregnancy, but don't overdo—marathon running, contact sports, and extreme workouts are not a good idea! As you grow larger, your balance may be affected, making exercise that involves balance, such as biking, skiing and horse riding a danger.

A walk in the fresh air every day provides the perfect level of activity.

Speaking of fresh air, don't neglect to sunbathe if weather permits. Folk wisdom says that sun on the belly nourishes the growing child.

Exercises that strengthen the abdomen and lower back will prepare you for the extra weight of the third trimester and make delivery easier. Be careful, however, with exercises that put stress and strain on the joints, such as excessive stretching and lunging. During pregnancy, your body produces a hormone called relaxin, which is designed to loosen the joints and make delivery easier. You may find that you have increased flexibility and range of motion, but this increased flexibility also makes you more prone to injury. If you couldn't touch your toes before pregnancy, don't try to do so while you are pregnant!

Swimming is a great activity during pregnancy—it strengthens breathing and relieves pressure on the abdomen. Unfortunately, most pools are heavily chlorinated, and chlorine is not a good chemical to be breathing in while you are pregnant. But if you have access to warm sea water, clean fresh water or a salt water-treated swimming pool, by all means swim as much as you like.

Gentle prenatal yoga is another good choice for exercise during pregnancy. Yoga squatting exercises can help prepare the pelvis for the birth.

An ideal activity during pregnancy is gardening, mainly because it involves squatting. The motion from standing to squatting with legs slightly apart helps move baby's head downward into the right position for birth. And gardening strengthens all the muscles in a relaxed and natural way—much better than trying to build up strength using exercise machines. Plus, it takes place in the fresh air and sunshine—all good for your baby-to-be.

And don't forget regular sexual intercourse with your partner as an important physical exercise during pregnancy. Studies indicate that long periods of sexual cohabitation with the father of a woman's child significantly decrease her chances of suffering preeclampsia.[6] The effect is credited to immune factors in the father's semen.[7] It also stimulates labor.

TREATING ANEMIA IN PREGNANCY

Pregnant women are usually checked for the presence of anemia—and this is an important blood test to take as anemia can have serious consequences. It's also a condition that you can do something about. Anemia in pregnancy not only makes the mother tired, but it can have adverse effects on the mental development of the child.

- Eat liver frequently, sautéed, or as paté or liverwurst.

- Make sure you are taking cod liver oil. Vitamin A is needed to absorb iron.

- Avoid refined carbohydrates and sugars.

- Take a B_{12} sublingual methylcobalamin tablet from Jarrow Formulas, one daily (see Sources).

- Blackstrap molasses, 2 tablespoons in a mug with hot water, is a good source of iron and makes an excellent afternoon pick-me-up. You may add 1 tablespoon coconut oil and 1/2 teaspoon ginger.

- Excess iron-loving pathogens, such as Candida, in the gut can cause anemia that is resistant to iron supplementation. In addition to the avoidance of carbohydrates and sugars, consume plenty of lacto-fermented foods. Of course, attention to getting the gut in balance should take place before pregnancy.

PRENATAL VITAMINS

Virtually all obstetricians, midwives and pregnancy nurse practitioners will recommend prenatal vitamins. Almost without exception, these vitamins pills are concoctions of difficult-to-absorb synthetic vitamins, artificial colors and other additives.

Consider the ingredients list of One-A-Day prenatal vitamins: Calcium Carbonate, Microcrystalline Cellulose, Magnesium Oxide, Ferrous Fumarate, Ascorbic Acid, Maltodextrin, Gelatin, dl-Alpha-Tocopheryl Acetate, Dicalcium Phosphate; Less than 2% of: Beta-Carotene, Biotin, Cholecalciferol, Croscarmellose Sodium, Cupric Oxide, Cyanocobalamin, D-Calcium Pantothenate, FD&C Red #40 Dye, FD&C Red #40 Lake, FD&C Yellow #6 Lake, Folic Acid, Hydroxypropyl Methylcellulose, Niacinamide, Polyethylene Glycol, Polysorbate 80, Potassium Iodide, Pyridoxine Hydrochloride, Riboflavin, Silicon Dioxide, Soybean Oil, Starch, Stearic Acid, Thiamine Mononitrate, Titanium Dioxide (color), Vitamin A Acetate, Zinc Oxide.

More "holistic" prenatal vitamin formulas contain additional ingredients. For example, Trimedisyn, advertised as "the most complete prenatal vitamin," contains in addition to folic acid, calcium and iron, "nineteen other essential vitamins and minerals, ten probiotics, CoQ10, DHA, ginger root, inositol, and choline—all in exact amounts to meet the needs of an expecting mother." The DHA in this formula comes from bio-engineered algae and the "vitamin A" is actually the precursor beta-carotene.

New Chapter Organic prenatal vitamins boasts the addition of herbs and sprouted seeds to their vitamin pills, along with "bacterially derived" vitamins. Unfortunately, the "vitamin A" is actually beta-carotene, and the formula also contains soy. Likewise, Vitamin Code Raw Prenatal contains carotene, not true vitamin A, and boasts B_{12}, even though it contains no animal products.

We cannot stress enough the fact that the nourishment for yourself and your growing baby needs to come from nutrient-dense food:

CALCIUM	Raw whole milk, yogurt, cheese, bone broths
FOLATE	Liver, beans, egg yolk, fish eggs, green vegetables
VITAMIN B_{12}	Liver, shellfish, fish eggs, meat, eggs
VITAMIN B_6	Raw meat, raw dairy, eggs, liver, bananas
DHA	Cod liver oil, fish eggs, egg yolks, liver
VITAMIN A	Cod liver oil, liver, egg yolks, butter
VITAMIN D	Cod liver oil, fish eggs, egg yolks, lard, butter
VITAMIN K_2	Cheese, poultry liver, meat fats, eggs
CHOLINE	Egg yolks, liver
ZINC	Red meat, liver, fish eggs
IRON	Liver, red meat, egg yolks, molasses
IODINE	Fish eggs, sea food, butter
PROBIOTICS	Lacto-fermented foods and beverages

By including liberal amounts of these foods in your diet, your baby will be getting what he needs. And remember, all these nutrient levels will be higher in the products of grass-fed animals.

If you are still concerned about getting enough nutrients for your baby, in addition to cod liver oil, Dr. Cowan recommends high-vitamin butter oil, Catalyn from Standard Process, 6 tablets per day, and B_{12}-Folic Acid from Standard Process, 3 tablets per day (see Sources).

Another choice is the multivitamin from Dr. Ron's Ultrapure (see Sources). It does not contain vitamins A and D and is designed to be taken with cod liver oil.

TRAVEL DURING PREGNANCY

There's no reason to avoid travel by car, bus or train (as long as you are able to bring nutritious food along), but travel by airplane should be minimized, especially during the first and third trimesters. Airplane cabin air, pulled from the engines, is poorly filtered and may contain some nasty chemicals; and on some international flights, passengers are sprayed with pesticides. Exposure to radiation while flying might have adverse effects, and cabin pressure changes can trigger early labor, much like women who go into labor during hurricanes.

Travel often involves long periods of sitting, which is not a good idea for pregnant women, so be sure to stand up and walk frequently if in fact you are required to fly.

VISITS TO YOUR PRACTITIONER

Once you suspect you are pregnant, you will prob-ably want to schedule a visit to a health care practitioner who focuses on pregnancy and delivery—in most cases this will be an obstetrician, but alternative physicians, nurse practitioners and midwives also offer these services. Readers of this book will most likely seek out someone open to the most natural and non-interventional approaches to pregnancy.

Unfortunately, the condition of pregnancy provides fertile ground for interventions of every description—blood tests, physical examinations, vaccinations, pharmaceutical drugs and high-tech screening. The vast majority of these interventions are not only unnecessary, but they also carry some risk; yet they are often foisted on pregnant women as though they have no choice in the matter.

The truth is, pregnant women have lots of choices, and in most cases the best choice is to just say "no." Actually, there's no reason to rush into your first prenatal exam—even conventional doctors tend to wait until at least eight weeks for the first visit—

FLU SHOTS FOR PREGNANT WOMEN

"If you're pregnant, a flu shot is your best protection against serious illness from the flu. A flu shot can protect pregnant women, their unborn babies, and even their babies after birth." This is the advice given on the Centers for Disease Control (CDC) website, advice that would have been unthinkable several decades ago, in the wake of the thalidomide-birth defect scandal. In fact, in years past, pregnancy was a contraindication to flu vaccine but today, the CDC recommends flu vaccine for women more than fourteen weeks pregnant.

Can flu vaccines harm your unborn baby? No one knows. The package inserts published by the flu vaccine manufacturers state that "Animal reproduction studies have not been conducted with influenza virus vaccine. It is also not known whether influenza virus vaccine can cause fetal harm when administered to a pregnant woman."

What is known are the risks to anyone taking the vaccine. The most common reactions are symptoms of the flu—fever, fatigue, painful joints and headache. The most serious reaction that has been associated with flu vaccine is Guillain-Barré syndrome (GBS) which occurs most often within two to four weeks of vaccination. GBS is an immune-mediated nerve disorder characterized by muscle weakness, unsteady gait, numbness, tingling, pain and sometimes paralysis of one or more limbs or the face. Recovery can take several months and can include residual disability—not something you want to risk while you are pregnant! And all for a shot that may not even be tailored to the current year's flu virus. According to one study, the shot covers only about 10 percent of the types of flu that are going around.[8]

Of course, flu during pregnancy needs to be taken seriously. As with all viral infections, the flu virus depletes vitamin A, particularly if you have flu with a high fever. If you contract the flu while pregnant, you should increase your dose of cod liver oil until all symptoms are passed, and take steps to keep your fever down (see Sidebar on Staying Cool During Pregnancy, page 67). Above all, stay in bed and take plenty of liquids, especially nourishing bone broths.

RH INCOMPATIBILITY

If you've ever had your blood type tested, you know that you're A, B, O, or AB as well as Rh positive or negative. The difference between positive and negative is a single protein called Rhesus (Rh) factor. If you have the protein sitting on the surface of your red blood cells, you're positive. If you don't, you're negative. If you're Rh negative and your baby is Rh positive, you have Rh incompatibility. If your body comes into contact with the Rh protein—a substance it's never seen before—it might begin making antibodies against it. For this reason, it may later mistake a fetus who is Rh positive for an unwelcome invader and develop an immune reaction that actually attacks it.

If you're Rh negative and your partner is Rh positive, there's a chance that your child will be positive, making incompatibility a concern. Rh incompatibility isn't usually a problem during your first pregnancy because blood from a developing fetus doesn't mingle with your own until the time of delivery. The immune system of an Rh negative mom must be exposed to Rh positive blood one or more times before it can develop a response that is strong enough to harm the baby. But during labor and delivery, you might be exposed to some of your child's blood. If you're Rh incompatible, your body might start making antibodies against this "foreign" protein.

These antibodies themselves are generally harmless until you have a subsequent pregnancy. If you become pregnant with a second Rh-positive baby, your antibodies may cross over into the baby's bloodstream and attack any cells they identify as foreign. This may cause your baby's red blood cells to swell and rupture—a condition called Rh disease. The illness can cause jaundice (yellowing of the skin and eyes), and anemia (low levels of red blood cells). In some cases, the disease can lead to brain damage, heart failure or even death. Modern medicine treats the risk of Rh disease with injections of a blood product called Rho immune globulin (RhoGAM). In other countries, women at risk get the injection within seventy-two hours of delivery, as did women in the U.S. until recently. Today doctors in the U.S. give the injection around the twenty-eighth week of pregnancy in order to prevent rare cases where a woman starts producing Rh antibodies months before delivery.

In recent years, women have begun to question the need for the RhoGAM shot (also called the Anti-D injection), especially during pregnancy as happens in the U.S. Since 2001, manufacturers have produced the vaccine labeled "thimerosol free," although traces of the mercury compound may remain; the shot definitely contains polysorbate and has been known to cause hepatitis and HIV infections in women receiving it. According to the package insert, the shot may cause side effects including severe allergic reactions (rash; hives; itching; difficulty breathing; tightness in the chest; swelling of the mouth, face, lips, or tongue); back pain; blood in the urine; dark urine; decreased urination; fast heartbeat; nausea; severe or persistent fever; shaking and/or chills; shortness of breath; sudden weight gain; swelling; unusual tiredness or weakness; wheezing; vomiting; and yellowing of the eyes or skin.

According to the March of Dimes, Rh disease affects four thousand infants each year and a mother with an RhD-negative blood type has approximately 0.7 percent chance of giving birth to a baby that suffers from the disease. If you receive the injection your chances decrease by 0.02 percent.[9]

The decision to refuse the RhoGAM injection is a difficult one to make, especially in a medical culture that accepts the treatment as self evident. It certainly should be refused during pregnancy, and only taken after the birth. A good resource to help you make the decision is *Anti-D in Midwifery, Panacea or Paradox?* by midwife Sara Wickham. Another helpful resource is http://blindedbythelightt.blogspot.com/2012/04/critical-look-at-rhogam-and-rhesus.html.

The role of nutrition in protecting your infant against Rh disease should not be neglected (although it usually is). Your diet of nutrient-dense foods, including liver and cod liver oil rich in vitamin A, can help mitigate the effects of the antibodies, strengthening the immune system of both yourself and your baby.

and when you do schedule an appointment, be well armed with information so that you can confidently refuse any unnecessary procedures. If your doctor insists on interventions you do not want, it's best to find another practitioner early in the game; failure to honor your wishes is a red flag that unwanted interventions will be foisted on you later in pregnancy and during delivery.

When making the kinds of decisions facing pregnant women, the Internet is your best friend. Never, never submit to a medical procedure without researching the benefits and side effects, especially when you are pregnant.

Typically the first prenatal visit involves an extensive medical history, physical exam, and weight and blood pressure measurements. Your physician may want to take a urine sample to test for urinary tract infections, and take a pap smear and a culture to check for chlamydia and gonorrhea. The pap smear and culture involve a pelvic examination. Some doctors do this with every visit; others let the whole pregnancy pass without a pelvic exam. If you prefer the latter course, be sure to ask about this when you make your appointment.

Typically blood is drawn to check for Rh status, anemia, syphilis, hepatitis B and immunity to rubella. In some cases the physician may also take blood to check for immunity to chicken pox and the presence of HIV, and order a skin test to see whether you've been exposed to tuberculosis.

Unfortunately, the really important measurements, such as blood tests to determine whether vitamins D, B_6, B_{12} and cholesterol levels are adequate, are rarely included in routine prenatal care. Sometimes doctors will do the tests for vitamins D and B_{12} if you ask for them. A do-it-yourself vitamin D test is available from the Vitamin D Council (see Sources).

Next on the list is the glucose tolerance test, to determine the presence of gestational diabetes. Doctors used to order the test only for those considered at high risk—now they order it for practically everyone. See page 69 for safer alternatives.

You will be offered or given a prescription for prenatal vitamins, which are not necessary if you are following our dietary guidelines. Remember that the prenatal vitamins are mostly synthetic, in a form not normally found in nature (see page 59).

If you decide to tell your doctor that you are consuming raw milk, eating liver and taking cod liver oil, be ready to stand your ground in the ensuing lecture!

The most important conventional tests for pregnant women are those that determine blood pressure and anemia. Blood pressure should be watched carefully during pregnancy (see page 71), and anemia is a serious condition that can affect the mental and physical development of your infant. (For dietary treatment of anemia during pregnancy, see Sidebar page 58.)

FLU SHOTS FOR PREGNANT WOMEN

You will almost certainly be offered a flu shot; be ready to just say "no" to that one. The flu is rarely a threat to a normal pregnancy and there is no convincing evidence that flu vaccines are effective during pregnancy anyway.

No studies have adequately assessed the risk of flu vaccine during pregnancy, not even in animals. Furthermore, many flu vaccines contain the mercury-based preservative thimerosal, which is classified as a human teratogen (meaning it causes birth defects), and even the "thimerosal free" vaccines may contain traces of mercury. Equally toxic aluminum often replaces mercury as a preservative in vaccines. The policy of routine flu vaccinations for pregnant women is not supported by the scientific literature and should be terminated.[10]

FETAL SCREENINGS

Modern medicine has devised a host of tests and interventions to determine whether your baby might be damaged or genetically defective in some way. While hailed as an important medical advance, fetal screening often leads to agonizing decisions based on incomplete knowledge. We can only describe each of these tests and present their pros and cons; we cannot make the decision for you of whether or not to take them. Such testing is completely pointless unless the parents would choose to terminate the pregnancy.

First trimester fetal screening involves a blood test called a "multiple marker screening" along with an ultrasound, the most controversial of all prenatal interventions.

Multiple marker screening is a blood test to determine the levels of three specific substances: alpha-fetoprotein (AFP), a protein normally produced by the fetus; human chorionic gonadotropin (HCG), a hormone produced within the placenta; and estriol, an estrogen produced by both the fetus and the placenta. The test is recommended for women who have a family history of birth defects, are age thirty-five or older, have diabetes and use insulin, or may have been exposed to harmful medications, drugs, viral infections or high levels of radiation during pregnancy.

High levels of AFP indicate the possibility of a neural tube defect in the infant; low levels may indicate Down syndrome. Abnormal levels of HCG and estriol may indicate other chromosome abnormalities. The key word here is "may." These tests do not provide a definitive answer as to whether your child has a deformity or chromosomal abnormality, only statistical indications. Should they indicate possible problems, additional testing may be recommended, such as amniocentesis or chorionic villus sampling (CVS).

The next step is ultrasound or sonography screening of the fetus, which uses cyclic sound pressure with a frequency greater than the upper limit of human hearing. The reflection signature can be used as a diagnostic tool to reveal muscles, tendons and internal organs. Doctors use ultrasound screening to determine the gestational age of the fetus, determine its location, assess the size and position of the placenta, determine the sex of the baby, determine the presence of twins, monitor fetal growth, check for fetal movement and heartbeat, and check for physical abnormalities.

The test lasts for ten to thirty minutes and is often given multiple times, sometimes even at every prenatal visit. If multiple marker screening indicates possible problems with the fetus, your doctor may recommend a high intensity, high resolution ultrasound, called a nuchal translucency screening, to determine the risk for Down syndrome. At high resolution, technicians can measure the clear (trans-lucent) space in the tissue at the back of the developing baby's neck. Babies with abnormalities tend to accumulate more fluid at the back of their neck during the first trimester.

Ultrasound or sonography is generally described as a "safe test" because it does not use mutagenic ionizing radiation, which can pose hazards such as chromosome breakage and cancer development.

However, in 2008, the *American Institute of Ultrasound in Medicine* published a report which stated that ultrasound indeed poses some potential risks. These include "postnatal thermal effects, fetal thermal effects, postnatal mechanical effects, fetal mechanical effects, and bio effects considerations for ultrasound contrast agents."[11] Think of the high-pitch operatic voice breaking a glass, only at the level of cells and chromosomes. In research conducted in 2001, in which an ultrasound transducer aimed directly at a miniature hydrophone placed in a woman's uterus, recorded a sound "as loud as a subway train coming into the station."[12]

In reality, a number of scientific studies have indicated considerable dangers from exposing the vulnerable fetus to ultrasound, especially to the developing brain. Additionally, frequent exposure to ultrasound is associated with a decrease in newborn body weight, an increase in the frequency of non-genetic left-handedness, delayed speech and potential speech impediments from damage to the inner ear.

Body temperature is critical to proper enzyme reactions; a core temperature of about 98.6 degrees F is the point at which many important enzyme reactions occur. Temperature affects the actual shape of the proteins that create enzymes, and improperly shaped proteins are unable to do their jobs correctly. If a condition of high heat lasts for more than a few minutes, enzyme reactions become less efficient until they are permanently inactivated, unable to function correctly even if the temperature returns to normal.

Since the fetus cannot cool off by sweating, it has another defense against temperature increases. Each cell contains what are called heat shock proteins, which temporarily stop the formation of enzymes when temperatures get too high. According

THE EFFECTS OF ULTRASOUND

- In a study of over fourteen hundred women in Perth, Western Australia, researchers compared pregnant mothers who had ultrasound only once during gestation with mothers who had five monthly ultrasounds from eighteen weeks to thirty-eight weeks. They found significantly higher intrauterine growth restriction in the intensive ultrasound group. Mothers who had received multiple ultrasound treatments gave birth to lower weight babies.[14]

- In a matched-case control study of seventy-two children two to eight years old presenting with delayed speech of unknown cause, researchers found that speech-delayed children were about twice as likely to have been exposed to ultrasound as the matched controls. The children were measured for articulation, language comprehension, language production, meta-linguistic skills, and verbal memory, all of which are sensitive measures reflecting sub-optimal conditions for development.[15]

- In 1993, a large study on ultrasound called the RADIUS study, found that routine ultrasound provided no benefit for mothers or babies in terms of pregnancy outcome. Ultrasound did not reduce the number of infant or maternal deaths nor lead to better care for the newborn. But it did expose the families to increased cost and risk.[16]

- When pregnant mice were exposed to diagnostic ultrasound, they manifested significant alterations in behavior, including decreased locomotor and exploratory activity and an increase in the number of trials needed for learning.[17]

- In another study by the same research team, mice were exposed to ultrasound, x-rays, and combinations of the two. The researchers found that repeated exposures to ultrasound or in combination with x-rays had negative effects on embryonic development, including impairment of adult brain function.[18]

- A 1997 study from Australia found that actively dividing cells of the embryonic and fetal central nervous system are most readily disturbed by prolonged ultrasound. Biologically significant temperature increases can occur at or near to bone in the fetus from the second trimester if the beam is held stationary for more than thirty seconds in some pulsed Doppler applications.[19]

- Another 1997 study found brain hemorrhages in mouse pups exposed in the womb to pulsed ultrasound at doses similar to those used on human babies.[20]

- A 2001 study found that exposing adult mice to dosages typical of obstetric ultrasound caused a 22 percent reduction in rate of cell division and a doubling of the rate of apoptosis of cells in the small intestine.[21]

- Other research has found that ultrasound induces bleeding in the lungs among other mammals, including newborns and young animals.[22]

- Exposure of mice to ultrasound waves for thirty minutes or longer caused a small but statistically significant number of neurons to remain scattered within inappropriate cortical layers and in the adjacent white matter of the brain. The magnitude of neuron dispersion was highly variable but increased with duration of exposure to ultrasound waves.[23]

to a 1998 article, when the heat shock response is activated in the fetus, normal protein synthesis is suspended, but survival is achieved at the expense of normal development.[13]

A complicating factor is the fact that ultrasound heats bone more rapidly than muscle, soft tissue or amniotic fluid. During the third trimester, the baby's skull can heat up fifty times faster than its surrounding tissue, subjecting parts of the brain close to the skull to continued heat after the ultrasound exam has concluded.

The truth is that the American Medical Association, the American College of Obstetricians and Gynecologists, and the American Academy of Family Physicians all advise against the routine or unnec-

essary use of ultrasound in pregnancy. And therein lies the dilemma: is it really necessary to determine your baby's sex, position, size and growth rate using ultrasound?

With the exception of sex determination, all this can be done by an experienced physician using hands-on skills and a fetoscope (a stethoscope designed to listen to the baby's heartbeat). And sex determination can now be very accurately accomplished at seven weeks with an over-the-counter blood test.

When ultrasound reveals a potential problem in the fetus, parents find themselves on an emotional roller coaster. Ultrasound technicians are wrong as often as they are right, and when a family is told that their unborn baby has some kind of defect, they

ULTRASOUND: AUTISM AND OTHER DEFECTS

In 1993, the FDA approved an eight-fold increase in the potential acoustical output of ultrasound equipment, greatly increasing the possibility of overheating and negative effects on the fetus. Sadly, we have no large, population-based studies examining the effects of ultrasound at the much higher intensities commonly used today.

What we do know is that since 1993, the incidence of autism has increased nearly sixty-fold. Critics of ultrasound are asking whether these two facts are related. They point out that autism has increased alarmingly during the last few decades in the very nations that use routine prenatal ultrasound on pregnant women—the U.S., Japan, Scandinavia, Australia, India and the U.K. In fact, in countries with nationalized healthcare, where virtually all pregnant women are exposed to ultrasound, autism rates exceed those in the U.S. Due to disparities in income and health insurance, and the fact that some women have enough distrust of medical interventions to refuse the ultrasound, some 30 percent of pregnant women in the U.S. do not undergo ultrasound scanning.

Over time, the number of ultrasound scans conducted during each pregnancy has increased, with low-risk women receiving two or more scans and high-risk women receiving many more. The range of time within which the fetus is scanned has been extended to include early pregnancy until late into the third trimester, and also during labor, sometimes for hours.

Consider also the fact that the ultrasound machine is often focused on the baby's genital organs in order to determine the baby's sex. Could the use of ultrasound in this way be a contributing factor to the increase in birth defects involving the genitals and urinary tract, now affecting as many as one in ten babies?[24]

The ultrasound machine is also often focused on the heart; serious defects of the heart increased nearly 250 percent between 1989 and 1996.[25]

These increases in birth defects have also paralleled the promulgation of disastrous dietary advice for pregnant women. Bad diet and the use of ultrasound could well be the deadly duo that has increased the incidence of congenital abnormalities and neuro-behavioral problems in our children to epic proportions.

will spend the rest of the pregnancy worrying, crying and in some cases may abort the baby because they are told it has an abnormality. And remember, having an ultrasound does not reduce the risk of birth defects—only sound nutrition and avoidance of environmental toxins can do that.

The most legitimate reason to undergo ultrasound screening is one in which the fetus is at high risk for abnormalities—due to the age of the mother, a family history of genetic defects, poor nutrition and exposure to toxins just prior to pregnancy. In such cases, it is best to limit the screening to one test only, and for the shortest duration possible.

Other tests for genetic defects include carrier screening, chorionic villus sampling (CVS) and amniocentesis. Carrier screening involves analyzing the DNA from blood samples or cells inside the cheek of both parents to determine whether your baby is at risk for genetic disorders like cystic fibrosis, sickle cell anemia, thalassemia and Tay-Sachs disease. If carrier screening indicates that both partners have a recessive gene for the same disorder, then further tests are recommended.

The chorionic villus is a portion of the placenta. A sample can be collected by putting a thin flexible tube or catheter through the vagina and cervix into the placenta. The sample can also be collected through a long, thin needle put through the belly into the placenta. Ultrasound is used to guide the catheter or needle into the correct spot for collecting the sample.

Amniocentesis involves collecting a small amount of amniotic fluid, which contains fetal tissues from the amnion or amniotic sac surrounding a developing fetus. The fetal DNA is then examined for genetic abnormalities.

Both CVS and amniocentesis are obviously highly invasive, the former requiring ultrasound throughout the procedure and the latter requiring a local anesthetic. They carry the risk of infection and miscarriage, not to mention damage of the fetus. And as with ultrasound, the results are not one hundred percent reliable. False positives may convince parents to terminate a pregnancy that is perfectly normal. Finally, many of the problems and weak-

NEW BLOOD TESTS FOR BIRTH DEFECTS

A simple blood test done on maternal serum early in the first trimester of pregnancy to determine whether a baby has Down syndrome or more severe genetic syndromes, is in the pipeline. The test, which analyzes fetal DNA in the mother's blood, has undergone a clinical trial showing it to be very accurate in detecting Down syndrome (Trisomy 21), Trisomy 18 (Edward's syndrome) and Trisomy 13 (Patau syndrome.) It can also detect Turner syndrome, a treatable condition in which girl babies are missing all or part of the X chromosome and face various health problems, including infertility.[26]

The study showed that Verinata's test accurately identified all 89 cases of Down syndrome, 35 out of 36 cases of Trisomy 18, and 11 of 14 cases of Trisomy 13. There were no false positives.

Most importantly, the test could replace older prenatal blood screening, such as Multiple Marker Screening, that is unreliable at predicting Down syndrome and other chromosomal abnormalities. These tests result in many false positives and often require further invasive tests such as amniocentesis, which carry a small risk of miscarriage.

The Verifi genomic test uses fast gene sequencing instruments combined with algorithms to analyze the mother's blood using a cell-free method that looks at DNA left over in blood samples in which cells have died. Approximately 20 percent to 25 percent of the DNA is from the fetus, which gives analyzers much more DNA to work with. Previous tests looked for a few fetal blood cells, perhaps 10 out of 200 billion in the sample, and those were fragile.

The test should also make the current plethora of tests and procedures less confusing, and provide more definite information to worried parents.

nesses found through these screening procedures, such as small kidney size, involve conditions that can be greatly helped through a nutrient-dense diet that supplies liberal amounts of vitamin A and other nutrients.

The bottom line is that these tests are not risk free, not completely accurate and definitely not something that makes life easier for prospective parents. They may be justified under certain conditions but their use in normal pregnancies is questionable. Worst of all, they come with a highly fatalistic attitude on the part of physicians, who assume that genes are destiny, that nothing can be done if we are dealt a bad hand in the genetic roulette of human reproduction—a view that is supported neither by science nor normal human emotions. Whether or not potential "defects" manifest in a child is due in large part on the presence or absence of a wide range of nutrients and the state of the uterine environment at conception and throughout the pregnancy. Thoughtful parents can exert a lot of control over both diet and environment, and the more diligently they prepare for conception and pay attention to the diet during gestation, the better their chances for a normal and optimally healthy child.

THE FETAL HEART MONITOR

After the twentieth week of gestation, a practitioner can easily hear the fetal heart beat, normally one hundred twenty to one hundred sixty beats per minute, with a fetoscope. Today, however, most physicians use a fetal heart monitor, a devise based on what is described as a Doppler technology, to magnify the heart beat so that both you and the physician can hear it.

The device contains a probe to detect high frequency sound waves produced by your baby's heart. To am-

---

STAYING COOL DURING PREGNANCY

If raised body temperature poses a threat to the developing fetus, what about things like hot tubs, steam rooms, saunas and hot baths? In a report on the effects of heat on fetuses, researchers warned that "hyperthermia during pregnancy can cause embryonic death, abortion, growth retardation and developmental defects."[27] A study published in the *Journal of the American Medical Association* found that women who used hot tubs or saunas during early pregnancy face up to triple the risk of bearing babies with spina bifida or brain defects.[28]

Hot tubs and prolonged hot baths present greater dangers than other heat therapies, such as saunas and steam rooms, because the immersion in water foils the body's attempt to cool off via perspiration. This does not mean that you cannot take regular baths and showers while pregnant; just don't linger or make them too hot.

While fever plays an important role in childhood (see Chapter 13), it is not such a good idea during pregnancy. If you develop a fever, it is important to take steps to keep your body temperature from going too high. One procedure to bring fever down is the application of "lemon socks." The gesture of the lemon is one of holding back or not assimilating warmth—it stays on the tree the whole season without ever becoming sweet. To make the lemon sock, squeeze one lemon into a bowl of tepid water. Dip a large cotton cloth in the water and squeeze it out so it is just damp. Wrap one foot with the cloth, starting from the toes and going to mid calf, then cover with a large sock. Repeat for the other foot and get into bed. Leave the socks on until the damp cloth has dried completely. This should help the body assimilate the fever in a healthy way.

The homeopathic medicine for bringing down fever is *Apis Belladonna* from Weleda or Uriel Pharmacy (see Sources). The dose is five pills sublingually every hour or two until the fever subsides.

Finally, an herbal tea of elder flower, lime flower, ginger and yarrow encourages sweating and can help lower a fever quickly.

plify the sound, a gel, oil or water solution is spread onto your belly. The probe is then moved around this area until the heartbeat is detected. Digital fetal monitors will then display the number of heart beats per minute on a screen. Fetal heart monitors can be purchased for home use, allowing parents to listen to baby's heart whenever they like.

What the glowing descriptions of fetal heart monitors do not reveal is the fact that these devises use ultrasound waves for detecting the baby's heartbeat. This is the same technology that has led to concerns about ultrasound devices that project images of the fetus on a screen. Even worse, the Doppler scans use continuous energy, rather than multiple pulsed energy of the diagnostic ultrasound.

There is sufficient evidence that multiple pulsed ultrasound scans, or as few as two continuous wave Doppler scans, or any ultrasound scan performed by an unskilled operator may cause harm. Why subject your unborn baby to anything that may cause damage, especially when a fetoscope works just as well?

According to a review study, "routine Doppler ultrasound in pregnancy does not have health benefits for women or babies and may do some harm."[29] A fetoscope works fine and that is what you should insist on.

GESTATIONAL DIABETES

Gestational diabetes is high blood sugar (diabetes) that starts or is first diagnosed during pregnancy. Usually there are no symptoms, or the symptoms are mild and not life threatening to the pregnant woman, although mothers with gestational diabetes do have an increased risk for high blood pressure during pregnancy. In severe cases, symptoms may include blurred vision, fatigue, frequent infections (especially of the bladder, vagina and skin), increased thirst, increased urination, nausea, vomiting and weight loss. Often, the blood sugar (glucose) level returns to normal after delivery.

Pregnant women with gestational diabetes tend to have larger babies at birth—having a baby over ten pounds always raises the suspicion of gestational diabetes. A large baby can increase the chance of problems at the time of delivery, including birth injury (trauma) because of the baby's large size; having a large baby also increases the chance of delivery by C-section.

(Actually, babies born to mothers following our nutrient-dense diet tend to be smaller than average, with denser bones. Doctors may interpret this as a problem with fetal growth as they are used to oversized babies. Often when baby is weighed, she turns out to be two or more pounds heavier than she looks.)

NATURAL TREATMENTS FOR IMPROVING GLUCOSE TOLERANCE

CINNAMON: A number of studies have confirmed the age-old tradition of cinnamon as an aid to glucose metabolism. So put cinnamon on your morning porridge or toast.

GYMNEMA: Known in Ayurvedic medicine as "sugar buster," this herb can be safely used by pregnant women. Mediherb makes a gymnema tablet that can be taken one tablet, two or three times per day to improve carbohydrate metabolism (see Sources).

ROSEMARY: Rudolf Steiner pointed to the use of rosemary as a help with diabetes. He described how rosemary awakens the ego or mental body, which is the part of us that can consciously affect our inner sugar balance. Rosemary can be used as an herb, and it can be taken internally, but Steiner specifically suggested rosemary oil baths for diabetes. Rosemary oil is available from Dr. Hauschka suppliers (see Sources). Add one tablespoon to a full warm bath, and soak for twenty minutes, two to five times per week. After the bath, one should wrap up in a warm blanket or towel and go directly to bed, to encourage the retention of the warmth. If you find the effect too stimulating for sleep, then take the bath in the morning, still keeping warm in bed for about twenty minutes afterwards.

Babies born to mothers with gestational diabetes are more likely to have periods of low blood sugar (hypoglycemia) during the first few days of life and there is a slightly increased risk of the baby dying when the mother has untreated gestational diabetes. There is also increasing evidence the diabetic state of the mother somehow imprints changes into the baby's system that place the child at higher risk for rapid weight gain and early childhood obesity.[30]

Your best protection against gestational diabetes is the diet we have outlined in the pages of this book, low in refined carbohydrates, containing adequate animal protein and rich in healthy fats, along with daily moderate exercise, all of which act together to keep the blood sugar stable. The diet should also include the fat-soluble vitamins, which your organs need to work properly. In particular, vitamin D is needed for insulin production. Your requirements for vitamin D increase during pregnancy, as vitamin D plays an important role in the building of the fetus; thus if your own intake is inadequate, pancreatic function may be sacrificed to the needs of the growing baby.

If you are following our dietary guidelines, your chances of developing gestational diabetes are low. But because gestational diabetes is a growing problem in the U.S., doctors now recommend routine testing for the condition between the twenty-fourth and twenty-eighth week of pregnancy. The problem is that the recommended diagnostic tool—the oral glucose tolerance test—is itself a risky procedure.

To take the test, the patient is given a sweet liquid containing glucose on an empty stomach. Then a blood sample is collected one hour later, at the time when blood sugar levels peak before beginning to drop. Unfortunately, that drop in blood sugar may go too low, putting the vulnerable pregnant woman in a state of hypoglycemia or low blood sugar.

Ironically, this dangerous test is mostly reserved for pregnant women. For the rest of the population, the main test used is the "casual plasma glucose test," in which a sample of blood is drawn without regard to the time of the last meal or the content of that meal. You are not required to abstain from eating prior to the test nor take a highly sweetened drink— the very worst thing a diabetic can do, especially a pregnant diabetic.

A glucose level greater than 200 mg/dL may indicate diabetes, especially if the test is repeated at a later time and shows similar results. Another test measures a protein in the blood called A1c, which indicates the levels of blood sugar over time.

If you have trouble controlling carbohydrate intake, have consumed a standard American diet for many years, are overweight or have a history of diabetes in the family, then you need to take the risk of gestational diabetes seriously.

If you manifest symptoms, you should have a casual plasma glucose test or the A1c test—not the dangerous oral glucose tolerance test—and then make a serious effort to get your blood sugar under control. This means eliminating refined carbohydrates and processed foods, and consuming more healthy fats—don't be afraid of putting loads of butter on everything you eat, including vegetables, meat and seafood.

Above all, it is important to ensure adequate intake of vitamin D, as vitamin D is critical to the production of insulin. That means consuming cod liver oil, grassfed butter and egg yolks, grassfed lard and seafood like shrimp and fish eggs.

RUBELLA AND OTHER VIRUSES

Rubella or German measles is characterized by a low fever, rash, swollen glands and achy joints. The illness is associated with a virus, which may or may not be the proximate cause. Many people said to be "exposed" to the virus—that is, the antibodies to the virus are found in their blood stream—do not develop symptoms.

Most children and adults fully recover from rubella with few complications. However, rubella infection in a pregnant woman during the first three months of pregnancy can result in miscarriage, fetal death or a baby with a birth defect, such as deafness, eye, heart, liver or skin problems, or mental retardation—a complex of abnormalities referred to as congenital rubella syndrome (CRS).

Conventional medicine treats the rubella problem with vaccines, calling for the rubella vaccine in children at twelve months of age. Whether due to the vaccine, improved hygiene or some other factor, the fact is that far fewer people now contract the disease in childhood, so we have many mothers becoming pregnant who have not been exposed to rubella, or for whom any immunity from the vaccination has worn off.

Conventional medicine suggests that a pregnant woman have a blood test to determine her immune levels. If found to have no immunity, she is advised to avoid people who have rubella and to get a rubella shot after delivery. Because the rubella vaccine (always given along with vaccines for mumps and measles) contains the attenuated (live but weakened) virus, the orthodox advice has warned pregnant women to avoid the vaccine; however, after a Centers for Disease Control (CDC) report showing no birth defects in children of mothers who had received the vaccine during pregnancy,[31] physicians have not felt the need to be so diligent in applying the precautionary approach. The CDC still does not recommend the rubella vaccine for pregnant women, but in today's vaccine-happy atmosphere, it may be offered in some medical practices. As with all medications during pregnancy, the safest response is still "no." The triple MMR vaccine—it is impossible to get a vaccine for rubella alone—has a long list of adverse side effects.

The focus on vaccines for rubella begs the question of why such a mild illness in pregnant woman is associated with birth defects. The orthodox explanation is that the rubella virus is capable of crossing the placenta and infecting the fetus, where it destroys cells or stops them from developing.

Little if any attention is focused on the nutritional status of the pregnant women who contracts rubella. The risk to the unborn child is high—miscarriage, still birth and birth defects occur in up to one percent of pregnant women who contract the illness; nevertheless, 99 percent of pregnancies are not affected. Surely a strong immune system, supported by good nutrition, plays a role in protecting the fetus.

Is it possible that vitamin A—which directs the development of the organs in early pregnancy—is depleted in the body's attempt to deal with the viral infection? Or that depletion of vitamin A in early pregnancy makes the pregnant woman vulnerable to a certain type of virus and its endotoxins?

Hilary Butler, author of *Rubella in Babies & Pregnant Women*, makes just such an argument, noting that viruses "pull vitamin A out of the system."[32] This applies not just to the rubella virus but also *Toxoplasma gondii*, HIV, cytomegalovirus and others. The link with birth defects stems from the fact that during the first few weeks, when a baby is forming, cells divide very quickly. Vitamin A is key to proper cell division, and if a mother contracts a virus, the body uses that vitamin A to fight the infection but the baby keeps on forming—minus one or more essential building blocks.

Surely taking cod liver oil and other vitamin A-rich foods is a better strategy than vaccines for preventing birth defects induced by the many known viruses—as well as viruses yet to be discovered.

SWELLING

A common complaint during pregnancy is swelling of the feet, ankles, fingers and hands. When you're pregnant, your body increases its supply of blood and other fluids by as much as 50 percent, softening and preparing the joints for childbirth. A lot of liquid surrounds the baby at all times, but swollen extremities are common starting around the fifth month.

This fluid has an important role to play in the upcoming birth, but it can also make you feel uncomfortable; some women experience pain in their legs and backs, others in their arms and hands.

Physical relief can be obtained with ice packs, Epsom salts baths and support hose—yes, support hose are made for pregnant women and can give considerable relief, especially if you need to be on your feet for any length of time.

It goes without saying that wearing high heels is not a good idea during pregnancy. This does not mean you necessarily need to wear matronly "sensible" shoes. Attractive flats with sturdy soles are the shoes of choice during pregnancy, especially in the later months.

Be sure to take time to rest your feet and legs by putting your feet up on a sofa or stool. And by the fifth month of pregnancy, you'll want loose, comfortable clothes for a number of reasons, including protection against swelling. Finally, don't let swelling prevent you from regular exercise, even if it only entails a daily walk around the block.

Conventional advice on swelling includes the suggestion to reduce salt consumption, but remember that you need salt for digestion, and baby needs salt for neurological development; however, avoiding all processed foods, which contain not only salt but also refined carbohydrates, the wrong fats and plenty of questionable additives, is certainly the first step for avoiding or reducing swelling. Raw milk, sipped throughout the day, is an excellent treatment for edema. Foods rich in potassium, such as bananas or potassium broth (see Recipes), can also be helpful.

PREECLAMPSIA, TOXEMIA AND ECLAMPSIA

Preeclampsia, characterized by sudden swelling in the hands and face, is caused by high blood pressure during pregnancy, often with accompanying toxemia, that is, a decline in liver and kidney function. Usually edema of pregnancy happens gradually, not overnight. But in preeclampsia, abnormally high blood pressure causes noticeable facial and hand swelling; if you experience sudden swelling, contact your doctor. He or she will monitor blood pressure and test for protein in the urine.

Preeclampsia is most common in first pregnancies, in women carrying twins or triplets, in women older than thirty-five, and in women with a history of obesity, diabetes, high blood pressure or kidney disease.

Mild cases are not dangerous but occasionally preeclampsia develops into full blown eclampsia, characterized by what is referred to as the HELLP syndrome—hemolysis (breaking of the red blood cells), elevated liver enzymes and low platelet count. In addition to swelling, other symptoms can include headache, nausea and vomiting, upper abdominal pain and vision problems.

This condition can have serious consequences, including permanent liver and kidney damage in the mother and death in the infant; the conventional treatment is to deliver the baby as soon as possible, even if premature. In most cases, however, the preeclampsia is mild, often manifesting simply as el-

evated blood pressure without any other symptoms. In these situations, bed rest is advised until the baby reaches term. Treatment with Epsom salts baths may help bring the blood pressure down.

Do make every effort to treat the condition at home with bed rest, frequent consumption of liquids and lots of good food; plenty of high-protein foods are recommended (see Sidebar, page 72) and no skimping on salt. Acupuncture treatments may be helpful.

In a hospital setting, you may be treated with blood pressure-lowering medications and steroids to hasten development of the baby's lungs.

Doctors may also suggest treatment with intravenous magnesium sulfate to lower blood pressure, reduce the risk of seizures and delay birth until the baby comes to term. This should be avoided except in extreme cases. Side effects of magnesium sulfate in the mother include muscle weakness, buildup of fluid in the lungs and blurred vision; rare side effects in the infant include low vitality at birth, low blood pressure and fluid in the lungs. Anecdotal evidence suggests that intravenous magnesium sulfate treatment may interfere with successful breastfeeding.

As with all other problems in pregnancy, the best defense is a good diet, devoid of junk food and rich in protein and saturated fats—saturated fats are highly protective of the liver. Preeclampsia is associated with low levels of selenium, vitamin D and protein—just one more reason to concentrate on animal foods rich in these nutrients, while avoiding carbohydrate-rich processed foods.

A STRESS-FREE PREGNANCY

One hundred years ago, pregnancy was viewed as a "delicate condition," which required special attention and care; today opinion has swung to the opposite extreme, one that assures pregnant women they do not need to curtail any activities until perhaps the last month or two.

The best course of action lies somewhere between these two extremes. Baring severe fatigue or morning sickness, pregnant women can and should continue their normal activities, including working outside the home. However, while the condition of pregnancy may not be "delicate," it is a time of

DIETARY TREATMENT OF PREECLAMPSIA

The factors involved in preeclampsia were elucidated in the 1950s and 1960s by an obstetrician, Dr. Tom Brewer. He discovered that the cause of preeclampsia was an abnormal blood volume, caused by malnutrition, or food deficiency, particularly protein deficiency.

The body's ability to nourish the growing fetus depends a great deal on its ability to increase the mother's blood volume. Normally, this blood volume is expected to increase by 50-60 percent over the course of the pregnancy. The liver makes albumin to facilitate this blood volume expansion. Albumin is similar to egg white. When it is in the mother's bloodstream, it creates osmotic pressure, which pulls extra fluid out of her tissues and back into the blood circulating in her blood vessels. The only way that the liver can make this albumin is from protein the mother eats.

However, if the mother is trying to restrict her weight gain to someone's "ideal" number, by going on a low-salt, low-calorie diet, much of the protein that she eats will get burned up for energy expenditure. Brewer found that when a woman ate one-third fewer calories than the twenty-six hundred calories he suggested, or about seventeen hundred calories, half the protein that she ate got burned for calories. In that case, only about half her protein intake would be available to make albumin (and baby cells, and uterine muscle cells), and she would probably have trouble expanding her blood volume adequately.

Salt also creates osmotic pressure to pull extra fluid out of the tissues and into circulation. Salt restriction is dangerous in healthy women. A healthy woman's taste buds are usually the most accurate indicator of the amount of salt that she needs, and studies have shown that it is not possible for a healthy pregnant woman to eat too much salt. Her kidneys simply excrete whatever extra salt that she eats. In fact, it has been shown that after just two weeks of "salt in moderation," the mother's blood volume begins to drop.

When the blood volume stops increasing, or drops, the body has no way of knowing that the mother is just eating less. All it knows is that the blood volume is less than it's supposed to be. So it starts the same processes that it uses when the blood volume is dropping due to hemorrhage. The internal organs must be preserved, at the expense of the limbs, if necessary. So the kidneys produce an enzyme called renin, which causes the blood vessels to constrict. During hemorrhage, this response is a very helpful stop-gap measure, decreasing the amount of blood in the limbs, to send more blood to the internal organs, while help is on the way. During pregnancy, however, when no hemorrhage is occurring, this blood vessel constriction causes a rise in blood pressure. Attempting to treat this rising blood pressure with salt restriction or weight restriction only causes the blood volume to drop even more, leading to further formation of renin and more blood vessel constriction. And the blood pressure continues to rise.

Meanwhile, the kidneys are desperately trying to increase the blood volume by reabsorbing as much water and salt as they can from the fluid that they have filtered out of the blood. They return this reabsorbed fluid and salt to the circulation. However, since there isn't enough albumin and salt in the circulation to hold this reabsorbed water, much of it leaks out into the tissues. The kidneys keep reabsorbing water at one end of the process, the water keeps leaking out of the capillaries at the other end, and the mother sees rapid swelling in her ankles and rapid weight gain (from the extra water in her tissues).

Many sources maintain that there is no known cause of toxemia, and therefore many practitioners continue to try to manage the situation by treating the symptoms alone, but they do so without success. The symptoms not only persist, but the mother also continues to experience one complication after another. The appropriate medical treatment for preeclampsia and eclampsia is IV albumin. Dr. Brewer would often tell of one woman who, unable to find a doctor who would give her IV albumin, brought her blood pressure down by eating fifty-two eggs and drinking six quarts of milk, over a period of three days.[33]

greatly increased hormone production and nutritional needs. Too much stress during pregnancy can use up vital nutritional stores, especially vitamin A. Worry and stress can be especially hard on the adrenal glands, leading to adrenal fatigue in both mother and baby.

Pregnant women need to set boundaries and be kind to themselves. Pregnancy is not the time to take on new projects, launch a business venture, organize a conference, accept a challenging assignment at work, get involved in politics, change jobs or remodel a house. (If you have to move house during pregnancy, try to time the move during the second trimester, not during early or late pregnancy.)

Pregnancy is a time for women to focus on their own needs, especially their need for optimum nutrition and adequate rest. Throughout the nine-month period, pregnant mothers should make a special effort to take the time to relax and engage in activities they like to do. And don't forget to maintain personal grooming—take time to be well-kept and attractive, and you will feel better about yourself and the coming birth.

Finally, don't be afraid to ask for help with chores like housekeeping, cooking, driving or care for other children. Sometimes even a little extra help can be a great relief.

With adequate rest, good nutrition and extra help from family and friends, the joy and excitement of that first "I'm pregnant" moment will last throughout pregnancy until the highly anticipated moment of birth.

Chapter 4
Your Baby is Born

Anthropologists tell us that among truly primitive cultures, childbirth is easy and painless, a simple and rapid process. In his visit to Alaska, Weston Price interviewed Dr. Joseph H. Romig, superintendent of the government hospital for Eskimos and Indians at Anchorage, Alaska.

"He stated that in his thirty-six years among the Eskimos," wrote Dr. Price, "he had never been able to arrive in time to see a normal birth by a primitive Eskimo woman." In fact, in many cultures, women give birth without any help. Dr. Price provides us with an outstanding example: "One Eskimo woman who had married twice, her last husband being a white man, reported to Dr. Romig and myself that she had given birth to twenty-six children and that several of them had been born during the night and that she had not bothered to waken her husband, but had introduced him to the new baby in the morning."[1]

All this changed with the advent of "civilization" and western foods. Wrote Price, "But conditions have changed materially with the new generation of Eskimo girls, born after their parents began to use foods of modern civilization. Many of them are carried to his hospital after they had been in labour for several days." Price cited the example of a hospital at the Six Nation Reservation at Brantford, Ontario, Canada, used "largely to care for young Indian women during abnormal childbirth."

Among "civilized" peoples, during the seventeenth and eighteenth centuries, between one and two births out of a hundred ended in the mother's death—from exhaustion, dehydration, infection, hemorrhage or convulsions. As the typical woman had five to eight pregnancies, her lifetime chance of dying in childbirth was one in eight.[2]

Pain in childbirth was considered God's punishment for Eve's sin of eating the forbidden fruit in the Garden of Eden. Not surprisingly, women regarded pregnancy with great fear, "the evel hour I look forward to with dread," as one American colonist wrote in her diary. And if a woman survived the birth, she often faced the death of her child in infancy. Typically, three children in ten died before the age of five.

Mortality rates reached very high levels in maternity institutions in the 1800s, sometimes climbing to 40 percent of women giving birth. The outcome was considerably better for home births with midwives assisting the delivery. One midwife, Martha Ballard, who practiced in Augusta, Maine between 1785 and 1812, delivered almost one thousand women with only four recorded fatalities.[3]

It was during the second half of the eighteenth century that men began to take an active part in a profession formerly the exclusive arena of women. Many well-to-do urban women chose male mid-wives and physicians, assuming that they would make childbirth safer and less painful. Physicians were more likely than midwives to intervene in labor with forceps and drugs, and also more likely to carry pathogenic germs from their work in the hospital morgues.

The mid-nineteenth century saw the introduction of ether and chloroform to relieve pain in childbirth. The practice of putting women to sleep during labor, along with newly instituted cleanliness protocols, contributed to the shift from home to hospital deliveries. In 1900 in the U.S., over 90 percent of all births occurred in the mother's home; by 1940, over half took place in hospitals and by 1950, 90 percent of births took place in hospitals. While sedation of the mother greatly reduced her suffering, many scientists, including Dr. Price, expressed concern about the effects of the general anesthetic on the oxygen supply to the infant. A paper presented to the American Medical Association in 1938 cited evidence that deficiency of oxygen caused microscopic changes in the infant brain and "various degrees of brain atrophy."[4]

A 1933 study by the New York Academy of Medicine revealed that mothers were better off delivering at home with the help of a midwife than in a hospital with the help of a physician. Researchers were surprised at the lack of improvement in death rates during the preceding twenty years; newborn deaths from birth injuries had actually increased. The report served as a jolt to obstetricians and galvanized the transformation of childbirth into a high-tech procedure involving fetal monitoring, blood transfusions, intravenous fluids, epidural or spinal anesthesia, drugs to speed labor, and—the most extreme intervention—delivery by Caesarean section. As much as we may decry these interventions, the medicalization of delivery coincided with a decline in death rates for women in childbirth, from one in one hundred births to about eleven per one hundred thousand, a difference of two orders of magnitude.[5]

Absent from historical accounts of childbirth trends is any mention of an amazing book, *Safe Childbirth*, by Kathleen Vaughn, published in Baltimore in 1937. Vaughn argued that ease of labor depended on a broad, well-shaped pelvis with a round opening. Weston Price noted that this "underdevelopment of the hips" paralleled the narrowing of the face that occurred with the introduction of processed food. Vaughn also argued that women should take steps to develop "flexible pelvic joints. . . [which] can be attained by correct exercises practiced during pregnancy so that the pelvis may expand at the joints (sacro-ilian and pubic symphysis) during the act of birth." She urged physicians to allow mothers to take the position "adopted instinctively by most women if left to do as they like at the time of confinement—squatting, crouching, kneeling."

Almost fifty years would pass before maternity wards would allow women to give birth comfortably by squatting or crouching, rather than in a prone position. But even a natural position during childbirth would not ensure success, said Vaughn, if the mother's pelvic opening were not large enough or her joints sufficiently flexible.

We provide this brief history in order to put modern childbirth practices into perspective. Most women today hope for a quick, natural childbirth, without interventions, without anesthetics. There is much to criticize about modern hospital deliveries, but critics usually fail to take into account the fact that most women giving birth today are laboring (literally) under the burden of several generations of poor nutrition. A nutrient-dense diet, appropriate preparation and a doctor or midwife with experience in natural childbirth can increase the odds for a successful outcome—indeed, many women who follow our dietary principles report a quick and easy birth that is almost painless.

But even those who consume a superlative diet during pregnancy may not be able to overcome the disadvantages of earlier dietary deficits. Her pelvic opening may be oval and narrow rather than round; endocrine imbalances may prevent the outpouring of hormones needed to soften the joints and speed delivery; and factors unknown may result in a baby getting stuck or presenting the bottom, feet or even shoulder to complicate the birth.

Observations of primitive peoples show us that rapid, natural and uncomplicated delivery for every woman is indeed possible; but the damage wreaked by several generations of poor diet may take several generations to reverse. In the meantime, many an expectant mother will end up submitting to interventions that she does not want, but which she will recognize as necessary to save her life and the life of her infant.

Fortunately, modern obstetrical practice has instituted a variety of improvements during the last few decades: the epidural is better for the baby than general sedation; the C-section is arguably safer than a forceps delivery in the hands of an inexperienced physician; improvements in surgical methods make recovery from C-section easier than before; and many hospital practices allow a more promising environment for mother and baby.

Natural positions during delivery, immediate maternal bonding, in-room arrangements for mother and newborn and many other baby-friendly practices are more widely available in hospitals today. And we now know a lot more about maternal and infant nutrition, knowledge that can minimize the negative consequences of these interventions.

While modern child delivery practices may not be ideal, birth is no longer an evil hour to be anticipated with dread; and fear of infant (or maternal) death no longer clouds the joyful arrival of your baby.

DECISIONS, DECISIONS

Long before baby arrives, prospective parents must make many important decisions. Obstetrician or midwife? Hospital, home birth or birth center? The ideal middle ground is a birth center, staffed by experienced midwives or nurse practitioners, one near to a hospital should things go awry. Deliveries that begin in a birth center are only 4 percent likely to end in C-section, compared to about 30 percent of those that begin in a hospital setting.[6] The problem is that birth centers are few and far between, especially in small towns. Also, a birth that begins in a birth center or at home with a midwife but ends up as a C-section in a hospital may not be covered by insurance—be sure to check with your insurance company on this.

High-tech interventions are avoided with a home birth—an option that requires a very experienced midwife and a family history of good health and easy delivery. While the medical profession has mounted a vigorous opposition to home births, studies show that a planned home birth with a certified birth attendant does not carry any greater risk than a planned hospital birth. Unattended home births and preterm home births *do* have a higher risk than a hospital birth, so if you go into early labor, or begin hard labor unexpectedly, get yourself to the hospital as soon as you can.

For the vast majority of women, the only choice is a hospital setting, but hospitals today offer a variety of options, including comfortable beds for delivery, rooming in after the birth and breastfeeding classes. Expectant parents should make a list of questions and organize an interview with enough time so that their concerns can be thoroughly answered.

If you take a childbirth class—something that is highly recommended—you will glean a lot of helpful advice from the instructor on practices at the various local hospitals and the suitability of various local obstetricians and midwives.

You will also want to query the hospital about postnatal practices. Does the hospital allow the presence of a birth assistant or doula? What about skin-to-skin contact of mother and baby immediately after birth to initiate breastfeeding, even after a Caesarean birth? Will they allow the complete drainage of the cord blood into the baby before the umbilical cord is cut? Will the hospital allow the waxy vernix caseosa to remain on the baby, or will it be dried off? Will baby be removed from the parents' sight at any time? Will baby be allowed to stay in the room with mom? What about routine interventions, such as vitamin K shots, sugar water in a bottle, antiseptic eye drops, circumcision—any problem if these are refused? Above all, can the hospital guarantee that baby will not be given any vaccinations after the birth? (See Chapters 5 and 6 for further discussion of these issues.)

And what about hospital food? Do meals contain real butter, eggs, meat, cheese? If not, can a friend or relative bring in nutritious food?

The challenge of the hospital delivery is the difficulty in avoiding unnecessary interventions during labor and afterwards to the newborn. A natural birth at a hospital is best accomplished by hiring the services of a doula, especially for your first child. A doula is a birth assistant who provides physical and emotional support during childbirth. She will visit you at your home during the pregnancy and give you advice on preparing for labor, delivery and caring for your new baby. When labor starts, she will come to your home to be at your side, assisting you during contractions and providing massage and other support. She will accompany you to the hospital and may remain at your side during the birth, acting as your agent in dealings with hospital staff and ensuring that interventions are withheld unless absolutely necessary. A postpartum doula may stay at your home for several weeks, providing breastfeeding support, help with cooking, newborn care, errands and light housekeeping.

In any event, the choice you make must be a choice you are comfortable with. Many women find the hospital environment to be highly unpleasant, one where the constant pressure to consent to various interventions sends the stress hormones coursing and the blood pressure soaring. Others become fearful at the very thought of a home delivery; such moms will feel most at ease in a highly structured hospital setting. The most important thing is to ponder all the upcoming decisions beforehand. Make a list, ask questions and think through the various choices that lie ahead so that you can make decisions before the fact, not during the heat of labor.

Another decision involves the father's presence at the delivery. Parents fought hard against a recalcitrant medical establishment for the father's right to see the birth. Today this is a routine practice—even an expected practice—but it is one that needs careful consideration. Many fathers lack the necessary skills in massage and relaxation counseling, many would simply rather remain in the waiting room— and many mothers would prefer to give birth with an experienced woman, such as a doula or midwife, rather than with the father present.

Michel Odent, a prominent obstetrician and expert on maternal hormones, argues that the presence of the father, for whom the birth process often produces an adrenaline rush, may make the mother tense and slow her production of the hormone oxytocin, resulting in a longer and more difficult labor.[7] In primitive societies, childbirth was a women's affair; in general men did not participate. On the other hand, the father's presence and participation may result in more involvement in the child's upbringing. After all, childbirth is a thrilling moment, and the father's presence may lead to bonding with mother and child that might not otherwise occur! And dad can be helpful making sure the hospital performs no unwanted interventions or vaccines.

ON THE HOME FRONT

Good preparation at home will make for an easier transition from pregnancy to motherhood. Baby will need a bed or cot, bedclothes, clothing and diapers. Make sure your car is outfitted with a car seat—it is illegal to drive with baby in a passenger's arms. Most mothers will want to invest in a baby sling or carrier. A baby seat that sits securely on the floor or counter top allows baby to safely observe goings on while his parents carry out daily activities like getting dressed, cooking or cleaning (for further information, see Chapter 8).

Most importantly, have food ready so you don't have to prepare meals during the first few weeks after the birth. A freezer full of frozen soups, stews and casseroles can lighten the load; frozen bone broth will help you revitalize after the birth; potassium broth makes an excellent post-birth tonic and should be on hand. And don't forget to have cod liver oil—the best post-natal support and breastfeeding superfood you can choose. If you participate in a food co-op or milk group, make sure someone can pick up your delivery for you until you are back in the swing of things.

It's good to have help at home, but that does not necessarily mean a prolonged stay by relatives. It might be better to arrange for in-laws to visit after you have had several weeks to adjust to your new status as mother. If relatives come to stay, they should be relatives you are comfortable with— having an experienced doula stay with you for the first week or two may be a better choice. Even if you don't think you will need help during the first weeks, you should have someone to call on in case you need to stay in bed after a difficult delivery or a Caesarean. Ideally your baby's father can take time off from work to assist in those first few weeks. Remember, you will be up frequently at night, and on call for breastfeeding throughout the day.

It's important to make sure that other children in your household are not neglected. Organizing some activities, classes or an afternoon babysitter for your new baby's siblings can be a wise move, one that gives mom some rest and brothers and sisters a diversionary outlet. Even better, as soon as you can, have someone look after the baby for a short period of time so that you can give a period of undivided attention to older siblings. If you already have a large family, do indeed invite a grandparent to stay and help out with family chores during the first few weeks.

CHILDBIRTH CLASSES

Pre-natal classes are an excellent way to prepare for labor and birth. The typical class includes up to eight weekly sessions and consists of lectures, discussion and exercises, led by a trained childbirth instructor. Usually the aim is to provide you with the tools you need to have a natural delivery, although classes at hospitals may be designed to vector you into medicalized interventions.

Classes should cover signs of labor, normal progress of labor and birth, your partner's role during labor, and when to contact your midwife or doctor. Most importantly, these classes should teach you breathing and relaxation techniques for coping with labor pains.

Some classes will cover complications, interventions and C-sections as well as breastfeeding techniques and newborn care. You will also find out about the pros and cons of the various local hospitals and birth centers.

Different techniques for dealing with the rigors of labor are available. Lamaze, Bradley method and hypno-birthing classes all teach various breathing and relaxation techniques to increase the chances of a birth free from routine medical interventions. Another choice is the Birth Works® childbirth classes, which provide information on a variety of methods to promote relaxation and facilitate labor.

The average American woman, preparing for her first child, is unlikely to have witnessed a childbirth. Some may have seen films of highlights of births that were edited for class. Many will have seen a birth on TV or in a movie. And almost every woman will have heard other women share their version of what happened to them. But how does this information help her in understanding what a normal childbirth is like?

You have no doubt heard women explain how different each birth is, that you never have any idea how it will go. That is true, to an extent. There are some variables that will cause labor to occur at different speeds or with different sensations. But for the most part, every woman experiences the same process for giving birth. Knowing the basic process of childbirth will help you understand and deal with any issues that may arise during your labor.

THE LAST MONTH

By the last month, most women will want to be off work—there is a real physiological reason for organizing your life so that your last month is as stress-free as possible. Under stress, we produce adrenaline, and adrenaline can inhibit the birth process. As preparation for a problem-free delivery,

---

PREPARING THE NIPPLES FOR BREASTFEEDING

Most modern advice to pregnant women insists that no preparation of the nipples for breastfeeding is necessary. Yet there are folk remedies for this very thing. One is to rub the nipples with diluted lemon juice, about once a day, starting several months before the birth. A similar procedure recommends rubbing the nipples with methylated spirits (denatured alcohol). You can mix the alcohol with equal parts of olive oil or almond oil. This certainly seems a simple precaution to avoid the very painful condition of sore and cracked breasts. In addition, your pregnancy diet will do a lot to prepare the breasts and nipples for pain-free nursing. Specifically, arachidonic acid in butter and meat fats creates strong cell-to-cell junctures and hence strong, healthy skin. Vitamin A from cod liver oil and liver is a critical nutrient for strong skin, as is zinc, from red meat and liver.

do your best to avoid situations that cause mental strain, frustration and worry. Instead, do the things you like to do and "go with the flow."

A rush of domesticity is common—during the last month or so, expectant mothers often develop a surge of enthusiasm for household chores such as cooking, cleaning out cupboards and organizing a room for baby. This is a great way to spend your last month, just be careful not to overdo. Be sure to continue your focus on nutritious, nutrient-dense food in preparation for delivery and never resist the temptation for a nap!

As your due date draws near, you will be monitored more frequently. At each appointment, your practitioner will measure blood pressure, weight gain and fundal height, that is, the distance of the top of the uterus from the pubic bone. This measurement gives a good idea of growth rates and may indicate potential problems such as a breech or sideways presentation. Your practitioner will listen to the baby's heart and note the pulse rate, which is normally one hundred twenty to one hundred sixty beats per minute. Your practitioner should use only a fetoscope; avoid

use of fetal monitors or ultrasound scans as much as possible (see Chapter 3).

THE GROUP B STREP TEST

At around thirty-five to thirty-seven weeks gestation, pregnant women are routinely given a swab test to determine whether they are "infected" with Group B Strep (GBS), a bacterium that approximately one in every three women carries in her vagina. Those who test positive are routinely given IV antibiotics during labor and delivery.

Here is yet another example of an intervention that has become routine, that is unnecessary, and that can carry unfortunate long-term consequences. At the very time when science is showing us the importance of healthy microbial life in the vaginal tract and on the bodies of pregnant mothers, along comes a practice that may disrupt normal flora— and normal flora can contain the Strep organism— so critical for programming the infant's intestinal tract at birth.

This bacterium poses little or no threat to the preg-

PACKING YOUR BAG FOR THE BIRTH

Here's a checklist for your hospital bag:

- Cosmetic case with items you use, such as shampoo, contact lens case and solution, glasses, tooth-brush and toothpaste
- Coconut oil or other massage oil
- Your own wash cloths and a large towel
- Waterproof pads for the car ride
- Any clothes of your own that you wish to wear as an alternative to hospital gowns, including warm socks and a warm, comfortable bathrobe
- Camera with extra film or battery charger
- List of people to call after the baby is born (include your childbirth educator)
- Snacks for labor support
- Nursing bras and pads
- Tee-shirt and blanket for baby
- Sanitary pads for after the birth
- Diapers—cloth or disposable
- Car seat with instructions
- Loose-fitting going-home outfit

nant woman, and most women who test positive for Group B Strep are able to deliver normal, healthy babies without complications.

Proponents argue that Strep B has the potential to cause very serious health consequences for the newborn baby. A few babies exposed to GBS may develop pneumonia or meningitis either immediately after birth or up to a week later. Some babies may have long term vision or hearing loss from the exposure, though this is quite rare.

But GBS infections occur in only approximately 0.0225 percent—that's one out of every 4444 babies—born to GBS-colonized women. And even in these cases, administration of antibiotics may not make any difference. In one review of babies with early onset GBS infections, use of IV antibiotics during labor "did not change the clinical spectrum of disease or the onset of clinical signs of infection within 24 hours of birth for term infants with GBS infection."[8]

Furthermore, routine antibiotic use poses real dangers to both mother and baby. Many women have reported severe allergies, asthma, ADHD and even autism in their children after mom received IV antibiotics during labor and delivery. These conditions can afflict children for years after the birth. Another danger is the increased occurrence of antibiotic resistant "superbug" infections like MRSA, as well as of sepsis and *E. coli*. Your risk of developing a superbug from IV antibiotics is much greater than the risk of your baby suffering from GBS infection. Yet, one in three women still receives antibiotics during labor and delivery.

If you are following our dietary guidelines, con-

BABIES ARE BORN WITH BACTERIA!

Scientists have long assumed that babies are born with sterile guts, picking up their first microscopic colonizers during the birth process or from their environment. However, new research indicates that babies pick up bacteria from their mothers while still in the womb. Indeed, it seems that babies even end up with bacteria carried on the father's sperm!

In 2007, researchers in Spain labelled bacteria with a genetic marker and fed milk containing them to pregnant mice. The mice then had their offspring delivered by Caesarean section in a sterile environment. The researchers found the labelled bacteria in the pups' meconium (first stool), suggesting that the bacteria had transferred from the mother's gut to that of the fetus during pregnancy.

Researchers have also identified bacterial communities in the meconium of human babies. The samples were dominated either by bacteria that produce lactic acid, such as *Lactobacillus*, or by a family of enteric bacteria, such as *E. coli*. Infants born with more enteric bacteria, for example, were at greater risk of eczema later on. Other studies have shown that certain types of gut bacteria are associated with either aggressive or gentle behavior in mice.

The type of bacteria present was linked to the mothers' lifestyles. Mothers with university educations all gave birth to babies dominated by lactic acid bacteria while women without a university education had babies whose guts were dominated by enteric bacteria. Smoking seemed to encourage an enteric microbiome while eating organic foods promoted lactic acid bacteria.

Researchers surmise that the bacteria find their way from mother to fetus via the placenta; bacteria have been found in the blood taken from the umbilical cord.

The obvious conclusion is that mothers need to take care to populate their own guts with the right kind of bacteria, especially just before and during pregnancy. That means plenty of lacto-fermented foods such as kefir, yogurt and sauerkraut while avoiding foods that feed yeasts and pathogenic bacteria, such as sugar and white flour.[9]

suming a diet rich in fat-soluble vitamins and ben-eficial bacteria from lacto-fermented foods, you and your baby will be highly protected against infection from pathogenic organisms, and the consequences of those infections should they occur. The fact that some infected babies end up with vision or hearing loss strongly indicates that deficiencies of vitamins A and D are involved. The healthy alternative to the Strep B test and IV antibiotics is a diet containing cod liver oil and the fats of grass-fed animals.

In Eastern Europe, it is the custom for women to apply yogurt or kefir to the vagina, starting about one month before birth; in principle, this practice will reduce the likelihood of Strep B infection.

The best defense against IV antibiotics is to just refuse the test. Even a healthy mother may test positive, and such tests are never fool proof—they may come back with a false positive when you do not actually carry the Strep B organism. Without a positive test result in your chart, medical personnel have a much weaker case for insisting upon IV antibiotics. If you have already taken the test and it came back positive, you can still refuse the antibiotic, but be prepared for a fight.

If for any reason you do receive an antibiotic during delivery—if you have a C-section, you cannot refuse IV antibiotics—it is very important to give your baby a bifidus bacterium supplement to colonize his intestinal tract with the right bacteria (see Chapter 7). Mom should take a probiotic supplement as well and make consumption of lacto-fermented foods a daily habit after the birth.

YOUR DUE DATE

According to the conventional view, childbirth usually occurs about thirty-eight weeks (266 days) after conception or approximately forty weeks from the last normal menstrual period. The World Health Organization defines the normal term for delivery as between thirty-seven weeks (259 days) and forty-two weeks (294 days) from conception.

Europeans consider forty-two weeks to be normal gestation. In biblical times, gestation was counted

---

TRADITIONAL METHODS TO SPEED CHILDBIRTH

Meriwether Lewis, of Lewis and Clark fame, recorded in his diary on February 11, 1805, that one of their party's interpreters administered crushed rattlesnake rattles to speed the delivery of Sacagawea's first child. Although this remedy may not be available to modern women, there are many natural methods that she can use to ease the pains of childbirth and speed delivery.

HERBS: A product called Eze-Birth Flower Essence, which combines thyme essence, citrine gem esence, clear quartz gem essence, silverleaf essence, squash essence, strelitzia essense and wild garlic essence, is designed to ease birth pains and speed delivery (see Sources).

HOMEOPATHY: Homeopathic remedies are available for the period leading up to labor and delivery, for first stage labor and then second stage labor.[10] A combination remedy called EZ Birth contains *Actaea racemosa*, *Caulophyllum*, *Arnica*, *Pulsatilla* and *Gelsemium sempervirens* (see Sources).

ACUPRESSURE: A fascinating description of acupressure points for easy delivery is available from www.maternityaccupressure.com. One of the easiest and most effective is in the web of flesh between the thumb and forefinger. Press firmly with the thumb and forefinger of the opposite hand, starting several weeks before your due date. This will help the cervix open slowly and gradually. Be wary of doing this too early in your pregnancy!

ACUPUNCTURE: Acupuncture is very common in China to get labor going or hasten it along. If you are approaching or surpassing forty-two weeks, by all means try acupuncture to help bring labor on.

as ten lunar months or 295 days, corresponding to forty-two weeks, the WHO upper limit for gestation.

Unfortunately, modern obstetrics now considers the due date to be the lower number, forty weeks from conception and in a conventional practice or hospital setting, nervousness often sets in after the thirty-eighth week. The result is that many babies are induced up to four weeks before they are truly full term and some even earlier than that.

To make things worse, dating the pregnancy from the last menstrual period often results in overestimating the length of gestation; and pregnancy with twins tends to go longer than pregnancy with a single child.

Today, only about half the women in America actually go into natural labor. Doctors would rather deliver a small baby than a large one, and many mothers want to get their pregnancy over with—but it is far better for your baby to be born with the lung development and extra pound or two that she gains during the last few weeks of gestation. If you carry your baby beyond forty weeks, be prepared for considerable pressure to come to the hospital and receive drugs that begin labor.

Barbara Katz Rothman, professor of sociology at the City University of New York and an eloquent defender of midwifery, believes that the research cited in defense of the forty-week due date is flawed. She notes that the surveys leading to this conclusion were conducted during the early 1950s when most women were told to restrict weight gain to about fifteen pounds and also to restrict salt, in other words, the research was carried out on a sample that was not normal. In normal, first-time pregnancies, the due date is more likely forty-one or forty-two weeks.[11]

Studies do show that after forty-two to forty-three weeks, there is a greater chance of still birth—of the baby being born dead. After forty-two weeks the rate doubles and after forty-three weeks the rate triples, usually because the placenta begins to wear out. Still, many pregnancies go safely beyond forty-two weeks.

Fortunately, inducing labor at forty-two weeks is generally safe—certainly safer than at forty-one weeks, when the cervix may not be ready to dilate. Forcing labor before forty-two weeks may result in a very slow labor or a failed induction, making a C-section more likely.

Unfortunately, most hospital staff think it is fine to induce labor or perform a C-section at thirty-nine weeks, or even earlier. This has resulted in a huge increase in what is referred to as "late preterm babies," babies born between thirty-four and thirty-seven weeks of gestation. Hospital wards today are filled with these babies, who often develop lung problems or infections, and who begin life at a distinct disadvantage.

There is no need to give in to pressure to induce delivery if you are at forty weeks and all signs are normal. (In fact, it's a good idea to have a conversation about this with your obstetrician early on. Find out whether he or she will let you go to forty-two weeks if that's what your baby and your body want.)

Of women at forty weeks, 65 percent go into labor within the next week; and of those at ten days beyond forty weeks, 60 percent will go into labor spontaneously within the next three days. If you come from a family with a history of normal but late deliveries, you may want to fudge a little about your date of conception to avoid the pressure to induce.

Most importantly, if for any reason your baby is going to be induced, or you know you will deliver by C-section, you should wait until at least thirty-nine weeks of gestation unless there is a serious medical reason to deliver sooner. With each week leading up to thirty-nine weeks gestation, the risk of respiratory problems, infection and death in your baby decreases. You should wait, even if you have gestational diabetes and your baby is very big. Just because a baby is big does not mean her lungs are sufficiently developed to survive a preterm delivery.

A NORMAL, NATURAL CHILDBIRTH

The process of childbirth actually starts weeks before you feel your first contraction. Your body will be preparing for the upcoming event in several ways you may or may not notice. The first of these events may be an increase of circulating blood volume, which can be recognized by mild or moderate swelling. Your body is designed to prepare for the blood loss after birth by providing you with more blood before labor begins. Because the blood must be held somewhere, the body will increase the capacity of the circulatory system by swelling tissues. This sometimes manifests as a glow in the facial features, which others will notice.

Long before delivery, you may experience small irregular contractions, called Braxton-Hicks contractions, sometimes referred to as "false labor." A better term is "pre-labor." As the day of delivery nears, these will increase in frequency. These contractions are important for strengthening the uterine muscle for the upcoming labor and birth. Most women find them painless, and they do not interfere in any way with regular activities.

Real labor begins when the contractions occur less than ten minutes apart, getting progressively closer together and progressively stronger. If you are unsure whether your contractions are those of real labor or simply more Braxton-Hicks, change your activity or eat something to see whether that has an effect on the contractions. If by changing your activity level or eating a small snack you find your contractions slow down or spread out, you will know that you are still in pre-labor, not real labor.

You may also notice that your breasts begin to secrete colostrum, a thick yellow fluid that will serve as your baby's first food. Usually the amount is small, and it will dry in the pores of your breasts.

Some women recognize when they have lost their mucus plug, others have no idea when or whether it has happened. The mucus plug is a grey "blob" of mucus (similar in texture to nasal mucus) that closes your cervix to protect the uterus during pregnancy. Seeing the plug in the toilet or in your underwear is an indication that your cervix has begun to dilate. That does not mean you are in real labor. You could lose your mucus plug and still have a few weeks to wait for labor to begin.

Another signal that labor is near is "bloody show," a small amount of blood-tinged mucus from the cervix as it thins and dilates. Usually the bloody show is a small amount of bright red blood, which may contain a few small clumps. You may find it in the toilet or in your underwear. There is no danger of

confusing this with vaginal bleeding, which is a profuse bleeding that may indicate a problem.

As the Braxton-Hicks contractions get closer together and last longer, you may also experience a mild diarrhea, a runny nose and an increased need to urinate. These are all "cleansing reactions" and further indications that you are moving closer to real labor.

Sometimes you can have all these signs of early labor, only to have them stop completely and then start again later, even as long as two days later.

Ideally, your contractions will get progressively longer, stronger and closer together. These contractions will help align the baby properly and push the baby and the bag of waters against the cervix to stretch it around the baby's head. If you are checked by your doula, midwife or physician at this time, he or she may determine that the cervix is dilated—that has opened up—two or three centimeters. But the progress of dilation is not uniform. Women have a habit of achieving several centimeters of dilation over very few contractions, and then waiting a few hours for the next change of dilation.

After a few hours, days or weeks of pre-labor contractions, your body will begin to have rhythmic contractions that are becoming longer, stronger and closer together. They will last for forty-five seconds to a minute and feel like pressure in the pelvis, menstrual cramping or a dull backache. These are all signs that you are moving from pre-labor into early labor. Still, at this point, most women are more comfortable keeping active through their contractions.

If you have planned for a doula or midwife to assist with a home birth, it is now time to let her know; most birth centers and hospitals want you to wait until the contractions are five minutes apart before you come in, especially if this is your first baby.

If at any time during labor your bag of waters breaks—there is no mistaking this because when it happens, a lot of clear liquid will come rushing out—it means that the birth could occur very quickly. Time to get to the hospital or birth center as soon as possible; if you are having a home birth, your doula or midwife needs to be at your side.

Once strong contractions begin to occur at uniform intervals, you can make an estimate of how long your labor will last. The average true labor lasts fifteen hours. If your contractions begin at less than eight minutes apart, you might expect your labor will be shorter than the average—shorter may mean anywhere from just a few hours to thirteen or fourteen hours. If your contractions start at twelve minutes apart or more, you can expect your labor to be longer than average. In general, labor is longer for first babies than for subsequent births.

As your contractions become stronger, they will demand more and more of your attention. You will want to stop what you are doing during the contraction and concentrate on relaxing. In the early stages, you can concentrate only on relaxing the abdomen; eventually you will need to concentrate on relaxing your whole body.

As labor continues and your body begins to focus its energy into the contractions, you may find that you have no desire for food. While it's fine to avoid food from this point on, it's important to stay hydrated during labor. Water with a pinch of salt and a squeeze of lemon added is your best bet, sipped between contractions.

Lots of interesting emotional changes occur as your contractions become more intense. While you may feel talkative as true labor begins, as it continues you may become very quiet, not wishing to speak with anyone. In addition, your modesty may decrease so that you don't mind if your doula, midwife, nurse or doctor sees you without clothes on.

During the period of real labor, your dilation will continue to increase. At this point, you will go into the "transition" stage of labor, when your body is completing dilation and you are preparing to push the baby out. Often considered the "worst" stage of labor, many women claim that it is not any more difficult than the rest of labor. Transition typically lasts for fifteen minutes to half an hour, but for many women, things happen so quickly that the transition period is over almost as soon as it has begun.

If the transition period is not rapid, many women

HEMORRHAGING DURING CHILDBIRTH

Hemorrhage during labor is most often related to bleeding associated with the placenta. A placenta previa or a low-lying placenta may bleed during labor as the contraction and relaxation of the uterine muscle interrupts the integrity of the placental tissue. In a complete placenta previa the pressure of the descending fetus will exert force on the placenta, which is blocking the fetus' descent.

A second condition, placenta abruption or premature separation of the placenta from the uterine wall, is another cause of bleeding during labor. When a placental abruption occurs the bleeding may be visible or it may be concealed between the uterine wall and the placenta.

Another cause of hemorrhage during labor is uterine rupture which may result in both internal and external bleeding. All of these situations of hemorrhage during labor have potential significant consequences for both mother and baby and require rapid intervention.

Our suggestion for mothers to take cod liver oil has raised concerns among some midwives that this could lead to abnormal bleeding during the birth. The Weston A. Price Foundation carried out a pregnancy survey to assess this risk and found that the proportion of women who reported vaginal bleeding during pregnancy and birth with or without cod liver oil was virtually identical. (There was a remarkable and highly significant lower odds of preeclampsia among womening using cod liver oil.)

One finding was that the majority of women were taking fish oil in addition to cod liver oil, thus resulting in an intake of EPA that could be too high. Fish oil (as opposed to fish liver oil) is a highly processed and rancid product that is *not* recommended for pregnancy. Taking fish oil in addition to cod liver oil can result in an excess of EPA, which thins the blood and blocks the body's clotting mechanisms, and could indeed lead to excess bleeding during pregnancy and birth.

wonder whether they can go on. Even women who have had several babies may feel at this point that they can't take any more. This is the time in labor when most women ask for something to help them with the pain.

Transition is also recognizable by various physical signs, which may or may not have been present during the labor, such as hot and cold flashes, cold sweats, nausea or vomiting, shivering or shaking, hiccups, burping and a general inability to feel comfortable in any position. This is the most common time for the bag of waters to break.

When you begin to show these signs, it does not matter whether you are dilated to one or ten centimeters, it means you are very close to pushing your baby out. If you are dilated only two or three centimeters, you will probably dilate the rest of the way in just a few contractions. In any event, transition can happen at any point of cervical dilation.

Sometimes when you enter the transition stage, the contractions spread out again. They generally move to about five minutes apart and may even stop completely, giving you a much needed rest. This occurs because once the baby passes through the cervix, the uterus may need to "catch up" to be snug against the baby. The contractions will only move the baby when the uterus is snug against the baby. Do not be alarmed if your contractions seem to have stopped or space out without an urge to push. That urge will come when the baby is in the proper position to be pushed out. It does you no good to push before you feel like pushing.

The urge to push is caused by the baby's head pressing on the nerves that signal the need for a bowel movement. In fact, as you begin to push, some feces may come out. You may feel this urge several times in one contraction, and then not feel it at all in the next contraction as the uterus catches up to the baby. Simply pay attention to your body and push when your body tells you to push and breathe when your body tells you to breathe. Above all, don't try to push when you don't feel like pushing.

Now is the time to take the position that is most comfortable for you. Some women like to squat; others like to sit on a low stool. Or you may want to be on your back in bed, propped up by pillows. You

may or may not feel like holding on to your legs to bring your knees nearer your chest.

Most women find that it is most comfortable to hold their breath while they push. Taking in air and holding your breath puts a pocket of air above the uterus to help align it properly, and many women find it lessens any discomfort they feel. Other women find no need to hold their breath, or prefer to exhale as they push, to allow them to remain relaxed.

Whichever method is comfortable for you, remember to breathe when your body calls for more oxygen. Women who are left alone to push as their body indicates generally push for six-second increments rather than the ten that is commonly asked for in maternity wards. If someone is asking you to push longer than is comfortable, simply smile politely and continue on about your work.

When you begin pushing, you will probably feel renewed excitement; but discouragement may follow if the pushing stage lasts a long time. Sometimes the pushing stage lasts no more than a few contractions, and you feel that you are quickly passing a bowling ball; sometimes it takes up to four hours. Either way, the important thing is to listen to your body, push when you feel like pushing and breathe in whatever way is most comfortable for your contractions. Eventually the baby's head will crown.

If you are flexible enough, you may be able to bend over and see your baby's head, at first a section only about the size of a quarter. You can also reach down and touch the baby. This thrilling moment may help you focus better on pushing. The baby may seem to take two steps forward and one step back until suddenly your skin begins to stretch and the widest part of the baby's head is passing through your vagina.

Crowning often creates a burning and stretching sensation. Some women remark that it feels as though their whole body is tearing in two, even if they do not tear! The skin does stretch, and it can be painful, but it is important to remember that the baby's head is putting tremendous pressure on the vaginal and perineal skin.

An experienced midwife or physician can help stretch the vaginal and perineal skin so that it doesn't tear, sometimes rubbing oil into the skin.

Fortunately, this pressure cuts off the circulation and numbs the surrounding tissues, dulling the sensation.

Sometimes the baby will just push right out with a whoosh, but if things are going more slowly, you can have more control over the whole process. When you feel your skin stretching, you can hold back from pushing, which will help prevent your skin from tearing.

Try to fully relax your pelvic floor muscle at this time to allow the most stretch possible for the baby's head and prevent tearing. Your physician or midwife will also be helping to stretch the skin around the baby's head. Even so, sometimes the skin will tear with a natural birth, or the doctor or midwife will perform a small episiotomy; that is, a surgical incision through the perineum made to enlarge the opening to the vagina. With the numbing pressure of the baby's head, you probably won't feel it.

Once the head is out, the baby will begin to turn to get the shoulders through the pelvis. Usually only one more push is required. As your baby comes out you will feel a gush of water as the rest of the amniotic fluid empties. Your baby is born!

Your baby will still be connected to the umbilical cord, and should remain connected for some time so that all the cord blood empties into the baby (see page 97). Your first instinct will be to put the baby near your breast, skin to skin, and that is exactly what you should do. In many cases, baby will actually squirm and root until he takes the breast.

After your baby is out, your uterus will continue to contract as it begins to work its way back to normal size. As the uterus shrinks, the placenta becomes detached from the uterine wall and is forced down towards the cervix and out the birth canal. Generally women feel the need to push gently as the placenta is expelled, or they may have an involuntary contraction.

The placenta may come out anywhere from five minutes to an hour after the baby. As long as you are not experiencing excessive bleeding, there is no need for alarm if there is a delay. Nursing the baby will encourage the expulsion of the placenta. While you wait, you can enjoy the eye-to-eye and skin-to-skin contact with your new baby. If you need stitches for an episiotomy, your midwife or doctor can do this with the help of a small amount of local anesthetic.

Your uterus will continue to contract for the next several days or even for several weeks. Each time you put your baby to the breast, expect to feel a good contraction. Little by little your uterus will return to pre-pregnancy size. During this time you will pass blood and will need to wear a sanitary pad. Use this bleeding—called lochia—as an indicator of whether you are doing too much. If the flow increases or the blood gets darker, it's a sign to cut back on your activity. You want the flow to gradually decrease and lighten in color until it stops.

A SYMPHONY OF HORMONES

The whole birth process is guided by a remarkable symphony of hormones. Four major systems are active before, during and after the birth process: oxytocin, endorphins, adrenaline and noradrenaline, and prolactin. In an undisturbed, natural childbirth, these work with exquisite balance and timing to bring the baby into the world. Indeed, when all goes well, the birth process culminates in a hormonally driven sense of ecstasy after a quick and relatively pain-free delivery.

The hospital setting with its many interventions, and especially the administration of drugs, can easily disrupt this natural hormonal process, leaving in its chaotic wake everything from stalled delivery, to lowered breastmilk output, to reduced feelings of bonding between mother and child.

Called "the hormone of love" or the "cuddle hormone," oxytocin is secreted during sexual activity, male and female orgasm, birth and breastfeeding, as well as in situations of love and altruism, including sharing a meal. Malfunction of the oxytocin system is implicated in conditions like schizophrenia, autism, heart disease and addictions.

Produced in the hypothalamus and stored in the posterior pituitary gland, oxytocin is involved in ejection reflexes—the ejection of sperm, the fetal ejection at birth, the placental ejection and the milk ejection or let-down reflex in breastfeeding. In addition, large amounts of oxytocin secreted during pregnancy enhance nutrient absorption, reduce stress and conserve energy by inducing sleepiness—in some women the urge to sleep is overwhelming, especially during the first and last months of pregnancy. Don't fight it! It's a sign that your oxytocin levels are high and that your childbirth may well be easy.

It's the hormone oxytocin that causes the rhythmic uterine contractions of labor; if the oxytocin system is working well, as the baby descends into the birth canal, stretch receptors in the lower vagina stimulate an even greater outpouring of the hormone.

The baby also produces oxytocin during labor; in fact, it's possible that baby's secretion of the hormone is the signal that initiates labor—labor should begin when baby is ready, not when mom wants it or when it is convenient for the doctors.

Immediately after birth, the levels in both mother and baby are very high. Skin-to-skin contact, eye-to-eye contact and baby's suckling all enhance the outpourings of oxytocin. During the months of lactation, oxytocin helps the mother remain relaxed and well nourished.

The second hormone, beta-endorphin, is a naturally occurring opiate, similar to Demerol, morphine and heroin. In fact, it works on the same receptors in the brain as these addictive drugs. Like oxytocin, beta-endorphin is secreted from the pituitary gland. High levels are present during sex, pregnancy, birth and breastfeeding. Under conditions of duress and pain, endorphins act as an analgesic; they also suppress the immune system, an effect that may help prevent a pregnant mother's immune system from acting against her baby.

Beta-endorphin levels are elevated during pregnancy and increase throughout labor, helping to transmute pain. They may even help the laboring mother

NUTRITIONAL SUPPORT FOR THE BIRTH HORMONES

Discovery of the various hormones responsible for the birth process has led to renewed emphasis on comfort and support for women in labor; but a focus on the nutrients needed for production of these hormones lags far behind. Yet, the huge outpouring of hormones during labor—and the coordination of these hormones—obviously calls for maximum nutritional preparation. Remember the easy and painless births described by Dr. Price and other anthropologists. This is how nature works in the context of superb dietary support.

Not surprisingly, the nutrients needed for production of the key birth hormones are the same nutrients supplied by the kind of nutrient-dense diet described in Chapter 1.

The receptors for prolactin, oxytocin, endorphins, adrenaline, and noradrenaline, as well as the prolactin and oxytoxin hormones, contain sulphur-containing amino acids—the kind found in meat, organ meats and egg yolks.[12,13,14,15]

The production of oxytocin, adrenaline, and noradrenaline is dependent on vitamin C,[16,17] which may explain cravings for oranges and other vitamin C-containing fruits during the last month of pregnancy. The production of these three hormones also requires copper, zinc and calcium,[16,18] minerals found in raw dairy products, bone broths, organ meats and red meat.

The production of endorphins also requires calcium.[19,20] The production of adrenaline and noradrenaline is also dependent on niacin, folate, vitamin B_6 and vitamin B_{12}.[21,22] Endorphin receptors require cholesterol.[23] The production of all of these hormones and receptors requires iron and magnesium,[24] available from red meat, liver, legumes and nuts.

Thus, the hormonal symphony depends on mom's diet throughout pregnancy. The diet that produces optimally healthy children also supports a quick, relatively pain-free and joyful birth.

A WATER BIRTH?

Water birth is an accepted practice in many parts of the United States, Canada, Australia and New Zealand as well as a few European countries, including the United Kingdom and Germany, where many maternity clinics have birthing tubs. Many independent birthing centers and many home-birth midwives offer water birth services. Water birth involves giving birth to the infant in the water or using it as a tool during the labor process. Proponents believe that this method is safe and provides many benefits for both mother and infant, including pain relief and a less traumatic birth experience for the baby. However, critics argue that the procedure introduces unnecessary risks to the infant such as infection and water inhalation.

Supporters of water birth claim that properly heated water helps ease the transition from the birth canal to the outside world because the warm liquid is thought to resemble the intrauterine environment. Many women report that water birth helps reduce tension and promotes relaxation. The buoyancy provided by water promotes efficient uterine contractions and better blood circulation. This results in better over-all oxygenation, combined with less pain for the mother. In addition, the umbilical cord pulsates longer, helping to remove damaged red blood cells from the baby's circulation, thus reducing neonatal jaundice. The interaction between mother and baby is increased and the warm moist air present in the birth room is beneficial for the baby's first breath.

However, the American Academy of Pediatrics' 2005 statement on water birth concluded: "The safety and efficacy of underwater birth for the newborn has not been established. There is no convincing evidence of benefit to the neonate but some concern for serious harm." Specifically cited is the danger of water inhalation by the infant. This statement is refuted by midwife Annie Sprague, who suggests this fear is not supported by current research, which has shown to the contrary that babies do not breathe underwater at the time of birth. Another concern is an increase in the risk of infection from the water. In a randomized controlled trial of the effects of water labor in Canada, no difference was noted in the low rates of maternal and newborn signs of infection in women with ruptured membranes.[25] Yet, in a 2004 study of the water of a birth pool following birth after filtration and more rigorous cleaning procedures (which had been put in place as a result of a study finding contamination between births) were instituted, high concentrations of *E. coli* and coliform contamination were found, along with staph and *P. aeruginosa*.[26]

A concern never mentioned in these arguments is the high level of chlorine needed to maintain hygiene in the birth pools. What are the effects on mother of breathing in the outgassed chlorine during the entire birth process? And on the child after the birth?

A 2003 review of the medical literature on water births concluded that the procedure showed no benefit to the infant and no clear evidence of reduced labor duration, risk of perineal tears, or use of pain medication.[27] There were sixty-four infants that experienced complications directly attributable to water birth, including bacterial infection, drowning, near-drowning and fever.

So despite glowing reviews, water birth should be embraced with caution. Water birth should not be attempted by any woman who does not want to be in the pool or who is afraid of being in the water, women who are less than thirty-seven weeks gestation or show increased maternal pulse rate, in situations of maternal fever or infection or persistent increased or decreased fetal heart rate; or if there is any concern for the baby's health, maternal preeclampsia, complicated pregnancy or presentation, active maternal herpes infection or for any women who have used a narcotic analgesic within the previous three hours.

For more information: *Water Labour, Water Birth: A guide to the use of water during childbirth*, by Anne Sprague.

enter an altered state of consciousness that some-times happens during an undisturbed birth.

Beta-endorphins work in a complex relationship with oxytocin. During labor, high levels will inhibit oxytocin release, thus slowing down contractions to give the laboring woman temporary relief from her labors. Beta-endorphins also support the release of prolactin during labor, which helps prepare mother's breasts for lactation. The hormone also aids in the final stages of baby's lung maturation. Beta-endorphin is released during breastfeeding and is present as well in breastmilk, inducing pleasure and mutual dependency in both mother and baby.

Adrenaline and noradrenaline—referred to collectively as catecholamines (CAs)—are fight-or-flight hormones secreted from the adrenal gland in response to fright, anxiety, hunger or cold, as well as excitement. These hormones shunt blood flow and energy from the organs to the muscles to facilitate swift reaction during dangerous and stressful situations.

High CA levels during the early stages of labor are associated with a longer labor and adverse fetal heart rate patterns. There is a real physiological reason for pregnant women to begin labor in a stress-free and comfortable environment. For most women, the sterile, brightly lit hospital setting increases adrenaline levels and predisposes the expectant mother to a long and tiring labor.

Towards the end of labor, however, these CA levels suddenly rise to activate the fetal ejection reflex. The mother may experience a sudden rush of energy along with several very strong contractions for a quick and easy birth. High CA levels explain the rush of alertness many mothers feel during the last minutes of labor.

A wonderful example of the way CAs work is given by an anthropologist working with an indigenous Canadian tribe. When a woman is having trouble with labor, the young people gather round and suddenly and unexpectedly shout out close to her. The shock stimulates an outpouring of CAs and triggers the fetal ejection reflex.

After birth, CA levels drop steeply, allowing oxytocin to predominate and reducing the risk of postpar-tum hemorrhage. But CAs are necessary to support the mothering process. Mice bred to be deficient in noradrenaline will not care for their young after birth unless the hormone is injected back into their systems. A certain level of anxiety makes for conscientious mothering!

The final hormone in the symphony is prolactin, called the "mothering hormone" because it is the major hormone for breastmilk synthesis and breast-feeding. Levels increase during pregnancy and again during labor and delivery, although other hormones, notably progesterone, inhibit milk production until the placenta is delivered. During breastfeeding, prolactin produces a certain amount of anxiety, which helps mothers put their baby's needs first. The baby also produces prolactin while in the womb and high levels are found in amniotic fluid. Prolactin also stimulates proliferation of oligodendrocyte precursor cells, ultimately responsible for the formation of myelin coatings on axons in the central nervous system.

Prolactin has a number of other effects: it contributes to surfactant synthesis of the fetal lungs at the end of the pregnancy and immune tolerance of the fetus by the maternal organism during pregnancy; it also decreases normal levels of sex hormones—estrogen in women and testosterone in men. It is this inhibition of sex steroids that is responsible for loss of the menstrual cycle in lactating women.[28]

CHILDBIRTH WITH INTERVENTIONS

A normal, natural childbirth represents the ideal, one all expectant mothers should strive to achieve. But sometimes our best-laid plans go awry; sometimes interventions are absolutely necessary. And when they are, good nutritional preparation can mitigate any side effects.

If you are having your baby in a hospital, even a hospital said to be supportive of a natural birth, it is imperative that you have someone at your side to speak up for your wishes—your spouse or partner, your own doula or a knowledgeable friend. (Hospital midwives and nurses may not always provide support for a drug-free childbirth, even if you have requested it.) As your labor progresses, you may lack the mental strength and clarity to stand your ground against the hospital staff. A person provid-

BREECH BIRTH

A breech presentation is the condition wherein baby enters the birth canal with the buttocks or feet first, as opposed to the normal head-first presentation. At full term, 3-4 percent of babies are born breech. The percentage is considerably higher for premature babies; most babies who are "upside down" entering the third trimester turn over to present head down by the time of the full due date.

Vaginal delivery of breech babies was the norm until 1959, when it was proposed that all breech presentations should be delivered by C-section "to reduce perinatal morbidity and mortality." Since that time, vaginal delivery of breech babies has become more and more rare, now accounting for only about 9 percent of breech deliveries.

The American College of Obstetrics and Gynecology has systematically condemned breech vaginal birth; for this reason, it is no longer offered as an option to most women in this situation. Opponents to vaginal breech birth cite one study by Mary Hannah, published in the *Lancet* in 2000.[29] The study found planned Caesarean section for breech births produced lower infant mortality and morbidity for babies in industrialized countries. There was no difference in maternal mortality or morbidity between vaginal and Caesarean groups. However, many have criticized the study as inherently biased and designed to minimize the difference in outcomes between the two groups.

The Hannah study contradicts a number of other studies, all of them from overseas. For example, a study out of Sweden showed no difference in outcome between elective Caesarean versus planned vaginal birth for term breech deliveries.[30]

Another study examined planned breech delivery in France and Belgium, finding no discernable difference in outcome with more than eight thousand breech patients studied.[31] Another study from France looked at more than five hundred patients and found no difference in outcome.[32] A study from the United Emirates found no clear difference in breech vaginal versus Caesarean, but did find more maternal morbidity associated with Caesarean section.[33]

The Malaysian Journal of Medical Sciences published a study in 2007 that concluded, "Most of the perinatal mortality was due to congenital abnormality and prematurity and there were no perinatal deaths related to mode of delivery or due to birth trauma."[34]

Breech babies do tend to have higher rates of birth defects but the preponderance of the evidence shows that there is no need to perform a C-section for a breech baby that is normal and full term. A skilled midwife can sometimes turn the fetus *in utero* so that the head will present downwards.

The problem is finding a physician or midwife who will do a vaginal delivery—with the blanket prescription to deliver all breech babies by C-section, very few have the skills or confidence to administer a breech birth. If you do find such a midwife or physician, both you and the pracitioner need to have full faith in nature's wisdom, allowing the labor to proceed at its own pace. The membranes should not be ruptured artificially and vaginal examinations should be restricted to avoid accidental rupture. Mom should be encouraged to give birth in an all-fours position—definitely not on her back. There should be no routine episiotomy and the third stage of labor should proceed without chemical or mechanical assistance. Often damage occurs by pulling on the baby once the torso and legs are out. If an arm is stuck, an experienced midwife will know how to pull it down.

For further information: *Breech Birth* by Benna Waites; "Breech vaginal birth is NOT an emergency," http://jeremyscorner-grifter.blogspot.com/2009/03/breech-vaginal-birth-is-not-emergency.html.

ing knowledgeable and supportive representation at your side can also help you assess the need for a more medicalized birth should that be necessary.

As you enter the hospital, you should have a list of your wishes written down so that there can be no confusion about doing routine interventions without your consent.

Remember that you should not go to the hospital unless your contractions are at least five minutes apart; but you may also be sent to the hospital from your doctor's office or birth clinic if tests indicate any problems to the mother or fetus.

The first intervention that usually occurs in the hospital setting is the fitting of an intravenous stent or IV lock in the crook of the elbow, "just in case" the hospital needs to give you pain-killing drugs or antibiotics. And that's exactly what you don't want— you don't want it to be easy for the staff to give you any drugs. Should drugs be necessary, the staff can fit the stent within minutes. The stents can be uncomfortable, especially if your labor lasts a long time. So just say "no" to a routine IV stent.

Once you are checked in, you will be assigned a bed in the labor ward, usually a private room or at least a bed behind a curtain to ensure privacy. The surroundings tend to be much more comfortable today than they were in days gone by. You should have plenty of pillows, a way to turn the lights down low, comfortable chairs available for your companions, and water with lemon juice and salt added to drink—not plain water, which can cause hyponatremic dehydration (not enough salt in the bloodstream) if consumed in excess. Some rooms are even equipped with a tub or Jacuzzi—probably to be avoided as the water will be almost certainly heavily chlorinated (see Sidebar page 89).

During the early stages of labor, you will be checked at intervals by a hospital nurse or midwife to listen to the baby's heart rate, assess the progress of dilation and ascertain your ability to handle the contractions.

The main reason for medical intervention is a very long or stalled labor. If your labor lasts more than about twenty-four hours, does not progress, or leaves you exhausted, the hospital staff will want to speed things up with drugs to increase contractions or by breaking the amniotic sack. If the contractions become unbearable, you will almost certainly agree to pain killers or anesthesia in the form of an epidural. This is the moment to be grateful for the benefits of modern medicine, which spares women the painful, sometimes fatal consequences of a birth that does not go as planned.

By the way, in days gone by, women in labor were not allowed to eat anything, "just in case" a C-section was later needed. Most hospitals have relaxed this policy—which is fortunate for those who get hungry. However, usually food is the last thing you will think about during labor.

It may be very difficult to restrict the hospital staff to listening to the baby's heart with a fetoscope. If the labor is long, or even as a routine matter, they will want to attach an external fetal monitor (see page 64). In the doctor's office, the external fetal monitor remains on only for a brief period, but the hospital staff will want to constantly monitor the baby's heartbeat. Remember that these instruments work on the principle of ultrasound, and can overheat the baby's brain. It may be necessary to remind your doctor that fetal monitors have not been shown to reduce neurological problems, and may actually increase them.[35] A U.S. Preventive Services Task Force study found that constant fetal monitoring for routine births made no difference in the outcome. The study concluded, "Routine intrapartum electronic fetal monitoring is not recommended for low risk women."[36]

For the monitor, you will be required to sit with knees and back partially elevated and with a cushion under the right hip, which moves the uterus to the left. In principle, you may sit in other comfortable positions as long as the uterus is shifted to the left for most of the time; but obviously, with the fetal monitor attached, your movements will be restricted.

Another way to monitor the baby is the nonstress test (NST), which measures fetal heart rate accelerations with normal movement. The monitor is attached on the outside in the same way as the fetal heart monitor—again, the monitor works on the principle of ultrasound. Baby needs to be awake and active for this test. If baby's heartbeat remains in the sleeping mode, you may be encouraged to eat something to stimulate fetal activity. Other ways to wake up baby include fetal acoustic stimulation (sending sounds to the fetus) and moving the fetus with a gentle placement of the hands on the abdomen.

The NST indicates whether or not baby is receiving enough oxygen because of placental or umbilical cord problems. The monitor measures the heart rate in response to baby's own movements. A healthy baby will respond with an increased heart rate during times of movement, and the heart rate will decrease at rest. When oxygen levels are low, the fetus may not respond normally.

A final method of externally monitoring your baby is the contraction stress test. The same monitors are used, attached to your abdomen. The test measures the ability of the placenta to provide enough oxygen to the fetus while contractions occur. If contractions are not occurring spontaneously they may be induced.

To induce contractions, your first choice is nipple stimulation. In this test, you will rub the palm of your hand across one nipple through your garments for two or three minutes. After a five-minute test, the nipple stimulation should continue until forty minutes have elapsed, or three contractions have occurred, lasting more than forty seconds within a ten-minute period. If a uterine contraction starts, you should stop the nipple stimulation.

The other method for inducing contractions is to give Pitocin, the synthetic form of oxytocin. This is the fateful moment when you go from a drug-free childbirth to one in which one or more drugs are used. If your contractions are not moving things along fast enough, if they have stopped, or if they have not even started but the baby seems to be in distress, your doctor will want to get contractions going—not only to administer the contraction stress test, but also to get your labor moving along.

The drug will be administered through an IV—this is the time to get that stent in the crook of your arm—until three uterine contractions have occurred, lasting forty to sixty seconds over a ten-minute period. Unfortunately, Pitocin sometimes moves things along very quickly, inducing very strong contractions close together within twenty minutes, interfering with the interplay of hormones that should regulate the progress of labor.

POSTPARTUM NUTRITIONAL SUPPORT

With all the excitement of the birth and arrival of the new baby, it's important for moms not to neglect their diet during the days and weeks after the birth.

In Asia, it is customary to present a new mother with jars of pigs feet simmered in a rich broth. The gelatin and collagen in this traditional dish provide the very nutrients mothers need for making a quick recovery after childbirth. In addition, if they can afford it, nursing mothers in Asia consume up to ten eggs per day for at least the first month of lactation.

It's a good idea to have plenty of bone broth and broth-based soups in the freezer for recovery after birth. A potassium broth made with potato skins will also speed recovery (see Recipes). Numerous eggs and egg yolks should be consumed, at least during the first few weeks, when extra nutrition for lactation is essential. Raw milk and/or raw cheese will supply available calcium and synergistic minerals for calcium- and mineral-rich breastmilk.

Cod liver oil will provide not only vitamins A and D for rich breastmilk, but the long-chain fatty acid DHA it contains will help protect against postpartum depression. The fetus rapidly uses up DHA from mother's stores during the last month in the womb, and breastfeeding uses up DHA even more.[37] Depletion of DHA, as well as vitamins A and D, explains the let-down of postpartum depression after the exhilaration of birth. With a focus on good nutrition, mom should sail through the postpartum weeks full of energy and joy, without a hint of depression.

A final way to monitor the fetus is the internal fetal monitor, which involves placing an electrode directly on the fetal scalp through the cervix. Only a few years ago, the internal fetal monitor was used routinely, making it very difficult for a woman even in normal labor to get comfortable. Today initial monitoring is done with the external monitor, but as decisions are made to use one or more drugs, you can expect the internal monitor to be used. It may cause some discomfort and carries a slight risk of causing infection or fetal scalp bruising. Most seriously, the internal monitor will position the beam of sound much closer to the fetus, putting it at higher risk. You should avoid the internal monitor if at all possible.

What the doctors will be looking for with the various types of monitors is a fetal heart rate between one hundred twenty and one hundred sixty beats per minute and a rise in heart rate with fetal movement. The fetal heart rate may drop slightly with each contraction, but should rise to baseline shortly thereafter. If the fetal heart beat does not rise with movement or return to baseline after a contraction, it may be a sign of cord compression (reducing blood flow to the baby), too little oxygen, incorrect positioning of the baby or other forms of fetal distress. Your doctor will want to hurry things along with more Pitocin, by breaking your waters or by performing a C-section.

Usually the first drugs given for pain are narcotics, taken orally. If these don't work and labor continues to stall, the next step is an epidural. A catheter is attached to the spine and the anesthetic injected; the pain of labor will quickly subside into numbness. A common reaction is a drop in blood pressure, which will be stabilized by fluids given intravenously and injections of ephedrine.

The relief from pain may cause the labor to go forward and your contractions to speed up; or it may make you fall asleep. If the labor does not go forward after a few hours, the next step is more Pitocin. Labor may then move forward. . . or it may not.

If it does go forward, you will be able to have a vaginal birth; you will give birth on your back under bright lights and can expect an episiotomy. Most likely, the doctor will need to help the baby out, possibly with the use of forceps.

Delivery with forceps can prevent a C-section, but also carries some risk if the doctor is not experienced. If the baby's head has not come down very far, most doctors today opt for a C-section rather than a forceps delivery.

Many women are upset at being unable to have a natural birth but these feelings pass as soon as your baby is born. Remember that you will be numbed only from the waist down. Whether you have a natural or a medicalized birth, you will be fully awake at the big moment and will immediately be able to take the baby into your arms, look into his eyes, and hold him to your chest. Make sure you let your doctor know ahead of time that this is what you want. If you have been following our dietary advice, you will be able to quickly clear the anesthetic and other drugs—and so will baby. This is the moment to be grateful for the miracles of modern medicine and to remember what many women had to go through in the past.

CAESAREAN SECTION

Today in the U.S. almost one in three babies is delivered by Caesarean section. Leaving aside women who schedule the day of their surgical delivery so that they do not have to undergo any labor—we assume that they are not the ones reading this book—the two main reasons for the C-section are stalled delivery and signs of fetal distress. Fetal heart monitors now provide obstetricians with clear signs that the baby might be in trouble—a heart rate that does not speed up with movement or does not return to normal after contractions.

The baby may not necessarily be in trouble, but the obstetrician must act as if she is. To do otherwise is to risk a punishing lawsuit; some of these lawsuits have cost hospitals so much money that they have had to close their obstetrics departments.

Sometimes babies just get stuck. The head may be turned sideways, or the pelvis simply has not expanded enough. In a normal, non-medicalized birth that stage may pass quickly but when the mother is medicated, progress may be very slow, or nonexistent.

If a woman has been in labor for hours and things have stalled, even with the help of Pitocin, even after her waters have broken, she normally readily agrees to a Caesarean, especially if the contractions become painful again—this can happen, even with the epidural.

With that consent, things move quickly. The Pitocin drip is turned off, the contraction monitor is removed, but the fetal heart monitor remains. You will be wheeled to an operating room. Today it is normal for your partner to remain with you, clad in scrubs, booties, mask and surgical cap. The anesthetic in the epidural is increased, your skin will be painted with antiseptic and your belly will be pricked to make sure it is completely numb—imagine having a Caesarean without modern anesthetics!

Caesarean methods have improved over the years, but the operation still requires cutting through the skin, the abdominal muscle, the peritoneum and the uterus. All this proceeds very quickly. Then the surgeon pulls the baby out—he may have to pull hard if the baby's head has descended into the birth canal. Finally, your baby is born!

The doctor then delivers the placenta through the opening. Thanks to the fact that C-sections are now performed with an epidural, rather than a general anesthetic, you can take the baby in your arms, just as you can in a normal birth. You can enjoy getting to know him, put him to your breast—and say a prayer of thanks for modern medicine. Have your partner or nurse hold the baby while you are being sewn up.

From the mother's point of view, the downside of a Caesarean is the fact that is it major surgery, one that requires a recovery period of considerable discomfort. She will need to stay in bed for at least a few days and be very careful of her activities for several weeks. Breastfeeding may be difficult, although many mothers who deliver by C-section breastfeed without problems.

From baby's point of view, the disadvantage of the C-section is twofold. One is that baby has not received the colonization of beneficial bacteria that happens with passage through the birth canal. All babies born by C-section should receive a supplement of bifidus bacteria, even if they are breastfed (see Sources).

Secondly, it is unlikely that your doctor will wait to cut the umbilical cord so that baby can receive all the cord blood—it is certainly possible to wait and allow the umbilical to drain after a Caesarean, but this often takes some negotiating to convince the staff to allow this. You can always ask, but it may be difficult to overturn hospital policy. (Just asking the question at the right moment could buy your baby a few seconds or even a minute of cord blood while you argue with the doctor!) If the umbilical is cut immediately, it will be important to watch baby's iron status carefully (see page 97).

But nevermind! Your baby is born! If you have followed our dietary guidelines, the likelihood is that you will recover quickly. You should take some cod liver oil as soon as you can and fortify yourself with all the bone broth you made during your last month of pregnancy. A vitamin B_{12} supplement for several weeks is also advised, as vitamin B_{12} can mitigate the toxic effects of anesthesia (see Sources).

FOR FURTHER INFORMATION

Easier, Shorter and Safer Birth by Lena Leino, www.easiershorterandsaferbirth.com.

Breech Birth by Benna Waites.

History of Childbirth in America, www.digitalhistory.uh.edu/historyonline/childbirth.cfm.

Chapter 5
Newborn Interventions

Modern medicine has provided us with lifesaving—albeit overused—interventions for childbirth. Unfortunately, the inclination to intervene has spilled over onto newborns, subjecting them to many types of unneeded and in most cases harmful interference with natural processes. It may take years before pediatrics recognizes the wisdom of nature in providing iron- and oxygen-rich blood from the umbilical cord, a coating to protect baby's immature skin, and a natural immunity that makes various shots and antibacterial treatments unnecessary.

Until non-interference becomes pediatric policy, parents who wish to give their newborn a truly natural start in life will need to make their wishes known to their midwife, doctor, hospital or pediatrician well before the birth; in fact, it's a good idea for parents to write their wishes down and have copies of their list of requests available for anyone who may become involved in the birth. Some states and some hospitals have forms to opt out of the various interventions, often requiring notarization. It's best to enquire early in your pregnancy and come to the hospital prepared. A letter from your attorney may be needed to ensure your wishes are granted.

CORD CLAMPING

Formed during the fifth week of development, the umbilical cord joins the fetus with the placenta, an arrangement that provides for the transfer of materials to and from the mother's blood without allowing direct mixing. Immediately after birth, the cord will pulsate for five to twenty minutes if left alone. This pulsation allows the rich placental blood to enter the baby.

Standard operating procedure in hospitals is to clamp the umbilical cord immediately after birth, before the cord blood has drained into the baby. Since the cord is composed of tough sinewy tissue, it requires a sharp instrument to cut it. The stump then dries over several days.

Some animals chew the umbilical cord to sever it and then eat the placenta; chimpanzees immediately nurse their babies with the umbilical and placenta still attached, allowing the umbilical cord to dry up and separate without intervention, usually within a day of birth.

Conventional medicine is beginning to recognize the benefits of delayed cord clamping, focusing on the iron status of the infant. A meta-analysis showed that delayed clamping of the umbilical cord in full-term neonates for a minimum of two minutes following birth is beneficial to the newborn in giving improved iron status and reduced risk of anemia for at least two months.[1]

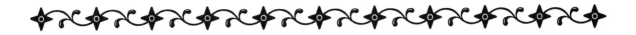

Those opposed to delayed cord clamping cite studies showing an increased risk of polycythemia (excess of red blood cells) although this condition appears to be benign.[2]

Scientists have recently discovered that the blood within the umbilical cord, known as cord blood, is a rich and readily available source of primitive, undifferentiated stem cells, leading to a thriving business in cord blood banks. These store the diverted umbilical blood should the child ever require the cord blood stem cells to treat conditions such as leukemia. Perhaps it would be better for the infant to get all those stem cells at birth!

(Blood can also be retrieved and banked from the placenta after the cord stops pulsating.)

George Malcolm Morley, MD, ChB, FACOG, an obstetrician of many years' experience, has been the primary voice calling for an end to immediate cord clamping, noting that left alone, the infant has a mechanism for ensuring that the right amount of cord blood drains into his body.

Morley does not mince words: "Most obstetricians, pediatricians and especially their academic peers have never seen a child close its own cord; they are totally ignorant of the physiology of the process. Institutional dogma and misinformation have obliterated scientific thought and method, and have changed a healthy, normal process into an imaginary disease. They then advise curing the imaginary disease with an injurious cord clamp. Amputating a functioning placenta destroys the organ that is keeping the child alive and is preparing the child for life outside the womb."

Noting that "Doctors are taught (and believe) that delayed cord clamping allowing placental transfusion gives the baby too much blood (hypervolemia)," Morely argues that this "excess" is actually normal in the newborn and especially important in the premature baby. "Neonatal intensive care units are filled with weak, fast-clamped newborns exhibiting signs of severe blood loss, pallor, hypovolemia (low blood volume) anemia (low blood count) hypotension (low blood pressure), hypothermia (cold), oliguria (poor urine output), metabolic acidosis, hypoxia (low oxygen supply) and respiratory distress (shock lung) to the point that some need

blood transfusions and many more receive blood volume expanders."

Morley describes the amazing mechanism whereby the newborn gets just the right amount of blood from the umbilical cord: "Before birth, the lungs are filled with fluid and very little blood flows through them; the child receives oxygen from the mother through the placenta and cord. This placental oxygen supply continues after the child is born until the lungs are working and supplying oxygen—that is, when they are filled with air and all the blood from the right side of the heart is flowing through them. When the child is crying and pink, the cord vessels clamp themselves. During this interval between birth and natural clamping, blood is transfused from the placenta to establish blood flow through the lungs. Thus the natural process protects the brain by providing a continuous oxygen supply from two sources until the second source is functioning well . . . during placental transfusion, blood may flow into and out of the child until the right amount of blood is attained after the child is breathing."[3]

When the cord is cut before the infant begins to breathe, the placental oxygen supply is instantly cut off and the child remains asphyxiated until the lungs begin to function. Blood that normally would have been transfused to establish the child's lung circulation remains clamped in the placenta, and the child diverts blood from all other organs—such as the brain—to fill the lung blood vessels.

In studies with monkeys, neurological disorders, memory and behavioral defects were produced through cord clamping. They did not occur in newborn monkeys that delivered without interference with the cord and placenta.[4]

After immediate clamping, the normal term baby usually has enough blood to establish lung function and prevent obvious brain damage, but it is often pale, weak and slow to respond.

Occasionally, a child will cry as soon as the head is delivered, and the uterine contraction that delivers the child may also squeeze in some placental transfusion before the fast clamp can be applied; however, cord clamping before the first breath always causes some degree of asphyxia and loss of blood volume, totally cutting off the infant brain's oxygen supply from the placenta before lungs begin to function. The result may be cerebral palsy, mental retardation or death.

Morley is especially scathing about the practice of immediate cord clamping when a baby is born showing lack of oxygen, usually from a knot in the umbilical cord. Such cases require a large transfusion of placental blood in order to prevent damage to the brain or the lungs.

Anemia in the infant can lead to mental retardation, behavioral disorders and learning disabilities. At birth, no newborn is anemic; adequate iron is supplied from the mother regardless of her iron status, and any newborn who receives a full placental transfusion through the umbilical cord at birth has enough iron to prevent anemia during the first year of life. The immediately clamped newborn may be missing one third to one half of its normal blood volume and is very prone to develop infant anemia.[3]

The small or premature baby is much more vulnerable to injury from immediate cord clamping than the robust term child. The brain is at an earlier stage of development and actively growing tissues are more easily damaged by lack of oxygen and lack of blood.

If you find that you will need to deliver prematurely, you should impress upon the delivering physician the importance of letting the baby have its cord blood. This can help prevent the numerous breathing and development problems associated with premature babies.

The importance of allowing the baby to receive the cord blood has been known for over two hundred years. "Another thing very injurious to the child, is the tying and cutting of the navel string too soon; which should always be left till the child has not only repeatedly breathed but till all pulsation in the cord ceases. As otherwise the child is much weaker than it ought to be, a portion of the blood being left in the placenta, which ought to have been in the child." This statement comes from Erasmus Darwin, grandfather of Charles Darwin, in 1801.

THE APGAR SCORE

The Apgar score was devised in 1952 by Dr. Virginia Apgar as a simple and repeatable method to quickly assess the health of newborns. Apgar was an anesthesiologist who developed the score in order to ascertain the effects of obstetric anesthesia on babies, but the results provide a useful assessment of baby's condition at birth.

The Apgar score is determined by evaluating the newborn baby on five simple criteria on a scale from zero to two, then summing up the five values thus obtained. The resulting Apgar score ranges from zero to ten. The five criteria are often listed as Appearance, Pulse, Grimace, Activity, Respiration as a mnemonic learning aid.

- Appearance: If body and appearance are pink, two points; blue in extremities, one point; blue or pale all over, zero points.

- Pulse: Pulse over one hundred, two points; less than one hundred, one point; no pulse, zero points.

- Reflex (Grimace): Cry or pull away when stimulated, two points; grimace or feeble cry when stimulated, one point; no response to stimulation, zero points.

- Muscle Tone (Activity): Flexed arms and legs that resist extension, two points; some flexion in arms and legs, one point; no flexion in arms and legs, no points.

- Breathing (Respiration): Strong, lusty cry, two points; weak, irregular, gasping breathing, one point; no breathing, zero points.

The test is generally carried out at one and five minutes after birth, and may be repeated later if the score is and remains low. Scores three and below are generally regarded as critically low, four to six fairly low, and seven to ten generally normal. Of course, every parent wants their baby to start out with a ten, and the best way to assure this happy outcome, even if anesthesia is necessary, is a nutrient-dense diet during pregnancy.

A low score on the one-minute test may show that the neonate requires medical attention but is not necessarily an indication that there will be long-term problems, particularly if there is an improvement by the stage of the five-minute test. If the Apgar score remains below three at later times, such as ten, fifteen, or thirty minutes, there is a risk that the child will suffer cerebral palsy or other types of longer-term neurological damage. However, the purpose of the Apgar test is to determine quickly whether a newborn needs immediate medical care; it was not designed to make long-term predictions about a child's health.

Babies born at high altitude are likely to score a one rather than a two on the Appearance test, due to what is called transient cyanosis. Usually this clears within a few minutes, in time for the second Apgar test.

If baby has a low score, he will surely be whisked away for further observation and interventions. But with good nutritional preparation, this is an unlikely scenario, and baby can move on to enjoy his first sensuous experience—skin-to-skin contact with mom.

MEETING YOUR BABY

Almost all mothers instinctively do the same things when meeting their babies for the first time: flushed with the excitement of the new birth, her levels of oxytocin and other hormones at high levels, she takes this strange new creature in her arms. She and baby look each other in the eyes. If the father has not participated in the birth, this is the moment for him to be called in, so both parents can say hello

LOTUS BIRTHING

Lotus birth, or umbilical nonseverance, is the practice of leaving the umbilical cord attached to both the baby and the placenta following birth, without clamping or severing, and allowing the cord the time to detach from the baby naturally. In this way the baby, cord and placenta are treated as a single unit until detachment occurs, generally two to three days after birth.

In Tibetan and Zen Buddhism, the term "lotus birth" is used to describe the birth of spiritual teachers such as Gautama Buddha and Padmasambhava (Lien-hua Sen), emphasizing their entrance into the world as intact, holy children. References to lotus births are also found in Hinduism, for example in the story of the birth of Vishnu. Although recently arisen as an alternative birth phenomenon in the West, delayed umbilical severance and umbilical nonseverance have been recorded in a number of cultures including those of the Balinese and of some aboriginal peoples such as the !Kung. Early American pioneers, in written diaries and letters, reported practicing nonseverance of the umbilicus as a preventative measure to protect the infant from an open wound infection.

Lotus births are rarely practiced in hospitals, but are more common in birth centers and in home births. Immediately postpartum, the umbilical cord pulsates as it transfers blood to the placenta from the baby, and vice versa. A natural internal clamping occurs within ten to twenty minutes postpartum.

Excess fluids are wiped off the placenta, which is then placed in an open bowl or wrapped in permeable cloth and kept in close proximity to the newborn. Air is allowed to circulate around the placenta to dry it, and to avoid its becoming malodorous. Sea salt is often applied to the placenta to help dry it out. Sometimes essential oils, such as lavender, or powdered herbs, such as goldenseal or neem, are also applied to encourage drying, to help to neutralize the smell of decomposition, and for their antibacterial properties. If drying aids are not applied, the well-aired placenta will develop a distinct, musky scent which can be halted by directly planting it in a garden or by refrigerated storage after the umbilical cord falls away. The umbilical cord dries to sinew and after a few days naturally detaches from the umbilicus. As it dries it becomes stiff; parents thus take great care to move the baby and the cord as little as possible to avoid causing it to detach prematurely.

Proponents of lotus births view the baby and the placenta as existing within the same auric field, with energy transfers continuing to take place gradually from the dead tissue of the placenta to the baby via the umbilical cord as the tissue of the placenta and umbilical cord dries out. For further information, see www.lotusbirth.net.

together. Baby will seem unexpectedly alert just after the birth, due to high levels of hormones in her bloodstream.

Then mom puts her newborn on her chest, skin to skin. A large and strong baby may actually wiggle up the chest, root around and find the nipple—almost always the left nipple. If this is your first baby, you may be in for a big surprise at the strength of the suckling reflex. Baby gets his first colostrum at this time. You may or may not feel a letdown reflex during the first few nursings.

The main thing is to enjoy the moment. Your midwife, doula and hospital staff should leave you in peace. And if you have made it clear you do not want any of the early newborn interventions, you should remain with your infant until you leave the hospital. Of course, baby needs to get weighed and measured, but this can and should be done right in front of your eyes.

THE VERNIX CASEOSA

The vernix caseosa (literally "cheese-like varnish") is the creamy white, viscous biofilm that covers a newborn's body. The vernix caseosa is produced during the last trimester of gestation as a remnant of the original fetal covering. It provides a temporary skin barrier that is suitable for the watery environment in the womb. The vernix has microvilli on the top of its surface and these work to transport substances between the amniotic fluid and the embryo. During delivery, the vernix caseosa acts as a lubricant.

After birth, the vernix continues to protect the skin from infection, as it contains a host of antimicrobial peptides. It also exhibits antioxidant, skin cleansing and temperature-regulating properties. Some research suggests that the vernix helps colonize the skin with beneficial organisms after birth. While the vernix appears as a messy, smeary coating, one we are tempted to immediately wipe off, it is actually a highly organized substance that serves many functions, including waterproofing, facilitation of skin formation and protection against inflammation and infection.

So amazing are the properties of the vernix caseosa that dermatologists are studying it to obtain a deeper understanding of its benefits. The results may be very expensive products for beautiful rash-free skin, even for wound healing. All these benefits come free of charge and evenly applied on the newborn. It may look messy but the last thing you want to do is wipe this wonderful natural cosmetic off your baby. Just leave this natural defense against dryness and infection there, and let it flake off naturally during the first week or so after birth, as baby's skin matures. Only when the vernix is all gone should you give your baby a bath.

EYE DROPS

It's common practice in hospitals to take the baby from you shortly after birth, weigh and measure him and apply an antibiotic ointment to his eyes—usually a preparation containing erythromycin.

The stated purpose of the eyedrops is to prevent any possible infection in baby's eyes from his trip down the birth canal. Eye infections used to be a major cause of blindness in children and were usually ascribed to the same bacteria that cause gonorrhea or chlamydia in women. When a woman is infected with these bacteria, they're present in her vagina, even if the woman has no symptoms of venereal disease. As a baby travels through the birth canal, he can pick up bacteria present in the mother's vaginal secretions or fluids.

Until quite recently, the compound used routinely was silver nitrate, a medicine that dates back to the 1800s. In fact, in most states, silver nitrate was required by law. Unfortunately, silver nitrate often caused red swelling in the eyes and in at least two cases caused blindness in the infant. Application of silver nitrate is painful to a baby, causing blurring of the vision and redness and conjunctivitis in almost half of all babies who receive it.

The antibiotic ointment used today does not cause swelling or redness and is considered to carry no risk. It is very hard to get out of this treatment in a hospital setting. Even if you test negative for gonorrhea or chlamydia, even if you have had a C-section, baby will be given the eye drops unless you take serious steps to prevent it. In some states it is actually mandatory, although most mandates allow exceptions.

So is there a downside? There might be. This will be baby's first antibiotic—administered in the eyes to be sure, not in the mouth, but why risk antibiotic resistance in any form? And the ointment will render the infant's vision a complete blur, just at that precious time when his elevated hormone levels allow him to see his parents clearly. How does the blurred vision affect those early bonding moments? And does the ointment have any longterm effects on vision, given at a time when the eye is developing rapidly?

Most disconcerting is the fact that the antibiotic will be resistant to only a few strains of bacteria in the vaginal tract. And will it kill beneficial bacteria on the skin around baby's eyes?

Of course, the rare complication of bacterial infection is blindness—the hospital staff will remind you of that fact. But the vast majority of babies do not go blind after birth, not even those whose mothers are infected with venereal disease. Whether a baby becomes blind after bacterial (or viral) infection almost certainly has to do with vitamin A status. Infection rapidly depletes vitamin A and a well-known consequence of severe vitamin A depletion is blindness. A pregnancy diet that provide generous amounts of vitamin A, along with co-factors D and K_2, is surely the best protection you can give your baby against infection, blindness or any other consequence of poor nutrition.

If your baby does develop an eye infection, a few drops of your colostrum or breastmilk, rich in immune factors, put into the eyes quickly solves the problem.

VITAMIN K SHOT

Another routine intervention is the vitamin K shot, which is given to support the newborn's blood clotting capabilities in order to prevent the very rare problem of slow bleeding into the brain in the weeks after birth—the risk in about one in every ten thousand live births. The shot also is supposed safeguard your baby in case you are involved in a car wreck on the way home from the hospital. Even a mild injury to a newborn could be life threatening if blood clotting capability is not adequate.

So why would any parent object to the vitamin K shot? For one thing, the vitamin K in the shot is a synthetic version of vitamin K, called phytonadione, and it is given at a dose that is one hundred times greater than the infant's Recommended Daily Allowance of this nutrient. It's easy to see that such a large dose of a synthetic vitamin, given during the infant's first moments of life, could easily cause imbalances.

In fact, studies have linked large doses of vitamin K with childhood cancers and leukemia. By some estimates, the chance of your child developing leukemia from the vitamin K shot is about one in five hundred, or twice as great as the risk of bleeding on the brain.[5]

In addition to vitamin K, the shot contains a number of questionable ingredients including:

- Phenol (carbolic acid, a poisonous substance derived from coal tar)
- Benzyl alcohol (preservative)
- Propylene glycol (better known as antifreeze and a hydraulic in brake fluid)
- Acetic acid (astringent, antimicrobial agent)
- Hydrochloric acid
- Lecithin (from soybean oil)
- Castor oil

The manufacturer's insert included with the shot includes the following warning: "Severe reactions, including fatalities, have occurred during and immediately after intravenous injection of phytonadione even when precautions have been taken to dilute the vitamin and avoid rapid infusion. . . ."

The liver of a newborn does not begin to function until three or four days after birth. As a result, your baby has very limited ability to detoxify the large dose of synthetic vitamin K and all other the dangerous ingredients in the injection cocktail.

The alternative to the vitamin K shot is vitamin K drops, which are safe and effective. They are given as one to two drops for the first twenty-four hours, one to two drops the first seven days from birth, and finally one to two drops twenty-eight days from birth. Although not approved by the FDA for this purpose, they are readily available, even without a perscription (see Sources).

Of course, baby's best protection is mom's vitamin K-rich diet throughout pregnancy—leafy greens for vitamin K_1 and cheese, liver, egg yolks and grass-fed meat for K_2, as well as daily portions of lacto-fermented foods so that your intestinal and vaginal tracts are populated with good vitamin K-producing bacteria. The vitamin K in your blood will transfer via the placenta to your baby before birth, and the good vitamin K-producing bacteria will transfer to baby during birth.

An overlooked source of vitamin K for baby is the cord blood, which will be rich in vitamin K if mom consumes plenty of vitamin K in her diet. According to one midwife who has delivered over eight hundred babies, all with delayed cord clamping, only one needed a vitamin K shot as a precaution, after having blood on the umbilicus every day up to day eight.[6]

HEP B VACCINE

If you have a hospital birth and are not careful, your baby will be given a hepatitis vaccine before you leave the hospital. There is probably no greater example of the extent and folly of newborn interventions than the shot against hepatitis B, an illness common among IV drug users, prisoners, prostitutes and other adults with multiple unprotected sexual encounters and—rarely—babies born to infected mothers.

The disease is hard to contract and not very dangerous—ninety to ninety-five percent of hepatitis B cases completely recover after a few weeks of symptoms, which include headache, nausea and fatigue. Pregnant women are tested for hepatitis B during pregnancy and unless they are positive carriers of the hepatitis B virus, their newborn should not even be considered for this vaccination. (Those who do test positive should not give the shot to their babies either, just redouble their efforts to consume a nutritious diet during the last weeks of pregnancy.) Yet in 2002, this shot was added to the recommended immunization schedule, often given to babies at just one day old.

Common reactions to the hepatitis B vaccine in children and adults include headache, nausea, fever and fatigue—the same symptoms as the hard-to-catch disease. Worse, the hepatitis B vaccine may cause a variety of immune and neurological problems.

Persistent reports tie the vaccine to sudden infant death syndrome (SIDS). Other reports indicate such adverse reactions as Guillain-Barré Syndrome (GBS), transverse myelitis, optic neuritis and multiple sclerosis, as well as immune system dysfunction including chronic arthritis. Autism cannot be left out of this list. The vaccine may contain neurotoxic mercury or aluminum or both. And there are reports of newborn and infant deaths immediately following injection of the hepatitis B vaccine.

So why in the world is this dangerous and unnecessary vaccine given to babies before they even leave the hospital? What is the logic here? Medical personnel argue that they are safeguarding the newborn, even in cases where the mother tests negative for hepatitis B. If baby does not catch hepatitis B from his mother, he may go home to live with chronic carriers of the hepatitis B disease. Another reason is simply to begin childhood immunizations while the child is there in the hospital in hopes of better compliance with the government's recommended schedule.

The truth is that the hepatitis B vaccine risks sacrificing the health of your innocent newborn baby on the altar of corporate profits. Merck, the maker of the hepatitis B vaccine, makes over one billion dollars yearly on the shot, the vast majority of it injected into babies. The biggest pusher of this vaccine, the Hepatitis B Coalition, receives the bulk of its funding from Merck itself.

Just say "no" to the hepatitis vaccine. There is no reason at all for your baby to have it, and it carries considerable risk. Make sure you fill out whatever form necessary to prevent hospital staff from giving it and insist that the words "No Hep B vaccine" be written clearly on your baby's chart. If you are questioned, just say, "We are delaying vaccinations." If baby is taken away from you in the hospital for any reason, your doula, partner or birth companion should stay with the baby at all times.

SUGAR WATER

In addition to vaccinations, eye drops and immediate cord clamping, many hospitals routinely give sugar water, usually between feedings or after a shot or heel prick, to calm crying. If you are breastfeeding and keeping baby in your room with you, there is little likelihood that the hospital staff will attempt to stick a bottle of sugar water in baby's mouth. But if your baby is not being breastfed and is kept on the ward, he is likely to be a target of this common practice.

Indeed, giving sugar water to babies is justified by several studies showing that the practice stops babies from crying. "A spoonful of sugar helps the medicine go down, but only a few drops of sugar-sweetened water quell the crying of newborn babies longer and more effectively than a pacifier does, a new study reports."
Advocates claim that sugar water is also useful for easing pain "among newborns undergoing medical procedures, such as blood collection and circumcision."[7]

"Sucrose or glucose along with other recommended physical or psychological pain reduction strategies such as non-nutritive sucking (NNS), breastfeeding or effective means of distraction should be consistently utilized for immunization," say advocates for sugar water.[8]

But there is a real downside to using sugar water. In a 2002 study carried out at McGill University, researchers found that repeated use of "sucrose analgesia" in premature babies put them at risk for "poorer neurobehavioral development and physiologic outcomes." Higher numbers of sucrose doses predicted lower sores on motor development and vigor, and alertness and orientation at thirty-six weeks, lower motor development and vigor at forty weeks and a higher neuro-biological risk score at two weeks postnatal age.[9]

THE SYNAGIS SHOT

A new intervention for all babies born at less than thirty-five weeks gestation is periodic shots of the drug Palivizumab, more popularly known as Synagis, in order to lessen the severity of Respiratory Syncytial Virus (RSV). RSV is usually a mild illness but can prove severe and even fatal under certain situations for premature babies.

Synagis is an immunoglobulin that must be administered in five separate injections, usually into the thigh muscle, at over one thousand dollars per injection. It is important to note that Synagis does not prevent RSV infection and only potentially reduces the severity of illness should RSV be contracted.

Doctors assure parents that Synagis is not a vaccine, and therefore safe. However, the shot contains a number of objectionable ingredients and can cause serious side effects, including high fever, ear pain or drainage, tugging at the ear; warmth or swelling of the ear; crying or fussiness, especially while lying down; change in sleeping patterns; poor feeding or loss of appetite; and easy bruising or bleeding.

The dark side of Synagis is the fact that this immunoglobulin is manufactured using recombinant DNA (rDNA) technology. What this means is that an artificial antibody that exists nowhere in nature was created using a composite of 95 percent human and 5 percent rodent (murine) antibody sequences in a process that involves the grafting of the rat antibody into the human antibody framework.

Recombinant DNA technology is the same genetic engineering process used to produce genetically modified rice and corn (see Sidebar on GM foods on page 31). No doubt, the high cost and generous profit margin of Synagis play a big role in the aggressive marketing in hospitals and doctors' offices to the emotionally vulnerable parents of premature babies—and it is highly likely that more such genetically engineered products are in the pipeline. But you should not let your baby serve as a guinea pig to genetic engineering. You can protect your baby from RSV infection with good nutrition, good sanitation and keeping him away from second hand smoke.[10]

No one likes to see a baby cry, especially the baby's mother. And that's just the point: mom should be with baby at all times for at least several weeks after the birth, protecting baby against interventions that make him cry, allowing baby to breastfeed whenever he is fussy, and gently rocking him to sleep if he is restless.

Breastmilk is naturally sweet with the right kind of sugar for baby—galactose—necessary for the infant's neurological development. That sweetness comes along with protein and fat to prevent blood sugar swings. But sugar water is naked sugar—tantamount to baby's first piece of candy and likely to set him up for sugar cravings throughout life.

BLOOD TESTS ON BABY

It is customary to perform a heel stick test on newborns, in order to draw a few drops of blood. This is sent to a laboratory to analyze for a variety of diseases and genetic disorders. If there are any positive results—which happen frequently—the test may be performed again. In some states, the test is required by law. In others it requires a parent's consent.

The three diseases the test most commonly screens are congenital hypothyroidism, PKU and galactosemia. Hypothyroidism occurs in one of every three to four thousand births. Conventional medicine treats the disorder with thyroid hormones, although we have reports of babies diagnosed with congenital hypothyroidism growing up perfectly normally on a nutrient-dense diet.

Phenylketonuria (PKU) is a recessive genetic disorder characterized by the inability of the body to utilize the essential amino acid phenylalanine. The treatment is a diet low in phenylalanine, which means a diet in which animal foods like meat, fish, poultry, eggs, cheese, milk and even beans and peas are absent. The recommended diet is one based on cereals, starches, fruits and vegetables, along with a "milk-free formula" based on sugar, modified food starch, vegetable oils, flavorings, artificial food colors and a host of amino acids and synthetic vitamins—in short a processed, synthetic diet for life.

You will be told that if undetected and untreated, PKU can lead to mental retardation and seizures. However, the diet is extremely difficult and will separate your child from the company of others for his entire lifespan—not to mention the fact that the diet itself may also retard your baby's development.

Should your baby test positive for PKU, you will be faced with a very difficult decision of opting for the PKU diet or taking your chances with a nutrient-dense diet. Some babies have a "variant" or "transient" form of the disorder, which means that they do not manifest symptoms, or "they grow out of it." Your best defense against disease in your children—even so-called genetic diseases—is proper nutritional preparation before and during pregnancy.

The third condition is galactosemia, an inherited disorder with a rate of around one of every seventy-five hundred live births. An infant with galactosemia is unable to break down galactose, the sugar found in milk and milk products. If undetected, newborns experience vomiting, liver disease and mental retardation. The recommended diet is a "milk-free diet under the supervision of a specialist."

That means your baby will be prescribed soy formula. A healthier alternative to soy formula is a modified version of our liver-based formula (see page 146) in which sugar replaces lactose and the whey is left out of the formula.

Very often parents will get a diagnosis of galactosemia when the baby shows no signs of problem whatsoever. False positives do occur in these tests; but the threat of mental retardation makes the parent's decision a very difficult one.

CIRCUMCISION

The practice of male circumcision, the surgical removal of some or all of the foreskin (prepuce) from the penis, is fraught with controversy and heated opinions. The practice dates back to ancient Egypt and those who learned it from the Egyptians, most notably the Semitic peoples. Today about one-sixth of all males in the world are circumcised, which is carried out either in infancy or as a rite of passage from puberty to adulthood.

The practice of non-religious circumcision commenced about 1900 in the United States, Australia and the English-speaking parts of Canada, South

THE TRADITION OF CIRCUMCISION[11]

Theories abound as to the purpose of circumcision among traditional cultures. Researchers have proposed the following reasons for the practice:

- As a religious sacrifice.
- As a rite of passage marking a boy's entrance into adulthood.
- As a form of sympathetic magic to ensure virility or fertility.
- As a means of enhancing sexual pleasure.
- As an aid to hygiene where regular bathing is impractical.
- As a means of marking those of higher social status.
- As a means of humiliating enemies and slaves by symbolic castration.
- As a means of differentiating a circumcising group from their non-circumcising neighbors.
- As a means of discouraging masturbation or other socially proscribed sexual behaviors.
- As a means of removing "excess" pleasure.
- As a means of increasing a man's attractiveness to women.
- As a demonstration of one's ability to endure pain.
- As a male counterpart to menstruation or the breaking of the hymen.
- To copy the rare natural occurrence of a missing foreskin in an important leader.

Researchers suggest that the custom of circumcision gave advantages to tribes that practiced it and thus led to its spread.

The Jews practice ritual circumcision on the eighth day after birth. Islamic scholars endorse circumcision for males but note that it is not a requirement for converting to Islam. The Roman Catholic Church formally condemned the ritual observance of circumcision and ordered against its practice in the Ecumenical Council of Basel-Florence in 1442. Today the Church maintains a neutral stance on circumcision as a medical practice.

Among traditional peoples, the Igbos of Nigeria traditionally practice circumcision of infants on the eighth day, often cited as evidence of a link between the Igbos and the Jews.

Circumcision is part of initiation rites in some African, Pacific Islander and Australian aboriginal traditions. In the Pacific, circumcision or superincision (involving a single incision along the upper length of the foreskin, exposing the glans without removing any tissue) is nearly universal among the Melanesians of Fiji and Vanuatu. Participation in the traditional land diving on Pentecost Island is reserved for those who have been circumcised. Circumcision or superincision is also commonly practiced in the Polynesian islands of Samoa, Tonga, Niue and Tikopia. In Samoa it is accompanied by a celebration.

Among some West African groups, such as the Dogon and Dowayo, circumcision is taken to represent a removal of "feminine" aspects of the male, turning boys into fully masculine males. Among the Urhobo of southern Nigeria it is symbolic of a boy entering into manhood. For Nilotic peoples, such as the Kalenjin and Maasai, circumcision is a rite of passage observed collectively by a number of boys every few years. Boys circumcised at the same time are taken to be members of a single age set.

A number of cultures practice the more painful penile subincision, in which the underside of the penis is incised and the urethra slit open lengthwise, notably in Australia, but also in Africa, South America and the Polynesian and Melanesian cultures of the Pacific, often as a coming-of-age ritual.

Indigenous cultures of the Amazon Basin also practice subincision, as do Samburu herdboys of Kenya, who are said to perform subincisions on themselves (or sometimes their peers) at age seven to ten.

Africa, New Zealand and to a lesser extent in the United Kingdom. There are several hypotheses to explain why infant circumcision became widespread. The germ theory of disease elicited an image of the human body as a conveyance for many dangerous germs, making the public "germ phobic" and suspicious of dirt and bodily secretions. The penis became "dirty" by association with its function, and from this premise circumcision was seen as preventative medicine to be practiced universally.

Many practitioners at the time, including John Harvey Kellogg, believed that circumcision was a method of treating and preventing masturbation. Circumcision was also said to protect against syphilis, infections and "excessive venery" (which was believed to produce paralysis).

By 1965, circumcision rates reached 85 percent in the U.S., and have since declined somewhat. Rates are also declining in the U.K. and Australia. The American Academy of Pediatrics does not recommend routine circumcision.

Proponents of circumcision cite studies showing a number of benefits including:

- A decreased risk of urinary tract infections.
- A reduced risk of sexually transmitted diseases in men.
- Protection against penile cancer and a reduced risk of cervical cancer in female sex partners.
- Prevention of balanitis (inflammation of the glans) and balanoposthitis (inflammation of the glans and foreskin).
- Prevention of phimosis (the inability to retract the foreskin) and paraphimosis (the inability to return the foreskin to its original location).
- Circumcision makes it easier to keep the end of the penis clean.

Those opposed to circumcision tend to disagree with the interpretation of studies showing positive effect, also noting that thousands of circumcisions need to be performed for even one to benefit.

Problems associated with circumcision include pain, bleeding and infection at the site of the circumcision, irritation of the glans, increased risk of meatitis (inflammation of the opening of the penis) and risk of injury to the penis. These injuries include concealed penis, urinary fistulas, chordee, cysts, lymphedema, ulceration of the glans, necrosis of all or part of the penis, hypospadias, epispadias and impotence.

According to the American Academy of Family Physicians, death from circumcision is rare, at one infant in five hundred thousand. The penis is thought to be lost in one in one million circumcisions.

In the West, most circumcisions are performed on babies one or two days old. The infants are strapped in a restraining device and subjected to one of three methods: the Gomco clamp, the Plastibell or the Mogen clamp.

With all these devices, the same basic procedure is followed. First, the amount of foreskin to be removed is estimated. The foreskin is opened via the preputial orifice to reveal the glans underneath and ensure it is normal. The inner lining of the foreskin (preputial epithelium) is bluntly cut away from its attachment to the glans.

With the Plastibell, once the glans is freed, the Plastibell is placed over the glans, and the foreskin is placed over the Plastibell. A ligature is then tied firmly around the foreskin and tightened into a groove in the Plastibell to cut off blood flow to the foreskin. The foreskin next to the ligature is cut away and the handle is snapped off the Plastibell device. The Plastibell falls from the penis after the wound has healed, typically in four to six days.

With a Gomco clamp, a section of skin is crushed with a hemostat (clamp to control bleeding) and then slit with scissors. The foreskin is drawn over the bell shaped portion of the clamp and inserted through a hole in the base of the clamp. The clamp is tightened, crushing the foreskin between the bell and the base plate. The flared bottom of the bell fits tightly against the hole of the base plate, so the foreskin may be cut away with a scalpel from above the base plate.

With a Mogen clamp, the foreskin is pulled dorsally with a straight hemostat and lifted. The Mogen clamp is then slid between the glans and hemostat, following the angle of the corona to "avoid removing excess skin ventrally and to obtain a superior cosmetic result" to Gomco or Plastibell circumcisions. The clamp is locked, and a scalpel is used to cut the skin from the flat (upper) side of the clamp.[12]

These gruesome operations are often performed without anesthesia, and by medical interns eager to "practice" a new procedure. Typically babies cry as if being tortured for the whole thirty minutes of the procedure, even when a topical anesthetic is used.

If anesthesia is to be used, there are several options: local anesthetic cream (EMLA cream) can be applied to the end of the penis sixty to ninety minutes prior to the procedure; local anesthetic can be injected at the base of the penis to block the dorsal penile nerve; and local anesthetic can be injected in a ring around the middle of the penis in what is called a subcutaneous ring block.

So why circumcise? Urologists do insist that serious infections are more common in uncircumcised men. Fungal infections and hygiene can be a problem in the uncircumcised.

Circumcision is said to lower sensitivity of the penis, but this may not be a bad thing during sexual intercourse. Slightly reduced sensitivity may give a man more control over the timing of his ejaculation, more ability to give pleasure to his partner. Some women decidedly prefer a circumcised man.

If you do decide to circumcise your baby boy, it's best to wait until the eighth day or later, and have the operation performed by an experienced physician or a Jewish *mohel* (one trained to perform circumcision as part of a religious ceremony), not a student doctor-in-training. An injected anesthetic should be used, followed by topical arnica cream and homeopathic arnica.

If you choose not to circumcise, your child should be trained to pull back the foreskin to clean the glans. This is easy to do in the bath. Little boys are usually only too happy to comply with the suggestion to play with their penis while in the water. Doing it themselves they rarely cause tears that lead to adhesions, which are the source of most infections. Because these tears cause pain, the boys avoid them and over time slowly work the foreskin back themselves, at that point cleaning the penis is no different than cleaning any other body part.

Chapter 6
Vaccinations

No subject in pediatric medicine evokes as much controversy as the subject of vaccines. During his years of practice, Dr. Cowan has seen the many effects of vaccines, both on the physical health of babies and children, and on the emotional and spiritual life of families. He has seen a healthy two-month-old child die inexplicably the day after a DPT shot—the vaccine was later exonerated for the death—and many other reactions, from mild to life-threatening. He has talked with parents who were paralyzed with indecision about vaccines, parents who literally divorced as a result of conflicts over vaccines, and even parents who have had their children taken away and then threatened with jail time as a result of their refusal to vaccinate. Clearly, this is a complex and highly emotional subject, exacerbated by government involvement and issues of freedom and personal choice.

Vaccination issues fall into three broad categories. The first is the central question of whether vaccines work; that is, do they truly prevent the illnesses they were designed to prevent? The second involves the toxicity of vaccine components—are these components understood and of greater consequence than the conventional medical world lets on? Third—and perhaps most important—do vaccines produce predictable medical problems independent of the toxicity issues, problems that might influence our decisions about whether or not to vaccinate?

VACCINATIONS AND EPIDEMICS

When parents bring a newborn child to their pediatrician to discuss the issue of vaccines, the doctor's arguments are based on the belief that while vaccines may present some minor problems, they are wholly responsible for eliminating many of the infectious diseases that caused so much suffering in children during previous eras. This assumption is reinforced by the fact that we rarely hear of modern children dying of polio, measles, smallpox or any of the illnesses for which we vaccinate. Today, it is extremely rare for a doctor to see a child with measles, an illness that was universal up to the 1960s, but which is now virtually extinct. Was this decline due to the introduction of the measles vaccine or to other factors?

While we have all been taught that vaccination ended the world's many deadly epidemics, an honest and careful review of original historical medical sources, publications and statistics from the past two hundred years reveals that infectious diseases declined at least 90 percent before vaccinations were ever introduced.

Experts attribute the cessation of epidemic diseases not to mass vaccination, but to a major sanitation reform movement that swept Europe and America during the late 1800s and early 1900s. During the nineteenth century, most large cities were pocketed

with smoldering garbage dumps and shanty towns; bathing was difficult, even for the well-to-do; public water supplies were filthy.

Public health reforms brought sewage systems, indoor plumbing, improved roads and cleaner water; new inventions led to refrigeration and the replacement of the horse with the car. Before the car came along, public health officials were in despair about what to do with all the manure that clogged the cities and contaminated public water supplies.

And cleaning up of water supplies was key. Until the end of the nineteenth century, the municipal water for the city of Chicago was drawn from the same place where sewage was dumped in Lake Michigan. The water supply for Bloomington, Illinois was fed by small streams clogged with garbage and human and animal waste.[1]

All the old terror diseases of plague, black death and cholera responded to these reforms, and epidemics declined long before the advent of vaccination. Even the Centers for Disease Control (CDC)

admits that the decline in infectious disease during the past century was due to improvements in sanitation, water and hygiene. Vaccination against whooping cough, diphtheria, measles and polio all occurred only at the very end of the life cycle of each epidemic, exposing the fallacy of the claim that vaccination ended epidemics.

The only exception to this decline in epidemic disease is smallpox, which, contrary to all we have been taught, actually increased with the advent of mandatory vaccination and decreased only after an organized uprising by parents and doctors forced European governments to end their mandatory vaccination programs. Even though the World Health Organization claims credit for the eradication of smallpox worldwide through vaccination, the fact is that smallpox declined in countries around the world whether the population was vaccinated or not.

Let's look at this issue another way. If we ask whether there are more cases of whooping cough (pertussis) today than one hundred years ago, clear-

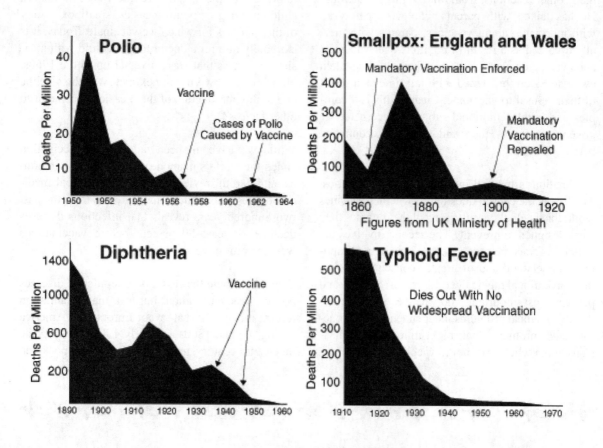

ly the answer is no; there were more cases one hundred years ago, many more. However, if we phrase our question differently and ask whether there are more problems with bronchial inflammation—an accurate description of whooping cough—now compared to one hundred years ago, we get a different answer. Asthma is a condition of bronchial inflammation, only one that is chronic rather than self-limiting. The child with whooping cough will feel miserable, but he will soon get well; but the child with asthma runs the risk of never overcoming the illness, and perhaps needing daily medication for a lifetime.

If we look back to our days in grade school, we may remember one or two children with asthma. Today, some 15 percent of school children suffer from asthma.[2] The point is, we haven't eradicated sickness with vaccines, we haven't even stopped inflammatory lung disease with the pertussis vaccine, we have just traded an acute, self-limiting illness for a chronic, never ending battle.

Actually, it is rare for a child who has had pertussis to contract asthma. You might say that pertussis actually "cures" a child of the tendency to get asthma. This phenomenon is not unknown or unreported in medicine. For example, chronic kidney disease in children—known as nephrotic syndrome—is often cured (meaning it goes away, never to return again) when the child contracts "wild" (naturally occur-ring) measles. But the measles vaccine does not help a child with nephrotic syndrome at all.

The point is, even if vaccines have no side effects whatsoever, and really were responsible for stopping epidemics of childhood diseases, there may be a real downside in preventing all infectious illness in our children.

TOXICITY

The second issue concerns the toxicity of the "excipients" contained in the vaccines. Although there is some variation from vaccine to vaccine, generally speaking vaccines consist of killed or attenuated (weakened) viruses, or toxoids (poisons made by bacteria, such as tetanus) that have been weakened so as not to cause overt disease. These active ingredients are then stabilized with a variety of substances to keep them from degrading into inactive fragments in the vial. The main excipients we are concerned with include thimerosal (a mercury cmpound), aluminum and formaldehyde. These three substances are neurotrophic, meaning they specifically seek out the nervous tissue to land in, and years of research has definitively shown them to be toxic to the nerves in which they take up residence. This is a very serious matter because most vaccinations are given during the first three years of life, the period of maximum brain growth and development.

VACCINATIONS AND AUTISM

According to vaccination defenders, vaccines are not the cause of autism. This claim became harder to justify with the 2010 publication of a study conducted by scientists at the University of Pittsburgh, which revealed that many infant monkeys given standard doses of childhood vaccines developed symptoms of autism. The researchers found that young macaque monkeys given the typical CDC-recommended vaccination schedule from the 1990s and in appropriate doses for the monkeys' sizes and ages, tended to develop typical signs of autism, while their unvaccinated counterparts developed no such symptoms. MRI and PET scans showed pathological changes to the amygdala, which performs a primary role in the processing and memory of emotional reactions.[3]

Included in the vaccine mix were several containing the mercury-based compound thimerosal, which has been phased out of some shots but is still present in batch-administered influenza vaccines. Also administered was the measles, mumps and rubella (MMR) vaccine, which has been linked many times with autism and other serious health problems. The study was presented at the International Meeting for Autism Research (IMFAR) in London, England, in May, 2012 and points to the need for more such investigations into the effects of immunizations. Vaccine safety testing is lax compared to testing for other drugs, and single vaccines have never been tested in combination with other vaccines.

Recently a neurologist from Canada, Russell Moulton, MD, has proposed an interesting concept to explain how these substances can cause damage. He claims that when these metals (mercury), heavy positively charged substances (aluminum) and neurotoxins (formaldehyde) enter the small capillaries of the brain, the body's immune system reacts to these invaders in the only way it knows how, which is to set up an inflammatory reaction in order to dissolve and then excrete the invader. Immune cells—mostly white blood cells—flood the area, but because they are unable to digest heavy metallic substances, a kind of congestion ensues, clogging the small capillaries in the brain. As the immune cells accumulate, this microcirculation is impaired, leading to a series of small vascular "strokes" in the brain of the young child. This can happen even with the first vaccine, and becomes a more likely scenario as one vaccine follows another. Moulton provides CT scan evidence showing that these vascular events are in fact taking place.[4]

Dr. Russell Blaylock has shown how vaccines cause brain injury by various mechanisms. He notes numerous studies showing that the toxins in vaccines, especially mercury and aluminum, can provoke a free radical storm in the brain. Free radicals are very reactive particles that can cause widespread damage, especially if unchecked by antioxidants and other protective compounds.[10]

THE SCIENCE OF VACCINES

In spite of claims to the contrary, scientists have carried out several longitudinal survey studies comparing the health of vaccinated versus unvaccinated children. These studies have clearly demonstrated the occurrence of statistically significant vaccinosis—illness produced in an individual after receiving a vaccine—in the vaccinated groups. The following summarizes a few of these:

- 1992 New Zealand Study: Four hundred ninety-five children were surveyed, with 226 vaccinated and 269 unvaccinated. "Results overwhelmingly showed that unvaccinated children suffer far less from chronic childhood conditions than vaccinated children." This included a ten-fold increase in tonsillitis (26) and tonsillectomies (10) in vaccinated children, as compared to three cases of tonsillitis and no tonsillectomies in the unvaccinated group. Similarly, the incidence of ear infections (56 versus 16), sleep apnea (14 versus 4), hyperactivity (13 versus 4), and epilepsy (4 versus 0) was statistically significantly higher in the vaccinated children than the unvaccinated.[5]

- 1997 New Zealand Study: Twelve hundred sixty-five children were surveyed. The vaccinated children experienced episodes of asthma (23 percent) and allergies (30 percent), as compared to no asthma or allergy incidences in the unvaccinated group.[6]

- 2000 Africa Study: The children of fifteen thousand mothers were observed from 1990 to 1996. Results showed that the death rate from diphtheria, tetanus, and whooping cough in vaccinated children was twice as high as that in unvaccinated children (10.5 percent versus 4.7 percent).[7]

- 2004 British Study: Thirty thousand children were compared. The vaccinated children had an increased risk of allergic asthma (5.04 percent) as compared to the unvaccinated children (0.36 percent).[8]

- 2011 German Study: This study of eight thousand unvaccinated children (which included medical documentation of each case), from newborn to nineteen years, revealed that vaccinated children have at least two to five times more diseases and disorders than unvaccinated children.[9]

In contradistinction, no scientific (peer-reviewed, placebo-controlled, double-blind) study has ever been conducted that supports the effectiveness of vaccinations. Despite the fact that Barbara Loe Fisher, president and co-founder of the National Vaccine Information Center, and her colleagues entreated the CDC, the NIH, and other federal agencies to "Show Us the Science" at the second NVIC conference in 2000, twelve years later no valid scientific research has yet been published proving the efficacy of vaccines.

In animal studies, vaccination increases the brain's inflammatory chemicals as well as inflammatory immune cells. The main immune cells in the brain are called microglia. In a resting state, these cells support growth and protection of brain cells and their connections. Once activated, they move around and secrete a number of harmful compounds, including inflammatory chemicals, free radicals and glutamate. These compounds are meant to kill invaders and when we have an infection, this system works for a few days to kill them off. During this process, we may suffer from "sickness behavior." This is why we may be restless, irritable, tired and have trouble sleeping when we are sick.

When a child receives a vaccine, the toxic adjuvants can cause an overreaction of the microglia, which can be very destructive to brain cells. This overreaction can persist for a long time, and the consequences of the destruction, the "sickness behavior," can manifest for weeks or even months after the vaccine.

In the elderly, elevated levels of inflammatory immune cells are associated with Parkinson's, Alzheimer's, anxiety and depression.

Mercury makes the brain more vulnerable to other toxins, such as glutamate and pesticides. If you are exposed to pesticides or eating processed food full of MSG, vaccines can put you at increased risk for adverse effects. Mercury increases brain free radicals, increases lipid peroxidation products, inhibits critical brain enzymes, inhibits antioxidant enzymes and impairs DNA repair ability.

Aluminum is a powerful cumulative brain toxin. Like mercury, aluminum can cause the microglia to overreact. With pressure to reduce the mercury content in vaccines, manufacturers are adding more aluminum.

Viruses and viral components can trigger the microglial cells. This is the explanation for dementia in AIDS victims and in those with severe viral infections. Up to 60 percent of vaccines are contaminated with foreign viruses and viral components.

In particularly vulnerable children, vaccines may cause autism, seizures and mental retardation; but for every severe reaction, vaccines may provoke numerous less acute but nevertheless problematic effects, such as confusion, language difficulties, memory problems, irritability, mood alterations, combativeness, difficulty concentrating and behavioral problems.[11]

Because a child's brain undergoes a period of rapid growth from the third trimester of pregnancy until age two years, their brains are at greater risk from vaccinations than the brains of older children and adults. A fully vaccinated child receives twenty-two vaccines during the first year of life; up to thirty-six by the start of school, including yearly flu shots.

By the way, beware of nasal flu vaccines, which

CENTERS FOR DISEASE CONTROL RECOMMENDED IMMUNIZATION SCHEDULE

Birth	Hepatitis B
Two Months	Hepatitis B, Rotavirus, DTP, Hib, Pneumococcal, Polio
Four Months	Rotavirus, DTP, Hib, Pneumococcal, Polio
Six Months	Rotavirus, DTP, Hib, Pneumococcal
Twelve-Eighteen Months	Hepatitis B, DPT, Hib, Pneumococcal, Polio, Flu, MMR, Chicken Pox, Hepatitis A
Two Years	Flu, Hepatitis B
Three Years	Flu
Four Years	Flu
Five Years	Flu, DTP, Polio, MMR, Chicken Pox
Six Years	Flu

Thirty-six shots by the age of six years. . . and sixty-eight by the age of eleven or twelve!

OPTING OUT

Once your child is born, the pressure to vaccinate comes from main two sources—medical authorities and school officials (not to mention in-laws and family members). Medically, you are free to make any decision at any time you feel is best regarding your child's vaccination schedule. However, if you opt out of vaccination, many doctors may lie about vaccines being mandatory or frighten you with exaggerated statistics about the dangers of not vaccinating; they may even refuse to treat your child. Unfortunately, the "bread and butter" of pediatric practice are the many "well baby" visits that include vaccination throughout your child's development.

However, it is the entry into day care or school that triggers the need for legal exemptions. There are three types of exemptions—philosophical, medical and religious. All fifty states allow medical exemptions, religious exemptions are on the books in all but two states (West Virginia and Mississippi), and philosophical exemptions exist in sixteen states. You can check the laws for your particular state at www. thinktwice.com or www.909shot.com/state-site/legal-exemptions.htm.

Private schools have their own rules and may reject children that have not been vaccinated (although there tend to be many unvaccinated children in Waldorf schools). Public schools, however, are required by law to accept your exemption when properly prepared according to the laws of your state. Home schooling sidesteps the issue entirely.

Once you check the laws for your particular state, you can choose the exemption type that is best for your situation. It is very important to submit the appropriate paperwork to the school so that your refusal to vaccinate cannot be interpreted as parental neglect. A philosophical exemption generally requires a short letter simply stating that you object to vaccination. The religious exemption also requires a letter, but some states stipulate that you actually belong to, and are a practicing member of, a religion that specifically objects to vaccination. The medical exemption is usually the most difficult to obtain because doctors are subject to review and censure by state medical authorities when they grant exemptions. In some cases medical exemptions may be obtained from the school nurse—and are often easier to obtain than from a physician.

Happily, simply signing and submitting the exemption is generally all that is needed. Some exemption letters must be notarized or drafted as a signed affidavit. And some School Immunization Records have an exemption section on the form itself, that you simply fill out. For examples of exemption letters for all possible scenarios and all states see www.vaclib.org/pdf/exemption.htm.

When discussing your decision to opt out, it is best to remain calm, courteous and diplomatic, even in the face of ignorance or resistance from authorities. Do not enter into arguments with authorities and draw attention to your decision. There is no need to attach documents to your exemption proving evidence of the problems with vaccination or explaining your reasons for opting out—you simply want an exemption for your child. If you encounter belligerent or arrogant authorities who intimidate you with threats of sending you to jail or taking your child away, try to sidestep their resistance in a non-confrontational manner and leave the situation as soon as possible. If you run into this kind of resistance, you should put your wishes in writing, escalate your exemption request to someone above that official, and demand a written response. You'll be surprised how quickly resistance from authorities can fade once they must put their illegal statements and intimidations in writing.

Above all, remember that no authority has the legal right to vaccinate your child without your permission. Should they do so, they open themselves up to legal liability and you have all the resources of the law behind you. While you may experience resistance, they are breaking the law, not you. Do not be coerced or intimidated into vaccinating your child—it is your choice and your right to do what you feel is best.

may be even worse because they introduce a live virus into the nasal passages, which then travels along the olfactory nerves, leading to the very part of the brain first and most severely affected by Alzheimer's disease.

The excipients or adjuvants in vaccines are designed to make them more potent; and because so many reports of vaccine failure have appeared in the literature—outbreaks of measles, mumps and whooping cough in populations fully vaccinated against these illnesses—manufacturers have added more immune adjuvants or made them more powerful. In those who are very young or very old, or who have nutritional deficiencies, these adjuvants can paralyze the immune system.

With natural infections, the immune activation occurs rapidly and once the infection is under control, it drops off. But the vaccine works differently, and the immune reaction may continue for months or even years, especially if more vaccinations are given. In the child, brain immune over-activation is particularly damaging to the amygdala and other limbic structures of the brain, and to the executive functions of the frontal lobes; in other words the workings of the mental body, the part of us that allows us to function in a complex world of ideas and social interactions.[12]

In regards to brain damage from vaccines, it is interesting to note that Rudolf Steiner predicted that the time would come when vaccines would make it very difficult to have any sense of a spiritual life. In 1917, he warned, "people are now vaccinated against consumption, and in the same way they will be vaccinated against any inclination towards spirituality."[14]

HERD IMMUNITY

Proponents of vaccines once argued that vaccines gave lifelong immunity; then when outbreaks of illness occurred in populations fully vaccinated for those illnesses—such as measles or whooping cough in children who had all received their inoculations for those diseases—booster shots were introduced to keep immunity from wearing off.

But even with booster shots, outbreaks still occur in children who have been fully vaccinated. The finger of blame is now pointed at unvaccinated children as causing these outbreaks. We need for everyone to be vaccinated, so the argument goes, to provide "herd immunity." This concept is based upon the idea that 95 percent (and some now say 100 percent) of the population must be vaccinated to prevent an epidemic.

In the original description of herd immunity, the protection to the population at large occurred only if people contracted the infections naturally. But naturally acquired immunity lasts for a lifetime, while vaccine immunity does not.

According to Dr. Russell Blaylock, the vaccine-induced herd immunity is mostly myth, which can be proven quite simply. "When I was in medical school, we were taught that all of the childhood vaccines lasted a lifetime. This thinking existed for over seventy years. It was not until relatively recently that it was discovered that most of these vaccines lost their effectiveness two to ten years after being given. What this means is that at least half the population, that is the baby boomers, have had no vaccine-induced immunity against any of these diseases for which they had been vaccinated very early in life. In essence, at least 50 percent or more of the population was unprotected for decades.

"If we listen to present-day wisdom, we are all at risk of resurgent massive epidemics should the vaccination rate fall below 95 percent. Yet, we have all lived for at least thirty to forty years with 50 percent or less of the population having vaccine protection. That is, herd immunity has not existed in this country for many decades and no resurgent epidemics have occurred. Vaccine-induced herd immunity is a lie used to frighten doctors, public-health officials, other medical personnel, and the public into accepting vaccinations."[13]

VACCINES AND THE IMMUNE SYSTEM

The final and most important issue concerning vaccines is the alteration that occurs with each and every inoculation with respect to our immune system. We now know that the immune system has two distinct arms. The first arm, the Th1, is the cell-mediated immune system, which responds to microbes by recruiting white blood cells, whose job it is to digest and eliminate invaders through various elimination channels available to the human body.

The second arm of arm immune system, called Th2 or humoral immunity, responds to invaders by making antibodies. These antibodies "remember" which microbes we have already been exposed to in order to give us long-term immunity. It is important to clearly understand that the symptoms we call sickness stem from the reactions of our own immune function, and only minimally from the microbes themselves.

When we encounter a micro-organism in childhood, say the virus associated with chicken pox, and we have no antibody memory of a previous encounter with this virus in the past, both arms of our immune system mobilize. The cell-mediated arm digests the microbes while at the same time causing symptoms

EXCIPIENTS: TOXIC ADDITIVES IN VACCINES[15]

Albumin from egg	Mouse serum protein
Albumin, human serum	MRC-5 cellular protein
Albumin or serum, bovine	Neomycin (antibacterial)
Aluminum hydroxide	Phenol (preservative)
Aluminum hydroxyphosphate sulfate	Phenol red
Aluminum phosphate	2-henoxyethanol (preservative)
Aluminum potassium sulfate	Pphosphate buffers
Amino acids	Polydimethylsiloxane (antifoaming agent)
Ammonium sulfate	Polymyxin B (antibacterial)
Amphotericin B (antibacterial)	Polyoxyethylene9-10 nonyl phenol (surfactant)
Benzethonium chloride (preservative)	Polyoxyethylated octyl phenol (surfactant)
Calcium carbonate	Polysorbate 20 and 80 (surfactants)
calcium chloride	Potassium chloride
Chlortetracycline (antibacterial)	Potassium glutamate
Cystine	Serum, bovine calf
Dextran	Sodium acetate
DNA	Sodium bicarbonate
EDTA (preservative)	Sodium borate
Ferric nitrate	Sodium citrate
Formaldehyde	Sodium deoxycholate
Gelatin	Sodium hydrogen carbonate
Gentamicin (antibacterial)	Sodium hydroxide
Glucose	Sodium phosphate
Glutamine	Sodium pyruvate
Glutaraldehyde	Sorbitol
Glycerin	Streptomycin (antibacterial)
Glycine	Sucrose
Histidine	Thimerosol (preservative, containing mercury)
Hydrochloric acid	Tocopheryl hydrogen succinate
Hydrocortisone	Tyrosine
Lactose	Urea (stabilizer)
Magnesium stearate	Xanthan gum
Magnesium sulfate	Yeast protein
Monosodium glutamate	

that we associate with being sick, such as aches and fever. Then the same cell-mediated arm eliminates the invaders and probably other toxic wastes through diarrhea, rash, mucus and cough.

These symptoms are the cleansing part of the process. You would never hesitate to remove garbage from your house (hopefully taking it to the compost pile); similarly, stopping or preventing the cell-mediated response to invaders leaves the garbage in your body—a big mistake.

As this cell-mediated reaction is taking place, the humoral arm is busy making antibodies to remember the organism that is making us sick. It is these antibodies that bind with the invading organisms and tell the white blood cells to digest and excrete them. This process is usually completed within six weeks, and the child is not only restored to health but has also exercised his cell-mediated response and cleansed his body of this particular organism and of other wastes as well. Most importantly, his body now remembers what happened, so he is stronger and more resistant going forward. In fact,

not only is the child restored to health, but he is likelier to be healthier than he was before the illness.

This is the whole point of natural illness in children; short-term illness actually improves longterm health. Like a snake shedding its skin, the process involves a certain amount of exertion and may carry some risk, but the key point is that one cannot be a healthy adult without having gone through some of the process we call sickness in childhood. To deny children the opportunity to be sick and then expect health in adulthood is like asking someone to lift a heavy weight without ever having lifted a weight before in their lives. Our immune systems, like our muscles, are built to work and that work makes us strong and resistant.

In contrast to this picture, consider what happens when instead of allowing our children to contract illnesses naturally, we force the experience of the vaccine. Vaccines are designed to provoke as little cell-mediated reaction as possible. After all, cell-mediated reaction is "sickness," and if vaccines make people sick, it's back to the drawing board to

THE DANGERS OF TYLENOL®

One of our best defenses against toxins in vaccines is dietary sulfur, from foods like egg yolks, liver, molasses and onions. Sulfur in the form of sulfate in the bloodstream is essential for disposing of vaccine components like aluminum and mercury. Sulfate is severely deficient in autistic children, at about one-fifth the level of free sulfate in the blood stream of normal children.

Often after a vaccination, a child develops a high fever, pacticularly after the triple MMR (measles, mumps, rubella) vaccine. Then Tylenol is given to lower fever, a huge mistake according to researcher Stephanie Seneff, PhD. Sulfate is needed to clear xenobiotics like acetaminophen (Tylenol), so less is available for getting rid of toxins like aluminum and mercury that are in the vaccine.[16]

This same detoxification pathway is necessary to eliminate excess adrenalin and dopamine from the brain. Impairment could lead to the formation of neurotoxic substances with psychedelic effects, as seen in severe reactions to vaccination with subsequent autism.

Autistic children are especially susceptible to asthma, and there has been a sharp increase in childhood asthma over the past thirty years. The timing corresponds with the aspirin scare in the 1980s when parents began giving Tylenol instead of aspirin to treat fever and illness. The bronchial tube epithelial cells produce cholesterol sulfate, which protects against asthma. Tylenol causes increased bronchial constriction and wheezing. In fact, eczema, asthma, leaky gut and susceptibility to infection are all explained by sulfate deficiency.

If it is impossible for you to avoid a vaccination for your child, be sure to fortify him with sulfur-rich foods for many days prior to the vaccine, and keep your child quiet and in bed after the shot. Never give Tylenol if he develops a fever. For natural treatment of fevers, see Chapter 13.

clean up the vaccine. The whole point of vaccines is to provoke memory without provoking a cell-mediated response.

There are two fundamental problems with this approach. The first is that the cell-mediated system is the only way we have of getting rid of toxins and micro-organisms, or even fragments of micro-organisms. So essentially we are injecting children with toxic chemicals, fragments of micro-organisms, dead or damped-down micro-organisms, while preventing the very reaction that allows us to get rid of these poisons. No wonder children get "poisoned" from this intervention. This accumulation of biotoxins and chemical toxins is literally the whole point of giving a vaccine. It is true we make an antibody response and will remember the encounter, but the real question is, at what cost?

That cost is serious chronic disease. Remember that vaccines activate the humoral immune system without activating the cell-mediated response. A partial list of adult illnesses that the scientific literature associates with elevated antibodies and an insufficient cell-mediated response includes all auto-immune disease including lupus, rheumatoid arthritis, Sjogren's syndrome and Hashimoto's thyroiditis, as well as asthma, cancer, eczema, type 1 diabetes, and probably many other chronic diseases, all of which make our lives miserable and may even cause untimely death.

In an important study published in the *Journal of Allergy and Clinical Immunology*,[17] the authors were able to show that asthmatic children have an imbalance in their Th1 and Th2 responses; specifically, these childern have a Th1-to-Th2 shift, meaning an accentution of their humoral or antibody-producing immune system.[18]

These findings correlate with the epidemiological trends of the past one hundred years; in any culture, within a few years from the advent of vaccinations, the incidence of chronic inflammatory disease and conditions of suppressed immunity such as cancer begins to increase. Undoubtedly there are other factors besides vaccines involved, including social factors, emotional factors, environmental degradation and poor nutrition. But vaccines most certainly contribute to this transformation.

Thus, to ensure optimal health in our children throughout life, we need to honor the wisdom of childhood illnesses rather than confront them with fear.

But the decision not to vaccinate should not be accompanied by insouciance about our children's health. The alternative to vaccines is a healthy diet. Good nutritional support is what prevents mild childhood illnesses from getting out of control and causing long-term injury. As always, the fat-soluble vitamins, especially vitamin A, play a key role in regulating the immune response and allowing our children to safely get sick. (See chapter 13 for more on diets for sick children.)

IF YOU MUST VACCINATE

- Delay vaccinations until age two.

- Give no more than one vaccine every six months.

- Never give more than one vaccine at a time.

- Avoid live virus vaccines.

- Never give a vaccination to a sick child.

- Avoid vaccines containing thimerosal. (In general, single-vial vaccines are thimerosal-free.)

- Supplement the child with extra cod liver oil, vitamin C, B_{12} and sulfur-containing foods such as liver and egg yolk before each shot.

IF YOU MUST VACCINATE

Ideally, both parents are of like mind in deciding not to vaccinate their child, and their relatives support their decision. That is the ideal. But as we all know, circumstances are not always ideal; sometimes vaccination may be the lesser of evils.

At the very least, vaccinations should be delayed until age two. Very few physicians will oppose that decision. When the question comes up at the hospital, pediatrician's office or with public health officials, a firm response, "We are delaying vaccinations until age two," is usually sufficient. If there is any likelihood of the hospital forcing a vaccine on your newborn—CDC guidelines call for the hepatitis B vaccine at day one—be sure to come armed with a written statement that no vaccinations shall be given at the hospital. It might even be a good idea to have such a statement written on your attorney's letterhead. Make it clear that you will hold the hospital or physician liable should any vaccine be given.

State laws differ on the choices that allow parents to decline vaccines. All states allow a medical exemption—and almost every family has a medical history that can justify exemption. A family history of neurological disorders, epilepsy, allergies, immune disease or severe reaction to a vaccination is sufficient for a doctor or nurse to provide a medical exemption.

All but two states allow a religious or philosophical exemption. Arm yourself with the facts and, above all, be prepared to stand your ground, politely but firmly, with any zealous medical personal.

If circumstance do require you to vaccinate—such as entanglement with social services, the possibility of divorce, child custody problems or family pressure—the provisions outlined in the Sidebar on page 118 will help minimize any adverse effects.

FOR FURTHER INFORMATION

Vaccines: Are They Really Safe and Effective? by Neil Z. Miller, 2002. Check his website for additional books, www.thinktwice.com.

Immunization, The Reality Behind the Myth, by Walene James, 1995.

Vaccination: 100 Years of Orthodox Research Shows that Vaccines Represent a Medical Assault on the Immune System, by Viera Scheibner, PhD., 2007, New Atlantean Press, (505) 983-1856.

How to Raise a Healthy Child in Spite of Your Doctors, by Robert Mendelsohn, MD, 1987.

What about Immunizations? Exposing the Vaccine Philosophy, by Cynthia Cournoyer, 2010.

The Vaccine Book: Making the Right Decision for Your Child by Dr. Robert Sears, 2007.

VACCINATION RESOURCES

www.novaccine.com is an excellent resourse, providing state laws on vaccinations, research on side effects, and reports showing the lack of effectiveness of vaccines. One excellent page on the website, www.novaccine.com/specific-vaccines/, provides an ingredient list for every vaccine by every manufacturer.

National Vaccination Information Center, www.909shot.com also provides information on exemptions in every state. Visit the page www.908shot.com/ResourceCenter/ResourceCenter.htm for a list of recommended reading.

California now requires a signed form by a doctor for vaccine exemptions, and other states may follow suit. The website www.askdrsears.com/topics/vaccines/find-vaccine-friendly-doctor-near-you posts a list of physicians who will provide such a form.

Homeopathic physicians who can give homeopathic treatments to build immunity to specific diseases are listed here: http://vaccinefree.wordpress.com/hp-supervision/.

Chapter 7
Nourishing Your Baby

It is assumed that any pregnant woman reading this book plans to breastfeed her baby. Mothers who recognize the importance of diet in the physical health of their infants will opt for mother's milk—a food uniquely designed for the infant—rather than commercial formula based on powdered milk, industrial oils, refined sweeteners, questionable additives and artificial vitamins.

The trend towards more natural methods of child-rearing began with a comeback for breastfeeding during the 1970s, as much a reaction to a medical establishment deemed paternalistic and insensitive to women's needs as a recognition, backed by many scientific studies, of breast milk's amazing properties.

For most women, breastfeeding comes easily. Immediately after birth, baby is put on mom's chest. He turns his head to the breast—he may even wiggle up her torso to the breast—roots his head back and forth to find the nipple and latches on. If the baby is healthy and strong, he will latch on with a tremendous, sucking grip, giving first-time mothers something of a shock. As baby sucks, mom feels a let-down reflex and the milk begins to flow. Baby nurses only a few moments at first, then longer and longer with each nursing. Within a few weeks, baby nurses for twenty minutes every two to three hours, steadily gains weight, and is contented between nursings. Mom and baby settle into a routine and all is well.

But for some women, even many women, all does not go well. Breastfeeding may be painful, mom may develop sores, baby may not latch on properly, and most seriously, baby does not gain weight, cries a lot and is obviously hungry. Or, mom may be exhausted or sick; breastfeeding may make her feel resentful, or even embarrassed; she may need to return to a work environment that makes breastfeeding difficult if not impossible. Or, she may not have any milk at all—due to illness, surgery or the fact that she has adopted her baby.

Most of this chapter will be dedicated to addressing these problems—not because we don't think breastfeeding is important, but because little needs to be said about normal, successful breastfeeding. After all, women have been breastfeeding for thousands and thousands of years. Those for whom breastfeeding goes smoothly will not even need this chapter; those who are struggling need detailed and specific advice.

Unfortunately, discussions about infant feeding today have become polarized, even acrimonious. Whereas fifty years ago, the medical community pressured women into giving formula as the scientific and modern thing to do, today many women feel pressured into continued breastfeeding even when baby is obviously not doing well. Breastfeeding literature tends to be judgmental—often implying that lack of breastfeeding success is the mother's fault, and that if she switches to formula, she is a bad mother.

We need to accept as a fact of life that breastfeeding is not always successful, in spite of the best efforts of the mother. In fact, it would be amazing that out of all the organs in the body, women's breasts had the unique property of working well under all circumstances.

Fortunately, we now have homemade alternatives to breast milk that are much healthier than commercial formula. The important thing is to provide the information needed to maximize either breastfeeding or formula-feeding success. Let's keep in mind that breastfeeding is not some kind of contest between moms to see who can do it longest and best, but a way of providing maximum nutrition to the infant; and that our role as parents, mentors, advisors and friends of a new mother is to provide information in a calm and rational way, and then to support her in whatever decision she may make.

THE AMAZING QUALITIES OF MAMMALIAN MILK

Under a microscope, the appearance of human or animal milk inspires wonder and awe. Although milk is a fluid, it has a structured appearance, with nutrients and bioactive components sequestered into various compartments. For example, the fats in milk are enveloped in a membrane, the milk-fat globule membrane, which is constructed in the milk ducts. Baby uses portions of this membrane to build his own cell membranes.

Often referred to as "white blood," milk contains a range of antibodies to protect the infant against pathogens. These antibodies are specific to the flora and antigens of the mother. Maternal antibodies derived from her gut and respiratory immune surveillance systems are transported to the mammary gland. In this way, baby receives immune factors to protect him against the antigens of the mother.

In addition, these immune factors are packaged with a component that protects them from stomach acids,

allowing the immune factors to reach the small intestine intact.

Other protective and immune-enhancing components in milk include lactoferrin, which binds to iron, thus making it unavailable to iron-loving pathogenic bacteria; lysozyme, which enhances the bactericidal activity of immunoglobulins; mucins, which adhere to bacteria and viruses and help eliminate them from the body; interferon and fibronectin, which have antiviral activities; leukocytes, which help build the immune system; and many others. Together these factors protect the immature infant from infection, create the immune system, weed out toxins and support the formation of a healthy gut wall.

In addition, the various proteins and enzymes in milk facilitate the absorption of fats, vitamins, including vitamins A, D, and B_{12}, and minerals, including calcium, iodine, magnesium, zinc and iron.

The wonders of milk include complex sugars, long thought to have no biological significance; however these sugars constitute the perfect food for the bifido strain of bacteria, the ideal bacteria for baby's gut. The sugars are similar to those found on the surface of human cells and are constructed in the breast by the same enzymes. Many toxic bacteria and viruses will bind to these sugars to be carried out of the body. Meanwhile the beneficial bacteria, thriving on the complex sugars, form a protective biofilm throughout the entire small intestine.

During the first week or so after birth, babies receive colostrum in their mother's milk. Colostrum has a very high concentration of protein and antibodies from mom's immune system, which protect the infant from illness for the first few days. It also acts as a laxative to help move the meconium—baby's first stools, composed of materials injested while in the womb—out of baby's digestive system.

High levels of some vitamins and minerals in colostrum may further protect the infant and may be important in the continued development of the heart, brain and central nervous system.

Milk composition changes according to the stage of breastfeeding and the age of the baby. The "hind" milk, the last milk out of the breast, is higher in fat than the foremilk. Over the first few weeks, the fat content in the milk increases while protein content declines.

BENEFITS OF BREAST MILK: CONFLICTING STUDIES

As science reveals the wonderful composition of breast milk, one would expect equally wondrous results in breastfed children compared to formula-fed children. Lower rates of asthma and allergies, fewer infections, fewer cavities, better growth and higher IQ are some of the claims made for breastfeeding. But to the surprise and disappointment of breastfeeding advocates, the scientific studies do not point to a resounding success for mother's milk. Studies comparing the results of breast and bottle feeding are conflicting; any benefit they show for breastfeeding is a small one, and some show no benefit at all.

For example, a study published in July 2001, found that breastfed children in Japan had more asthma than bottle-fed infants.[1] A study from New Zealand found that breastfed children were significantly more likely to be allergic to cats, dust, mites and grass pollen.[2] A European study found that breastfeeding was not positively related to iron status in one-year-old children. Those with the best iron status were those who received iron-fortified formula.[3]

A Swedish study found that breastfed infants were just as likely to develop childhood cancer as formula-fed babies.[4] In fact, babies breastfed for one month or more had a higher risk of non-Hodgkins lymphoma, although this finding was based on a small number of cases.

A study from Norway found that breastfeeding did not provide protection against frequent ear infections.[5] A report in *Pediatric Clinics of North America* noted that many breastfed babies suffer from failure-to-thrive and dehydration.[6] The author warned: "Those who enthusiastically promoted breastfeeding for its many health benefits must confront the reality of breastfeeding failure and implement necessary changes in medical education and support services to foster successful outcomes in breastfed infants."

Only one study carried out during the past few years found a clear-cut benefit for breastfeeding. Researchers at the Harvard Medical School found that children who were breastfed were much less likely to be overweight as adults.[7]

Studies on the relationship between breastfeeding and cognitive skills are mixed. Some studies have shown that breastfed infants are more intelligent while others show no difference.[8] Critics contend that better cognitive scores in breastfed infants are due to the fact that mothers with higher levels of educational attainment are more likely to breastfeed.

Formula manufacturers are quick to use the lackluster performance of breastfed children as proof that formula is "just as good" as breast milk. Breastfeeding advocates retort that the studies were designed to give results that benefit the formula makers. Our interpretation is the following: the diet of modern American women is so appalling, and their preparation for successful breastfeeding so lacking, that their breast milk may provide no better nourishment for their infants than factory-made formula.

THE ROLE OF NUTRITION

"Breastfeeding mothers do not need to worry about their diets. As long as they are getting enough calories, their milk will be fine." This is the dogma of many groups promoting breastfeeding throughout the world. "The message that diet has an influence on milk quality will discourage mothers from breastfeeding," they contend.

When books on breastfeeding do include nutrition advice for lactating women, that advice is usually woefully lacking: "Include fruits, vegetables, grains, meat or meat alternative and lowfat milk products in your diet every day. Avoid caffeinated beverages and alcohol." Lactating women are advised to eat "vitamin-A rich foods" such as "carrots, spinach, sweet potatoes and cantaloupe." Above all, say the so-called experts, "don't worry too much about what you eat. Your diet does not have to be 'perfect' to nourish your baby well."[9] Some breastfeeding advocates even insist that "breast milk is never deficient in nutrients."

Those who claim that diet has no effect on the quality of mothers milk cite one study, which found no difference in certain immune components of breast

CAN BREASTFEEDING PREVENT DENTAL DEFORMITIES?

Does bottle feeding contribute to poor palate development? Many insist that it does, that the breast acts as a kind of orthodontic apparatus. The theory is that bottle-fed babies have significant mechanical and structural challenges due to the abnormal muscular action bottle feeding imposes on the tongue. According to this point of view, when babies are breastfed, the infant obtains milk by a natural peristaltic, or wave-like motion of the tongue in order to compress the soft breast nipple against the hard palate, which in infants is actually quite malleable. This natural tongue movement is said to mold the palate into a "U" shape and support the proper development of the jaw.[10] By contrast, according to this theory, the bottle-fed infant must employ a more forceful squeezing or "piston-like" tongue movement to obtain milk or formula from an artificial nipple, leading to a narrow and unnatural "V-shaped" hard palate. Bottle-feeding is also said to disrupt normal swallowing habits.

Proponents of this theory point to a 1981 study published in the *American Journal of Preventive Medicine*, "Does Breastfeeding Protect Against Malocclusion? An Analysis of the 1981 Child Health Supplement to the National Health Interview Survey."[11] This study did find an association of bottle feeding with malocclusion: children breastfed twelve months or more had a reported malocclusion incidence of about 16 percent, whereas those breastfed zero to three months had a reported malocclusion incidence of 33 percent. A serious flaw with the survey is the fact that the incidence of malocclusion was self reported by the parents, not determined by an orthodontic examination. The authors cite another study, carried out in Czechoslovakia, which found a slight association between bottle-feeding and dental occlusions: among those breastfed less than three months or not at all, 36.4 percent had anomalies; among those breastfed four to six months, 32.1 percent had anomalies; and among those breastfed longer than six months, 24.2 percent had anomalies.[12]

By contrast, an informal survey of WAPF members or children of WAPF members who were adopted and fully bottle fed found that six out of seven had naturally straight teeth. The holistic dentist Raymond Silkman of Los Angeles reports little correspondence between cranio-facial development and the length of time the child was breastfed. He has seen severe dental malocclusion in some fully breastfed children, noting that this usually occurs when the mother is a vegetarian or vegan.

The problem with the published surveys is that it is impossible to separate the physical effects of bottle feeding from the nutritional deficiencies of the formula. The real question: is it the bottle that causes dental deformities or what's in the bottle? Clearly bottle-feeding does not necessarily condemn a child to having a narrow palate—nor does breastfeeding guarantee normal development. The experience of mothers feeding nutrient-dense raw milk baby formula to their adopted infants indicates that the key factor to normal facial development is nutrition, not the physical action of sucking on a bottle.

When properly nourished, a child will grow to conform to the genetic blueprint of a U-shaped palate and wide jaw. This pattern can be interrupted by the application of constant pressure—think of foot-binding in Asia or the custom of flattening the baby's head with a board in South America. However, bottle feeding is not a constant activity and when the baby is well-nourished, it is unlikely to contribute to palate deformation; but when the baby is not properly nourished, the physical action of bottle feeding may be a contributing factor, especially if the baby also sucks his thumb or a pacifier for many hours of the day. However, regarding thumb sucking, at least three large studies found no significant difference in thumbsucking habits between bottle-fed and breastfed infants.[13]

The wide variation in dental malformations does not point to bottle feeding or thumb sucking as a major cause of palate malformation, in spite of what the dentists might believe. It is interesting to note that most baby mammals suck on a very narrow nipple, not a full breast, yet malocclusion is rare in the animal kingdom.

milk between mothers of "marginal nutritional status" and those of "poorer nutrition status." These factors are the immune-protecting compounds sIgA, lysozyme and lactoferrin.[14] Another study found that postpartum vitamin A supplementation did not increase milk concentrations of these immune factors in Bangladeshi women.[15]

One could question whether there is any great difference between "marginal nutritional status" and "poorer nutrition status," but even if maternal nutrition status has little effect on the concentrations of certain immune factors, there can be large variations in other nutrients depending on what the mother eats. As early as the 1940s, Weston Price observed a decline in the quality of human breast milk, as evidenced by the extensive dental problems he found in his breastfed patients.[16] Today dentists are reporting narrow palates, severe crowding and extensive decay in fully breastfed children, noting that these problems are most common in the fully breastfed children of vegetarian mothers.

FATS IN HUMAN MILK

A mother's diet has a significant influence on the fat content of her milk. Traditional dietary fat in mom's diet increases milk fat as well as the enzymes lipase, esterase and alkaline phosphatase—all necessary for baby's optimal assimilation and digestion.[17] *Trans* fats found in processed and commercial fried foods will lower the fat content of mother's milk, a discovery made in research on mice.[18] In humans, margarine containing *trans* fat reduces milk fat in lean women whereas butter consumption increases the levels of antimicrobial short- and medium-chain fatty acids as well as cholesterol in breast milk.[19] So important is cholesterol to the developing infant that mother's milk contains a special enzyme to ensure that baby absorbs one hundred percent of it.[20] Cholesterol is critical to the formation of the brain and nervous system, as well as the "second brain"— the digestive tract.

Mother's milk contains long-chain polyunsaturated fatty acids that babies need for the development of their nervous systems. These special fats accumulate in the brain and retina. If they are absent in the infant diet, the child is likely to suffer from learning disabilities and reduced visual acuity. The most important of these are arachidonic acid (AA or ARA) of the omega-6 family and docosahexaenoic acid (DHA) of the omega-3 family.

The presence of AA and DHA in the tissues of growing infants is largely determined by the levels in the milk the baby consumes.[21] The recognition that these fatty acids are vital for the optimal development of the infant has led to their inclusion in commercial formula.

What is less well known is the fact that the levels of AA and DHA in human breast milk greatly depend on the mother's diet. An important 1997 study compared the fatty acid composition of breast milk of mothers in two Chinese provinces with that of Canadian mothers.[22] Mothers in the traditional province of Chongqing had higher levels of milk fat than those from westernized Hong Kong, and higher levels of AA, due to a period of special feeding for the first four weeks after the birth, during which Chongqing mothers consume up to *ten* eggs per day and large amounts of chicken and pork. The diet of Hong Kong mothers was much lower in fat and calories, but because of high fish consumption, their levels of DHA were as high as those of Chongqing mothers. But breast milk levels of AA and DHA in both provinces were much higher than those of Canadian mothers eating a westernized diet.

The Chinese breast milk study proves that the levels of important fatty acids in mother's milk are strongly influenced by the mother's diet. Likewise, harmful fats will show up in breast milk if the mother is consuming industrial fats and oils. Eurcic acid, a long-chain monounsaturated fatty acid considered harmful, increased in the milk of Chongqing mothers during the later weeks of lactation, reflecting a dietary switch from animal fats to rapeseed oil. Adversely high levels of omega-6 linoleic acid were found in the milk of Hong Kong mothers, reflecting their use of high-omega-6 vegetable oils derived from corn and soy.

Ideal breast milk contains high levels of saturated fat as well. Adequate DHA, AA and saturated fat can be obtained by consuming high levels of animal fats plus eggs, cod liver oil and oily fish throughout the lactation period. Saturated fats in mother's milk stimulate the immune system and work synergistically with DHA and AA to maintain them in the tissues where they belong.[23] Levels of fat in a mother's milk will decrease with each baby unless she takes special care to consume high levels of nutrient-dense fats between pregnancies, during pregnancy and during each lactation.[24] Babies born to vegetarian women have lower levels of DHA and AA in their blood.[25]

Dietary carbohydrates can be converted to beneficial short- and medium-chain fatty acids. This conversion takes place in the breast. So, while women should not overdo carb consumption during breast-feeding, some carbohydrate intake is beneficial. Women whose diets are based largely on carbohydrates tend to have lower levels of calories in their milk, due to lower levels of fat.[26]

When the meat and dairy products in a mother's diet come largely from pasture-fed animals, her milk is likely to be rich in conjugated linoleic acid (CLA), believed to have a positive effect on the immune system in the prevention of excess weight gain.[27]

While protein levels in human milk remain constant from the third week onward, at about 11 percent, levels of fat—essential for the development of the nervous system—vary widely. Levels of lactose—also essential for nervous system development—also have a wide range.[28] Even the various anti-inflammatory and antibacterial compounds in a mother's milk vary markedly according to her diet.[29]

VITAMINS AND MINERALS

A recent study found that breast milk did not meet the minimum requirements for many nutrients.[30] Vitamin D was especially low. A study in Nigeria found that calcium and potassium levels in human milk varied by a factor of two, magnesium and copper by a factor of three, chloride levels by a factor of four, iron and selenium by almost five, iodine and sodium by almost seven, and zinc, which is vital to the nervous system, by over seven.[31] In other words, some mothers had seven times more zinc in their milk than others.

Another survey found large variations in the levels of B vitamins.[32] Vitamin B_6 concentrates in breast milk, and B_6 requirements are increased in lactating women.[33] More B_6 is required if the woman is exercising—an important reason to refrain from heavy exercise during the nursing period. The same study found that vitamin C ranged from 0 to 11.2 mg per 100 grams and vitamin A from 15 to 226 IU per 100 grams of breast milk.

Levels of choline in mother's milk are dependent on her dietary intake.[34] Choline is essential for the development of the brain and nervous system. The best sources are egg yolks and liver.

Vitamin D levels are so low in the milk of some women that their breastfed infants develop rickets. Adequate intake of vitamin D can increase breast milk concentrations to 400 IU per liter.

Dr. Catherine Gordon of Children's Hospital Boston recommends regular supplementation of vitamin D to nursing mothers after finding widespread deficiency in mothers and cases of rickets in their breastfed infants.[35]

Vitamin A is vital for the development of the infant. Vitamin A is found only in animal fats. Mothers can convert some of the precursors in fruits and vegetables into true vitamin A, and these will then show up in their milk, but adequate supply can only be met with consumption of animal foods rich in the true form of this nutrient.[36] A 1992 study carried out in Indonesia found that mothers who received vitamin A supplementation had higher levels in their blood and milk than those who received a placebo, and that the infants of the supplemented group were less likely to be vitamin A deficient.[37] Deficiency was measured by the presence of conjunctivitis in the eyes. Incidence of conjunctivitis fell in infants nursing from mothers taking a vitamin A supplement.

The authors noted that vitamin A status was lowest in women who were thin and who had had many babies—a warning not to lose weight too quickly after the birth of a baby and to put sufficient space between children so that vitamin A stores can be rebuilt.

Confirmation of the importance of adequate vitamin A and child spacing comes from a recent European study, which found that one-third of women with short birth intervals or multiple births had borderline deficiencies in retinol. "If the vitamin A supply of the mother is inadequate," they warned," her supply to the fetus will also be inadequate, as will later be her milk. These inadequacies cannot be compensated by postnatal supplementation."[38]

Adequate B_{12} is essential for the development of the infant. One study found a B_{12} deficiency in the breastfed infant of a strict vegetarian.[39]

Magnesium concentrations in breast milk vary over a wide range, from 15 to 64 mg per liter.[40] Levels of trace minerals, such as iodine and selenium, can be extremely variable. Iodine levels depend on maternal dietary intake. Iodine is critical during periods of brain development.[41] The best sources of selenium are animal foods like pastured beef and dairy; iodine is obtained from seafood and butterfat.

Thus, the science makes it abundantly clear that a mother's diet has a profound effect on the quality of her milk.

BAD THINGS IN BREAST MILK

Trans fats from partially hydrogenated vegetable oils are present in margarine, shortening, processed foods and fried foods. The accumulated evidence indicates that *trans* fats are bad news indeed. They interfere with many enzymatic processes, cause reduced learning ability, disrupt the endocrine system,

and contribute to allergies, asthma and many other diseases.[42] However, small amounts of one form of *trans* fats naturally occurring in butter and meat fats are beneficial, not harmful.[43]

If exposure to *trans* fats is bad for adults, it is even worse for babies and children during their growing years. Formula makers know better than to put *trans* fats into baby formula—yet human milk will contain *trans* fats if the mother consumes margarine, fried foods and commercial baked goods. The Chinese study described above found that Canadians had thirty-three times more *trans* fats in their milk than the traditional Chongqing mothers who did not consume processed foods! Hong Kong mothers had four times more *trans* fats in their milk than the Chongqing mothers, reflecting the inroads that processed foods have made in westernized Hong Kong.

Many other bad things can end up in mother's milk, including pesticides, flame retardants, fabric treatments like Scotchgard, Teflon from nonstick pans, mercury from amalgam fillings, and high levels of phytoestrogens, if the mother is eating soy foods or animal foods fed a lot of soy (such as chicken)—however, phytoestrogens in the milk of mothers who eat a lot of soy are still about three thousand times less than levels in soy-based formula.[44] Failure to thrive on mother's milk may be due to the presence of environmental toxins.

MYTHS AND TRUTHS ABOUT BREASTFEEDING

MYTH: Every woman can breastfeed successfully.
TRUTH: Even in traditional societies, a portion of the women did not have adequate milk supply. Babies of mothers with inadequate milk supply were nursed by other women in the village or given milk of cows, goats, sheep, water buffalo, camels, reindeer or llamas.

MYTH: Most diets provide adequate nutrition for nursing mothers. There is no need for nursing women to add special foods to their diets. All human milk is equally nutritious.
TRUTH: Human milk will be lacking in vitamins A, D, B_{12} and many other nutrients if the mother's diet is poor. Human milk will also lack long-chain fatty acids if these are not present in adequate amounts in the mother's diet. In addition, mothers on calorie-restricted diets will have lower levels of fat and lactose in their milk. Weston Price found that in traditional societies, women continued to consume special nutrient-dense foods during the lactation period.

MYTH: Breastfeeding can prevent dental problems such as cavities, crowded teeth and underdeveloped jaw.
TRUTH: The development of the face and jaw depends on the nutrients available to the child from preconception through childhood. Breastfed children can have dental deformities if their nutrition in the womb and the breast milk they receive provides inadequate nutrients.

One study discovered peanut proteins in mother's milk and warned that lactating women who eat peanuts may cause peanut allergies in their infants![45] Even mother's milk can cause allergies. Many mothers report fussiness in their babies after mom eats certain foods, especially foods containing MSG or gluten.

Thus a superlative maternal diet, one that contains plentiful amounts of nutrient-dense foods and is devoid of foods likely to contain industrial fats and oils, pesticides, MSG and empty carbohydrates, is essential if baby is to obtain maximum benefit from breastfeeding. Those who assure nursing mothers that all breast milk is equally nutritious have done a great disservice to a whole generation of children.

SUCCESSFUL BREASTFEEDING

First and foremost, continue with the nutrient-dense diet described in Chapter 1. Optimal nutrition is the fundamental requirement for optimal development in the breastfed baby.

A number of other practices can contribute to successful breastfeeding. Mom should insist on keeping baby with her immediately after the birth, with no separation for any exams or interventions. Even if parents opt for various interventions, these can wait until after the first breastfeeding. Immediate skin-to-skin contact facilitates a flood of oxytocin and other hormones that tell mom to produce milk. Baby should be allowed to root, latch on and nurse for as long as he wishes.

These practices have been confirmed by studies demonstrating that early skin-to-skin contact improves bonding between mother and infant, and that infants who have early maternal contact nurse more effectively at the first feeding. In one study of infants separated from their mothers during the early stage of the hospital stay, only 37 percent were still breastfeeding at three months compared with 72 percent of infants not separated from their mothers.[46] Even premature infants benefit from skin-to-skin contact with the mother. To prevent heat loss during this bonding period, cover baby's back and head with a blanket.

It's important to let baby root out the breast on her own rather than force her to nurse. So be patient as baby roots around and finally latches on without assistance—baby's first accomplishment! This may take up to an hour—all the better for maternal bonding to take effect.

There are many positions that mom can use to breastfeed her baby, none of which has been shown

---

SIGNS OF SUCCESSFUL BREASTFEEDING

- On-demand schedule of eight to twelve feedings per twenty-four hours.
- Infant mouth opens wide before latch-on.
- Latch-on includes entire nipple and most of the areola.
- Infant tongue placed under the nipple.
- Brief pauses in sucking with audible or visible swallowing.
- Infant breathing coordinated with suck and swallow cycle.
- Visible movement of jaw joint during active nursing.
- Wet diapers at least six to eight times per day.
- Baby seems content, with little crying.
- Adequate infant weight gain, with the following approximate milestones:
    Return to birth weight by two weeks;
    Weight gain of 4-7 ounces (112-200 grams) a week during the first month;
    An average of 1-2 pounds (1/2-1 kilogram) per month for the first six months;
    An average of one pound (1/2 kilogram) per month from six months to one year;
    Growth in length by about one inch a month (2.5 cm) during the first six months.

to be better than any other for breastfeeding success. You should try a variety of holds to find the one that is most comfortable. Lightly brushing the breast against the cheek of your infant should provoke the rooting reflex followed by latch-on. If you are feeling nervous about the procedure, be sure to get help from your doula or midwife; in a hospital setting you can call on the services of a lactation consultant.

One very good reason for a natural childbirth, without anesthetics or drugs, has to do with the negative effect these drugs have on breastfeeding success. As early as 1961, researchers demonstrated that anesthetics given to the mom resulted in disorganized behavior in the infant and a delay in effective breastfeeding and weight gain.[47] These effects are greatest when the drugs are administered more than one hour before delivery (and hence in mother's bloodstream longer).[48]

Such drugs are delivered in spades during a C-section. Nevertheless, if an infant is put to the breast within the first two hours following delivery, long-term breastfeeding success is unaffected.[49] If you end up needing a C-section, be sure to insist on the same postpartum bonding that you would be afforded in a normal delivery.

Some women have reported that administration of magnesium sulfate (for the prevention of seizures in preeclamptic patients) hinders breastfeeding, although no study data is available to evaluate these observations. Many more infants are exposed to Pitocin (synthetic oxytocin), used to induce labor; fortunately the drug has not been shown to interfere with breastfeeding.

Women who have a long labor have lower milk volumes five days after delivery;[50] likewise women who score higher in an exhaustion scale following labor have similar difficulties.[51] All the more reason to prepare yourself for labor with superlative nutrition and some of the techniques outlined in Chapter 4, so that labor is short and energy levels remain high.

During the first few days after birth, frequent breastfeeding leads to better long-term success.[52] This is best accomplished by having baby remain in mom's room for the entire postpartum stay, a practice referred to as rooming-in. Mom should nurse baby as often as baby indicates. In the case of a birth at home or a birth center, help at home during the first week or two allows mom to devote herself to nursing baby, eating well and getting enough rest. In some countries, home help is provided for one month after the birth. Exhaustion and stress can definitely have a negative effect on milk supply.

With rooming-in, mom can put a stop to any attempts by hospital staff to give a pacifier or bottle to her baby. Pacifier use has been associated with a fourfold drop in breastfeeding rates at six months compared to nonusers.[53] It is thought that both bottles and pacifiers cause "nipple confusion" and con-

NATURAL CANNABINOIDS IN BREAST MILK

In recent years, scientists have made the amazing discovery that the body produces cannabinoids, the same compound that is found in marijuana; and cannabinoids have been detected in human breast milk as well as bovine milk.[54]

Cell membranes in the body are naturally equipped with receptors which, when activated by cannabinoids, protect cells against viruses, harmful bacteria and cancer. The cannabinoids also stimulate hunger and promote growth and development. Other attributes of these natural feel-good chemicals include boosting immune function, protecting the brain and nervous system, relieving pain and protecting against inflammation.

There are none of these helpful compounds in infant formula. Breastfeeding supplies your baby with these appetite-stimulating yet soothing biochemicals, which the body assimilates and then clears without side effects; and if you can't breastfeed, a formula based on raw milk will supply them as well.

tribute to breast refusal and less efficient sucking, especially when given in the very early days.

Signs of successful breastfeeding include a good latch-on, visible sucking and swallowing by the infant, frequent wet diapers and, most importantly, adequate weight gain. A small amount of weight loss after birth is normal. Infants should begin to regain weight by the fourth or fifth day of life and should exceed their birth weight by days ten to fourteen. If you have any doubts or concerns about weight gain, purchase or rent an infant scale and weigh your baby each day. Be sure to weigh your baby at the same time every day, without diaper or clothes, and

under the same circumstances, for example after a wet diaper and just before nursing.

DIAPER WATCH

Baby's bowel movements can give a good indication of whether she is getting enough to eat and digestion is proceeding normally. For the first few days after delivery, the baby passes meconium, a dark green, almost black substance composed of materials ingested while in the womb.

Meconium is passed during the first few days, and by the third day, the bowel movements start be-

SOME NATURAL REMEDIES FOR BREASTFEEDING PROBLEMS

Most important for breast health is a diet rich in saturated fats. Saturated fats will keep the nipples and breast tissue strong, resilient and resistant to infection. Arachidonic acid (AA) in animal fats helps create tight cell-to-cell junctures, so important for healthy skin.

ENGORGEMENT: Nursing after a hot shower can help with engorgement that causes poor milk flow. Massage breasts with thumbs toward the nipple as baby nurses to work out any lumps. If engorgement results in too much milk, a very strong sage tea can reduce the flow of milk. It is taken sip by sip, up to three cups a day. (See sidebar on Oversupply, page 137.)

MASTITIS

* Tincture of propolis, 10 to 15 drops twice a day.

* Tincture of echinacea, two dropperfuls, as often as twelve times a day. Continue taking echinacea for at least a week after all symptoms have cleared.

* Tincture of poke root (*Phytolacca americana*), no more than two drops of the tincture daily. May be combined with echinacea for acute and severe infections.

POULTICES, COMPRESSES AND SOAKS FOR SORE BREASTS: A poultice consists of fresh or cooked herbs placed directly on the breasts. A compress is prepared by soaking a cloth and applying it to the breasts. A soak is the application of hot water to the breasts.

Hot water alone has beneficial effects for women dealing with sore breasts, no matter what the cause. Hot water stimulates circulation and eases the tension in taut, swollen breast tissues. Herbs infused in the water used to compress or soak increase the effectiveness. Soak the breasts in a sinkful of warm water. Fill the sink, lean over, and immerse one or both breasts. You can massage the milk out while soaking to further relieve engorgement and ease pain.

When applying external remedies, frequent, consistent, short applications work better than sporadic, lengthy treatments. That is, six or seven treatments of five minutes each spread over the day will be more effective than one treatment lasting for thirty minutes. If infection is present, discard any plant material and wash the poultice cloths after each use so as to prevent the spread of the infection.

For a compress, place a handful of fresh or dried parsley or comfrey leaves in a clean cotton diaper and tie it closed with a rubber band. Put in a pan of water and simmer for ten to fifteen minutes. Apply the

coming lighter. Usually by the fifth day, the bowel movements take on the appearance of the normal breast milk stool.

The normal breast milk stool is pasty to watery, mustard colored, and usually has little odour. Curds from digested milk should be visible, in fact, the stool should look like yellow cottage cheese. There may be variations in color and consistency, but a baby who is breastfeeding only, and is starting to have bowel movements which are becoming lighter by the third day of life, is doing well.

Without becoming obsessive about it, monitoring the frequency and quantity of bowel motions is one of the best ways of knowing whether your baby is getting enough milk. After the first three or four days, the baby should have increasing bowel movements so that by the end of the first week he should be passing at least two to three substantial yellow stools each day. Many infants have a stained diaper with almost every feeding.

Some breastfed babies, after the first three or four weeks of life, may suddenly change their stool pattern from many each day, to one every three days or even less frequently. Some babies have gone as long as fifteen days or more without a bowel movement.

SOME NATURAL REMEDIES FOR BREASTFEEDING PROBLEMS

hot (fresh) parsley as a poultice or use the (dried) herbs still tied in the diaper as a compress to ease swollen and painful breasts.

A cold poultice of grated raw potato can draw out the heat of inflammation, localize infection and un-block clogged tubes. Grated raw potato is applied directly to the breasts and covered with a clean cloth. When dry, it is removed and replaced with fresh grated potato.

Marshmallow roots can soothe tender tissues and sore nipples, open clogged ducts and tubes, power-fully draw out infection, and diminish the pain of engorged, inflamed breasts. Steep two ounces of dried marshmallow root overnight in half a gallon of water just off the boil. The texture of the finished brew should be slippery and slimy. Heat as needed, pouring the hot liquid into a sink or basin and soak your sore and aching breasts.

Infused herbal oils—such as those made from the flowers of calendula, elder or dandelion, or from the roots of yellow dock—can ease the pain of tender breasts and sore nipples. Buy them ready-made, or make them yourself: Gently warm a handful of dried or fresh blossoms in just enough olive oil to cover; keep warm for twenty minutes. Strain, cool and rub into nipples and breasts whenever there is pain or sensitivity.

SORE NIPPLES

- Crushed ice wrapped in a wet cloth, or a frozen gauze pad, applied to the nipples is a good local pain killer.

- Comfrey ointment softens and strengthens nipples at the same time. It is exceptionally soothing to sensitive nipples and rapidly heals any fissures or bruises.

- Yarrow leaf poultices—or yarrow infused oil—provide almost instantaneous pain relief and heal cracked nipples rapidly.

- Any of the poultices described for painful breasts may be used advantageously. Comfrey and marsh-mallow are especially effective. Many brief poultices work better than one or two lengthy sessions.

- The gel from a fresh aloe vera leaf will soothe and heal sore and cracked nipples.

- Calendula ointment is an old favorite to heal and strengthen the nipples.

SOURCE: www.susunweed.com

As long as the baby is otherwise well, and the stool is the usual pasty or soft, yellow movement, this is not constipation and is of no concern. No treatment is necessary or desirable. However any baby between five and twenty-one days of age who does not pass at least one substantial bowel movement within a twenty-four-hour period should be seen by a pediatrician. Generally, small, infrequent bowel movements during this time period mean insufficient intake.

BREASTFEEDING CHALLENGES

Even if you have a plentiful milk supply, there are numerous challenges that breastfeeding moms may face. We describe a few of the major ones below.

WEAK SUCK

Premature or very small babies may have a weak sucking reflex, due to overall weakness or respiratory problems. The breast may continually come out of the baby's mouth, particularly when the mother shifts even slightly. Also, milk may leak out of the baby's mouth while he is nursing. Assisting the baby to have a stronger suck and increasing the flow of milk are the keys to overcoming a weak suck.

Aside from ensuring that the baby's latch-on and positioning are correct, cheek and jaw support are essential. You will need to hold baby's face right up to the breast and help close the mouth onto the nipple. If baby really is too weak to suckle, you can give expressed breast milk with a syringe or eye dropper until he gains enough strength to breastfeed.

One cause of weak suck is the condition of tongue tie. When a baby has a restrictive or tight frenulum (tongue tie), it can impair the ability of the tongue to move properly to effectively breastfeed. The frenulum is a piece of tissue that attaches the tongue to the floor of the mouth.

A tight frenulum can be remedied with a procedure called a frenotomy, in which the frenulum is

WHEN BREASTFEEDING MAY NOT BE BEST

GALACTOSEMIA: This is a rare genetic disorder in which the infant cannot digest galactose. The child will die if it is breastfed. A cautionary note: If your baby has been diagnosed with galactosemia, be sure to have the test done again. False positives from this test are common. Our liver-based formula, made with sugar instead of lactose, can be used for cases of galactosemia.

VEGANISM: The milk of vegan mothers will be lacking in vitamin D, vitamin B_{12} and important long-chain fatty acids. If a vegan mother insists on breastfeeding, her baby's diet should be supplemented with cod liver oil, egg yolks and liver, all animal foods.

JUNK FOOD DIET: Junk foods full of *trans* fatty acids will reduce the fat content of mothers' milk and cause *trans* fatty acids to be present in mothers' milk. Homemade whole food baby formula will be more nutritious than the milk of mothers on a junk food diet.

INSUFFICIENT MILK SUPPLY: This is uncommon, but not as rare as is indicated in the medical literature. A supplemental homemade formula should be given using the Lact-Aid breastfeeding aid (www.lact-aid.com).

ADOPTED BABIES: It has been reported that breast milk has been stimulated in nonbiologic mothers, but this phenomenon is rare. Strong hormonal drugs that stimulate breast milk can be given, hormones that can come through the milk—not a good idea! Adopted babies should be given homemade baby formula.

IN VITRO PREGNANCY: Many hormones are given to mothers who get pregnant by these high-tech methods, and these hormones can pass into breast milk. As with adopted babies, babies born from in vitro fertilization should be given the homemade formula.

clipped. It can be performed in the pediatrician's office and often results in immediate resolution of the latch-on problem.[55] Dentists report that the tongue tie is best dealt with in the newborn period.[56]

POOR LATCH-ON

This is a common breastfeeding challenge. A baby who does not take the breast correctly will not get as much milk and mom will probably end up with sore nipples. If baby has poor latch-on, you will need to help her. Sit in a relaxed, comfortable position and position baby's head and body to face your breast with her mouth at the level of your nipple. Pull her in close so she does not have to turn her head or strain her neck to reach your nipple.

Cup your breast in your hand, with your fingers and palm underneath and thumb on top, well behind the areola. Avoid holding the nipple itself between your two fingers as this will interfere with latch on. Express a few drops of milk. Using your milk-moistened nipple, gently massage your baby's lips, encouraging her to open her mouth wide. As she opens wide, direct your nipple slightly upward and toward the center of her mouth while pulling her close to you, so that her mouth will close down over your areola. The important thing is to get baby's mouth on the nipple when the mouth is wide open and then keep baby pressed close to you so that the nipple is still in the mouth when she closes it.

Make sure your baby feeds from the areola, not just the nipple. To prevent painful breastfeeding, her gums should take in a one-inch radius around the nipple as she latches on.

CLOGGED MILK DUCTS

If you develop a tender lump somewhere in your breast, it may mean that a duct leading from the milk-producing glands to the nipple is blocked with milk. This is a condition that needs immediate treatment as a clogged milk duct can easily become in-

---

WHEN BREASTFEEDING IS FINE, IN SPITE OF CONTRARY MEDICAL ADVICE

PHENYLKETONURIA: This is a rare genetic disorder in which the infant must avoid phenylalanine, an amino acid. With careful medical supervision, these children have been successfully breastfed in combination with a phenylalanine-free protein substitute.

HIV POSITIVE: Mothers who test HIV positive are told not to breastfeed. But a South African study found that the HIV virus is much less likely to be passed to breastfeeding infants when the mother's diet contains sufficient vitamin A.[57] So cod liver oil is a must if you have HIV and are nursing an infant. Other studies indicate that breast milk antibodies help neutralize HIV.[58]

DIABETES: Although diabetic mothers are often warned not to breastfeed, breastfeeding actually diminishes complications in the infants of diabetic mothers. Once again, adequate maternal nutrition is vital.

JAUNDICE: Breastfeeding actually helps clear juandice in the infant. As long as bilirubin levels are less than 20 milligrams, no special supplements are needed. You should not be put off by any suggestions to stop breastfeeding for a day or two or that your milk is somehow bad for your baby. As long as your baby is otherwise healthy, jaundice is short-lived and harmless. If your baby's jaundice is related to other health problems, your milk is very valuable for him and you should continue to breastfeed.

BREAST INFECTION: Going for long stretches between nursing or failing to empty the breast completely may contribute to mastitis. In most situations, breastfeeding can continue even though there is a breast infection—in fact breastfeeding may help to clear up the infection faster. For dietary suggestions and other holistic remedies, see pages 130-131.

LYME DISEASE: Women with Lyme disease are told they can pass the illness on to their babies if they breastfeed. But several studies show that the Lyme organism is not passed through human breast milk.[59]

fected. To treat a clogged duct, apply a warm moist washcloth to the area for a few minutes before feeding.

Breastfeed on the sore side first as baby is more likely to dislodge the plug at the beginning of a feeding when her sucking is strongest. As baby nurses, gently massage the area down toward the areola to encourage the plug to clear.

Plugged ducts often occur when your infant is nursing less frequently, for example, when you start back to work, or when baby sleeps longer at night. Even if you are nursing less frequently, be sure to completely empty the breasts by expressing milk or using a breast pump. Avoid tight bras and sleeping on your stomach, as both can put unnecessary pressure on your breasts.

CRACKED AND SORE NIPPLES

In the case of sore nipples, an ounce of prevention is worth a pound of cure. A suggested preventive measure for cracked and sore breasts from the old days is the daily application of rubbing alcohol (methylated spirits) or diluted lemon juice to the nipples, starting about a month before the birth. If you can, expose the nipples and breasts to sunlight each day, gradually increasing from thirty seconds to three minutes. Olive oil, sweet almond oil, lanolin or comfrey ointment rubbed into the nipples throughout the later part of pregnancy can also help. Most importantly, do not wash the nipples with soap, which can cause drying, chapping and tearing.

Breastfeeding may be uncomfortable during the first few days, but it should not lead to cracked and sore

---

PROBIOTICS FOR BABY

Probiotics are beneficial bacteria that proliferate in the digestive tract. In a healthy human being, the entire digestive tract is lined with a biofilm composed of billions of beneficial microorganisms. These play many important roles, protecting the digestive tract, preventing the absorption of pathogens and toxins, protecting against infection, and aiding in digestion and the production of nutrients. In fact, digestion is impossible without beneficial bacteria.

Before birth, baby's digestive tract is thought to be sterile. During a normal birth, to a mother with healthy intestinal flora, baby's gut is colonized by the beneficial bacteria he picks up in the birth canal. Mother's milk also provides beneficial flora, plus factors that encourage the growth of this flora, including special sugars, called oligo-saccharides, that the bacteria feed on.

Colic, fussiness, poor digestion and frequent bouts of infectious disease in infants may be signs of inadequate intestinal flora. Infants born by C-section or to mothers who have used antibiotics, suffer from Candida overgrowth or who otherwise have less-than-healthy intestinal flora may need a probiotic supplement. In the premature infant, use of probiotics greatly reduces the incidence of serious infection[60] and encourages weight gain.[61]

In a recent study, one week of supplementation with a probiotic microorganism called *Lactobacillus reuteri Protectis* reduced crying time in colicky babies by 74 percent, compared with 38 percent with placebo. These results are in line with other studies.[62] Thus, for the colicky baby, a good probiotic supplement should be the first line of treatment. They are also recommended for babies suffering from diarrhea and other digestive disorders, as well as frequent infections. In response to a growing body of evidence demonstrating the effectiveness and safety of probiotics for infants, some formula makers are adding them to commercial infant formula. Our own homemade formula contains probiotics specifically beneficial to infants.

When choosing a probiotic for your baby, be sure that the supplement is designed for infants, who have a different balance of organisms in their guts than adults (see Sources).

nipples. A common cause of persistent nipple pain is poor latch-on by baby. Make sure that baby takes your breast with her mouth wide open and closes it on the entire aerola, not just the nipple. Be sure your baby's tongue is between his lower gum and your breast—if you pull down gently on baby's lower lip, you should be able to see her tongue. A lactation consultant can often help with latch-on problems that lead to nipple pain. Avoid using creams containing steroids, antibiotics and painkillers, as these can have a negative effect on both mother and baby. For natural remedies, see sidebar on page 131.

BREAST INFECTIONS

Breast infections—called mastitis—commonly occur between two and six weeks after birth, but they may appear at any time after delivery, or even before delivery. Typical symptoms of mastitis are painful engorgement, hot and tender breasts, redness, fever, an overall flu-like feeling, headache and reduced milk supply. The best treatment for breast infections is prevention through diet—with liberal amounts of saturated fat, strictly limiting sugar and including lacto-fermented foods on a daily basis.

Although mastitis can be painful, mom can continue nursing in spite of the infection. There is no danger of the infection being passed on to the infant through nursing. In fact, continued nursing will benefit the mother, as infections tend to clear up more rapidly when breastfeeding is continued. However, occasionally the infant may not want to nurse at the affected breast because the milk tastes sour. In such cases, mom can still nurse from her unaffected breast and express or pump the milk from the breast with mastitis.

The conventional treatment for mastitis is antibiotics, but there are also dietary and herbal remedies (see pages 130-131). Get plenty of rest, increase your dose of cod liver oil and drink bone broths frequently. A tablespoonful of coconut oil added to a mug of broth is an excellent remedy. You may also benefit from taking a natural form of vitamin C.

In addition, make sure your bra gives full support. You will be most comfortable if your infected breast is properly supported in a nursing bra. When you nurse, offer your infected breast first so that it is emptied fully, reducing pressure from fullness. Do not suddenly wean because of a breast infection as this may contribute to the formation of an abscess, complicating the mastitis and possibly even requiring surgery.

BREASTFEEDING JAUNDICE

Jaundice, also known as hyperbilirubinemia, causes a yellow tinge in the skin and eyeballs of newborn infants, especially during the first week or two. Jaundice happens because babies are born with more red blood cells than they need. When the liver breaks down these excess cells it produces a yellow pigment called bilirubin. Because the newborn's immature liver can't dispose of bilirubin quickly, the excess yellow pigment is deposited in the eyeballs and skin of the newborn. Jaundice tends to be more common in breastfed babies and to last a bit longer, but this is no reason to discontinue breastfeeding. Jaundice is also more common in premature infants, who are less able to cope with excess bilirubin.

Most cases of jaundice are not harmful and will clear on their own. Once the newborn's bilirubin-disposal system matures and the excess red blood cells diminish, the jaundice subsides, with no harm to the baby.

In some situations, such as an incompatibility of blood types between mother and baby, jaundice may be the result of problems that go beyond the normal breakdown of excess red blood cells. In rare instances, the bilirubin levels can rise high enough to damage baby's brain. For this reason, if the physician suspects that something more than normal physiologic jaundice is the cause of baby's yellow color, bilirubin levels will be monitored more closely using blood samples. If the bilirubin level gets too high, your doctor may try to lower the bilirubin level using phototherapy, special lights that dissolve the extra bilirubin in the skin, allowing it to be excreted in the urine.

In most cases, however, it is not necessary to treat jaundice when bilirubin levels are less than 20 milligrams, and you can continue to breastfeed. In fact, it helps to breastfeed as frequently as possible. The more often you breastfeed, the more quickly bilirubin will exit your baby's body via his stools. Resist any attempts to give your baby bottles of sugar water. The practice has been shown to be ineffective and may even aggravate the jaundice, because babies whose tummies are full of glucose solutions may nurse less often, reducing their milk intake and the opportunities for bilirubin excretion in stools.

If high bilirubin levels make phototherapy treatment necessary, talk to your healthcare provider about alternatives to placing baby in the hospital nursery under phototherapy lights. For most babies a photo-optic bilirubin-blanket (phototherapy lights that wrap around the baby) works well (see Sources). You can hold and breastfeed your baby at home while the lights dissolve the bilirubin.

Brief daily exposure to the sun, with baby in diaper only, is also very effective.

FUSSINESS, GAS AND SPITTING UP

Babies are sometimes fussy after eating. They may spit up, have gas or discomfort, or may squirm as they have a bowel movement.

The most important way to prevent discomfort is to burp your baby! Yes, even the most experienced baby nurse or lactation consultant may forget to tell new mothers about this old fashioned but most important practice. Place a towel or diaper on your shoulder and place baby upright against your body with her head facing over your shoulder. Gently rub baby's back until she burps. She may also spit up a small amount. None of this is anything to worry about and the burping will quickly ease most discomfort.

Another important tip: be sure that baby empties your breast when he nurses. The hindmilk is much richer in fat than the foremilk, and that fat will keep baby contented for longer. If mom has lots of milk, she should only nurse one breast per nursing. If mom is struggling with supply, she can nurse both breasts, but she should be sure that each breast is completely emptied.

Babies may be fussy because of something mom has eaten. Some mothers find that baby will be fussy after they have eaten garlic or crucifers like cabbage, or gluten-containing foods like wheat. If you eat processed food, the MSG it contains may well make baby cranky—just another reason to avoid processed foods! Pasteurized dairy in mom's diet can also cause lots of gas and spitting up.

Babies are often fussy at certain times of the day—often in the late afternoon or evening when mom may be tired also. Having someone else to hold and walk around with baby may offer welcome relief during this "witching hour." Baby may want to nurse more frequently at this time, or, she may just want to observe the goings-on in a busy household. A baby seat on the kitchen counter where baby can watch you prepare a meal may be just the ticket. (Be sure baby is strapped in and *never* turn your back on baby. If you must leave the room momentarily, place the baby seat on the floor.) On the other hand, some babies may become overloaded with unfamiliar sights and sounds. Too much activity and noise during baby's day may make him fussy by evening.

COLIC

If baby cries loudly after feeding, it's a sign that he is either still hungry or in pain.

If you know that baby is getting enough milk, but cries vigorously for long periods of time, despite your best efforts to console, baby may be crying due to the pain of colic. Often the crying occurs around the same time each day or night, usually after feedings. Baby may show signs of gas, discomfort and abdominal bloating or have a hard, distended stomach. She may cry with knees pulled to the chest, clenched fists, flailing arms and legs, and an arched back.

Experts disagree on the causes of colic. The best explanation is that the newborn digestive system is not mature enough to function properly. Muscles that support digestion have not developed the proper rhythm for moving food efficiently through the digestive tract. A lack of benevolent bacterial flora may exacerbate the problem.

To make matters worse, infants often swallow air while feeding or during strenuous crying, which increases gas and bloating, further adding to their discomfort.

Gentle rubbing of baby's stomach may ease her pain. Rub gently from the lower right hand side of the abdomen up to the bottom of the rib cage, the across to the left and down, in the direction of the colon; or, put baby on your shoulder and rub her back.

Mom may find that avoiding certain foods like onions or garlic helps relieve the cry of colic in her baby. Pasteurized dairy in mom's diet can lead to colic. Sometimes increasing probiotic foods in mom's diet can help, even taking a probiotic supplement. (One suggestion is to put the probiotic powder, mixed with a little water, on your nipple while you are breastfeeding.) And while some mothers will need to avoid gluten-containing grains, soaked and cooked grains such as oats in mom's diet have relieved fussiness in their nursing babies in more than a few instances. Mom should be on a full diet while breastfeeding, not a diet that eliminates important carbohydrate foods, such as the GAPS diet.

A homeopathic remedy called Colic Calm Gripe Water, available online and in select health food stores and health practitioners' offices may help with baby's colic (see Sources). Be sure to avoid products containing sodium bicarbonate as this will raise the natural pH of baby's stomach acid and make digestion more difficult. In addition, products containing essential oils should not be taken internally.

Gentle chiropractic treatment can help with colic in some cases.

Whatever the cause, colic usually resolves by twelve to sixteen weeks.

MILK SUPPLY

Persistent crying after nursing, or at any time, should raise the suspicion of inadequate or under-

OVERSUPPLY

Although concern about not having enough milk is the number one reason that mothers wean their babies early, having too much milk can also be a problem. When you consider the fact that many women can't produce enough milk for their babies no matter what they do, then having too much milk is a relatively good breastfeeding problem to have, and is usually fairly easy to resolve.

Babies whose moms have too much milk will often exhibit symptoms such as fussing, pulling off the breast, colicky crying, gassiness, spitting up and hiccupping. They may want to nurse frequently, and they may gain weight more rapidly than the average baby, or they may gain weight more slowly than the average baby. Their stools may be green and watery, and their bottoms may be red and sore. The mother's letdown reflex may be so forceful that the baby chokes, gags and sputters as he struggles with the jet of milk that sprays too quickly into his mouth.

Mothers who produce too much milk may suffer from full, engorged breasts, plugged ducts and mastitis. Sometimes they feel a few seconds of intense pain as the letdown reflex occurs, because it is so forceful.

When mom has an oversupply of milk, baby may end up getting too much foremilk, which is rich in lactose, and not enough hindmilk, which is rich in fat. The overabundance of lactose may be hard for baby to digest, leading to gas and fussiness; and the lack of fat may lead to low blood sugar, crankiness and the need to nurse frequently. The solution is to give one breast only during a feeding so that it is emptied completely. You may want to express a small amount of milk before nursing so that your letdown reflex is not so strong.

A suggested herbal remedy is sage tea, which contains a natural form of estrogen that can decrease your milk supply. Discontinue use when your supply begins to level out.

Moms who produce a lot of milk may want to donate to a milk bank or even give or sell their milk to mothers who do not produce enough. For information on donating milk, contact the Human Milk Banking Association of North America at www.hmbana.org. Moms with bountiful supply should also keep some on hand frozen for emergencies.

nutritious milk supply. You would cry also if you were not being fed enough or not receiving adequate fat and other nutrients and had no other way to express yourself.

According to most breastfeeding proponents, insufficient milk supply is rare. The problem, they say, is not a deficiency in the mammary gland, but a "shared belief" among women or health workers "that insufficient milk is a common phenomenon." Baby's frequent crying, they say, should not be interpreted as a sign of insufficient or poor quality milk—even though this is what a mother's instincts tell her. According to a La Leche League handbook, "The word 'insufficient' is like the word 'inadequate'—once it has been directed at a mother it can never be retracted, and her confidence in her body's ability to nurture and nourish at the breast often plummets."

Yet ancient medical literature abounds in treatments for lactation failure.[63] Concern about milk supply is not a modern phenomenon, inculcated by evil formula manufacturers in order to sell more formula—although the formula makers are indeed quick to exploit this concern. Most traditional cultures use special foods or "galactogogues" in the belief that they increase milk flow, ranging from powdered earthworms in India, to fish soup in China and Japan, to a variety of special teas. Soup made from roosters is a galactogogue used in several areas of the world. Weston Price recorded the practice of special feeding for pregnant and lactating women. The foods given were animal foods rich in fat-soluble vitamins and, in a few cases, soaked cereal gruels.

Mothers from all societies and in all ages have naturally been concerned about having enough milk for their infants. An 1885 votive painting from Japan depicts a mother praying for an abundant milk supply for her newborn infant.[64] The adjoining painting shows her prayer answered, as milk flows from her breast to a bowl. If adequate milk were automatic for all women, they would have no need to offer prayers. In fact, there is a large variation in the amount of milk that women produce—some women can squirt their milk across the room while others manage to extract only a couple of ounces total after using a breast pump throughout the day.

Until recently, breastfeeding literature dismissed the notion of galactogogues as mere superstition, but these attitudes are changing. Many websites now recommend herbs like fenugreek and milk thistle to increase milk supply, and galactagogue herbal formulations are widely available.

The production of milk is a complicated process governed by a complex interaction of hormones, involving the hypothalamus, pituitary gland and thyroid gland. It would be amazing if this were the one system in the body that functioned well at all times; the claim that most, or almost all women can successfully breastfeed their babies is especially inappropriate in this era of industrial food and ubiquitous endocrine disruptors.

Thyroid hormone and iodine are essential to initiate breastfeeding, and the need for thyroid hormone and iodine is increased during pregnancy. If you have a history of poor thyroid function, breast milk production may indeed be inadequate. Foods that support thyroid healing include cod liver oil (for vitamin A, needed for the production of thyroid hormones), butter (a source of iodine) and seafood, including seaweed (also sources of iodine). You may need treatment with thyroid hormone to get breast milk flowing.

The two hormones that govern the last stages of milk production are prolactin and oxytocin. Milk production occurs in the epithelial cells of the mammary gland in response to prolactin activation of prolactin-receptors. Prolactin production is inhibited by a number of compounds including bromated pharmaceuticals and dopamine antagonists.[65] Women under stress and fatigue produce more dopamine, norepinephrine or both, which inhibit prolactin production. This is why the environment for the nursing mother should be as relaxed and as stress-free as possible; but for many women, burdened by domestic strife or financial worries, a stress-free environment may be impossible to achieve.

The other important hormone involved in milk ejection or the let-down reflex is oxytocin. When the newborn begins suckling, oxytocin is released from the posterior pituitary gland—or should be—after synthesis in the hypothalamus; its physical effects in women include uterine contractions to facilitate labor. During the first few weeks of breastfeeding,

THE SCANDAL OF COMMERCIAL FORMULA

In addition to the slew of industrially produced macro-nutrients in commercial formula, manufacturers have begun adding compounds claimed to render formula more like breast milk. Two of these are the long-chain fatty acids DHA (an omega-3 fatty acid) and arachidonic (AA or ARA, an omega-6 fatty acid). High levels of these fats in mother's milk are associated with optimal brain development; unfortunately, the DHA and ARA added to commercial formula are extracted from algae and soil fungus using chemicals such as hexane, acid and bleach. Formula makers insist that no traces of these chemicals have been found in the infant formula to which they are added. However, the real concern is rancidity. DHA and ARA are extremely fragile and likely to be highly damaged during the manufacturing process. This may explain high rates of diarrhea observed by nurses in babies put on these formulas. And there is no evidence whatsoever that these additives will make babies smarter, as the formula makers imply.

According to FDA edict, all formulas today contain added iron, which is contraindicated in the first six months because it competes with zinc, needed for neurological function and the formation of many important enzymes. Another potential source of toxins in formula is the packaging. Lining of the cans may contain bisphenol-A (BPA), shown to alter hormone levels. BPA can leach into both liquid and powdered formulas, although much lower levels are found in powdered formulas. A final concern is contamination with pathogens. There have been many recalls of commercial formula, due to contamination with harmful microorganisms and other substances—including broken glass! Listed below are the ingredients in two popular brands of formula:

"MOM-TO-MOM MILK-BASED INFANT FORMULA WITH IRON. "This formula provides complete nutrition for my baby's first year." Essential Nutrition Based on Milk with DHA & ARA, nutrients found naturally in breast milk; Prebiotic dietary fiber to support babies' immune system; Meets FDA Requirements: Nonfat milk, lactose, vegetable oil (palm olein, soy, coconut and high oleic safflower or sunflower oil), whey protein concentrate, maltodextrin, galacto-oligosaccharides. And less than 1%: mortierella oil (a source of arachidonic acid ARA), crypthecodinium oil (a source of docasahexaneoic acid DHA), vitamin A palmitate, beta-carotene, vitamin D_3, vitamin E acetate, mixed tocopherol concentrate, vitamin K_1, ascorbyl palmitate, thiamine hydrochloride, riboflavin, vitamin B6 hydrochloride, vitamin B_{12}, niacinamide, folic acid, calcium pantothenate, biotin, ascorbic acid, choline chloride, inositol, calcium carbonate, calcium chloride, calcium hydroxide, magnesium chloride, ferrous sulfate, zinc sulfate, magnesium sulfate, cupric sulfate, potassium bicarbonate, potassium iodide, potassium hydroxide, potassium phosphate, sodium selenite, sodium citrate, taurine, l-carnitine, monoglyerides, soy lecithin, nucleotides (adenosine-5'-monophosphate, cytidine-5'-monophosphate, disodium guanosine-5'-monophosphate, disodium inosine-5'-monophosphate, disodium urisine-5'-monophosphate). $4.99 for 8 ounces, 227 grams, about two days' worth."

"SIMILAC ADVANCE INFANT FORMULA, Complete Nutrition for your Baby's 1st Year. Closer Than Ever to Breast Milk. Nonfat milk, lactose, high oleic safflower oil, coconut oil, galacto-oligosaccharides, whey protein concentrate. Less than 2%: C cohni oil (a source of docasahexaneoic acid DHA), alpine oil (a source of arachidonic acid ARA), beta-carotine, lutein, lycopene, potassium citrate, calcium carbonate, ascorbic acid, soy lecithin, potassium chloride, magnesium chloride, ferrous sulphate, choline bitartrate, choline chloride, ascorbyl palmitate, sodium chloride, taurine, m-inositol, zinc sulphate, mixed tocopherols, d-alpha-tocopheryl acetate, niacinamide, calcium panothenate, l-carnitine, vitamin A palmitate, cupric sulfate, thiamine chloride hydrochloride, riboflavin pyridoxine hydrochloride, folic acid, manganese sulphate, phylloquinone, biotin, sodium selenite, vitamin D3, cyanocobalamin, calcium phosphate, potassium phosphate, potassium hydroxide and nucleotides (adenosine-5'-monophosphate, cytidine-5'-monophosphate, disodium guanosine-5'-monophosphate, disodium inosine-5'-monophosphate, disodium urisine-5'-monophosphate). $13.29 for 12.4 ounces, 352 grams, about three days' worth."

THE TRAGEDY OF SOY INFANT FORMULA

Just say NO to infant formula based on soy. Soy is a toxic plant, with many entries in the FDA toxic plant database.[66]

- High levels of phytic acid in soy reduce assimilation of calcium, magnesium, copper, iron and zinc. Phytic acid in soy is not neutralized by ordinary preparation methods such as soaking, sprouting and long, slow cooking, but only with long fermentation. High-phytate diets have caused growth problems in children.

- Trypsin inhibitors in soy interfere with protein digestion and may cause pancreatic disorders. In test animals, soy containing trypsin inhibitors caused stunted growth.

- High levels of oxalic acid in soy can cause kidney stones, or stones anywhere in the body.

- Soy phytoestrogens disrupt endocrine function and have the potential to cause infertility and to promote breast cancer in adult women.

- Soy phytoestrogens are potent antithyroid agents that cause hypothyroidism and may cause thyroid cancer. In infants, consumption of soy formula has been linked to autoimmune thyroid disease.

- Vitamin B_{12} analogs in soy are not absorbed and actually increase the body's requirement for B_{12}.

- Soy foods increase the body's requirement for vitamin D. Toxic synthetic vitamin D_2 is added to soy milk.

- Fragile proteins are over-denatured during high temperature processing to make soy protein isolate and textured vegetable protein. Thus the protein in soy is less available to the infant.

- Processing of soy protein results in the formation of toxic lysinoalanine and highly carcinogenic nitrosamines.

- Free glutamic acid or MSG, a potent neurotoxin, is formed during soy food processing, and is present even if not labeled.

- Soy formula contains high levels of aluminum, which is toxic to the nervous system and the kidneys.

- Babies fed soy-based formula have 13,000 to 22,000 times more estrogen compounds in their blood than babies fed milk-based formula. Infants exclusively fed soy formula receive the estrogenic equivalent of at least four birth control pills per day.

- Male infants undergo a testosterone surge during the first few months of life, when testosterone levels may be as high as those of an adult male. During this period, baby boys are programmed to express male characteristics after puberty, not only in the development of their sexual organs and other masculine physical traits, but also in setting patterns in the brain characteristic of male behavior.

- In animals, studies indicate that phytoestrogens in soy are powerful endocrine disrupters. Soy infant feeding—which floods the bloodstream with female hormones that inhibit testosterone—cannot be ignored as a possible cause of disrupted development patterns in boys, including learning disabilities and attention deficit disorder. Male children exposed to DES, a synthetic estrogen, had testes smaller than normal on maturation and infant marmoset monkeys fed soy isoflavones had a reduction in testosterone levels up to 70 percent compared to milk-fed controls.

- Almost 15 percent of white girls and 50 percent of African-American girls show signs of puberty, such as breast development and pubic hair, before the age of eight. Some girls are showing sexual development before the age of three. Premature development of girls has been linked to the use of soy formula and exposure to environmental estrogen-mimickers such as PCBs and DDE.

- Intake of phytoestrogens even at moderate levels during pregnancy can have adverse affects on the developing fetus and the timing of puberty later in life.

For more information and references: www.westonaprice.org/soyalert

this dual action of oxytocin can cause mildly painful contractions in the uterus.

Oxytocin analogues like Pitocin are sometimes used to encourage uterine contractions and to help placental coagulation after the baby is delivered. Pharmaceutical oxytocin inhibitors do exist—used in some countries to suppress premature labor—so it is safe to assume that oxytocin production and release can be inhibited in a variety of ways, starting with problems in the hypothalamus. Oxytocin nasal sprays are marketed for the treatment of fearfulness and anxiety, with the suggestion that they could be used to stimulate the letdown of milk for easier breastfeeding.

Consumption of *trans* fats lowers the overall fat content of mother's milk.[67] The poor quality of the American diet, including *trans* fatty acids in commercial foods, is another reason why so many mothers abandon breastfeeding after the first few weeks—even if milk flow is abundant, baby is not happy with the quality of milk that she is getting from the breast.

A Norwegian study found that higher levels of testosterone in women during pregnancy and postpartum negatively affect the development of glandular tissue in the breast, leading to lower milk output.[68]

According to a University of Rochester Medical Center study, exposure to dioxins during pregnancy harms the cells in rapidly changing breast tissue, leading to lower milk supply. Researchers found that dioxin alters the induction of milk-producing genes, which occurs around the ninth day of pregnancy, and decreases the number of ductal branches and mature lobules in the mammary tissue. When exposure occurs very early in pregnancy, but not

later, sometimes the mammary glands can partially recover from the cellular injury.[69]

According to B. Paige Lawrence, PhD, an author of the study, three to six million mothers worldwide are either unable to initiate breastfeeding or unable to produce enough milk to nourish their infants.

According to Marianne Neifert, MD, author of *Great Expectations: The Essential Guide to Breastfeeding*, about fifteen percent of women experience inadequate breast milk supply. She notes that about four percent of women experience lactation failure due to insufficient glandular tissue in the breasts. Absence of typical breast changes during pregnancy and failure of postpartum breast engorgement are signs of congenital inability to breastfeed. It's important—and usually a relief—for these women to understand that lactation failure is not due to poor technique.

According to Neifert, "Preserving the 'every woman can nurse' myth contributes to perpetuating a simplistic view of lactation and does a disservice to the small percentage of women with primary causes of unsuccessful lactation."[70]

According to Diana West, IBCLC, a coauthor of *The Breastfeeding Mother's Guide to Making More Milk*, "We're seeing a dramatic increase in the number of women who have primary problems, possibly because of environmental contaminants. Lactation consultants around the world are reporting increases in the numbers of women who can't produce enough milk." West also notes that interventions are allowing women to get pregnant when they wouldn't otherwise, causing babies to be born to women who might not have fully functional reproductive systems. For example, women with

---

RECIPE FOR LACTATION TEA

1 ounce blessed thistle, dried
1 ounce raspberry or stinging nettle leaf, dried
1 teaspoon per cup aromatic seeds such as anise, caraway, coriander, cumin, dill or fennel

Place the leaves in a half gallon jar and fill to the top with boiling water. Cap tightly and let steep overnight. Strain and refrigerate the liquid. Before nursing, heat 1 cup of the brew to near boiling and pour over 1 teaspoon of any of the aromatic seeds. Allow to brew for five minutes. Sip slowly during the nursing period.   SOURCE: www.susunweed.com

polycystic ovarian syndrome (PCOS) tend to have lower amounts of functional breast tissue.

Even women who start off with a good supply of milk may have ups and downs. When your period starts again, milk supply may drop, and also drop before the beginning of each period; it soon picks up again. Sometimes babies have a growth spurt when they are ravenously hungry, and it may take a few days for mom to catch up. The important thing is to keep nursing, keeping the breast stimulated, and, if need be, pump to encourage more production. You can also give the homemade formula using a breastfeeding aid. With the breastfeeding aid, the formula is put into a plastic bag that has a small tube which allows the baby to suck both from the tube and the breast (see Sources).

INCREASING BREAST MILK SUPPLY

Your baby has a very good way of telling you that she is not getting enough to eat: it's called crying! Crying may also be baby's way of telling you that she not getting enough nourishment from your milk, even though your supply may be good. If baby cries after nursing, and in addition is not gaining weight, it's a sure sign that either the amount or the quality of your milk is inadequate—a situation that calls for immediate attention.

Increasing caloric intake—especially intake of good fats—and nursing frequently can sometimes solve the problem, especially during the first few weeks after birth. Nurse every hour if need be, and at least once at night. Remember that the hindmilk, the last milk out of the breast, contains the most fat and therefore is the most satisfying milk for baby. In addition, it is important for the breast to completely drain in order to stimulate increased milk production.

Carry your baby a lot to get the oxytocin flowing, but not to the point of exhaustion.

Manual expression of milk may help get milk flowing. In the case of a small baby with a weak suckling reflex, expressed milk may be given with an eyedropper or a syringe until baby becomes stronger and can nurse effectively.

To express milk manually, gently massage the breast to start the milk moving down the ducts. Work evenly around the breast, stroking repeatedly downward toward the areola. Then, starting about halfway up the breast, run your thumb firmly down. As it reaches the edge of the areola, press in and up and the milk will squirt from the nipple. You will want a scrupulously clean container to catch the milk. You can even express milk directly into baby's mouth as she nurses, to increase your supply. Repeat all the way around the breast. Do not squeeze the nipple as this will close the ducts, nor continue expressing until you think the breast is empty. Stop when the milk starts coming in drips rather than jets.

Don't hesitate to call in the help of a gentle and understanding lactation consultant—some consultants can leave mothers in tears, with the impression that low milk supply is due to faulty technique. But a good lactation consultant can be just the ticket to increasing your confidence and ensuring that the breastfeeding goes smoothly.

THE BREAST PUMP

In situations of low breast milk supply, the breast

DONATED BREAST MILK

One solution to inadequate supply, or for babies who have been adopted or whose mother has died, is shared human breast milk. Unfortunately, the human milk in breast milk banks is pasteurized, but there are many informal sharing networks that can help you find direct donations of breast milk (see Sources).

The downside is that the donating mother's diet may be very poor and her milk, albeit plentiful, inadequate to fully nourish an infant. You will want to make inquiries about the mother's diet before using her milk, and you should carefully observe her baby. If baby is rosy and robust, it's a sign that mother's milk is nutrient-dense. But if baby is pale and whiney, it's best to look for another source or use our homemade formula.

COW'S MILK FORMULA

Makes 36 ounces.

Our milk-based formula takes account of the fact that human milk is richer in whey, lactose, vitamin C, niacin and long-chain polyunsaturated fatty acids compared to cow's milk but lower in casein (milk protein). The addition of gelatin to cow's milk formula will make it more digestible for the infant. Use only truly expeller-expressed oils in the formula recipes, otherwise they may be rancid and lack vitamin E.

The ideal milk for baby, if he cannot be breastfed, is clean, whole raw milk from old-fashioned cows that feed on green pasture, produced in clean conditions. For sources of good quality milk, see www.realmilk.com or contact a local chapter of the Weston A. Price Foundation. For a video on formula preparation, visit westonaprice.org/childrens-health/recipes-for-homemade-baby-formula.

INGREDIENTS
- 1 7/8 cups filtered water
- 4 tablespoons lactose[1]
- 2 teaspoons gelatin[1]
- 2 teaspoons coconut oil[1]
- 1/4 teaspoon high-vitamin butter oil (optional)[1]
- 2 cups whole raw cow's milk, preferably from pasture-fed cows
- 1/4 cup homemade liquid whey (See recipe for whey, page 45) Note: Do *not* use powdered whey or whey from making cheese (which will cause the formula to curdle). Use only homemade whey made from yogurt or kefir.
- 1/4 teaspoon *Bifidobacterium infantis*[1]
- 2 or more tablespoons good quality cream (preferably not ultrapasteurized), more if you are using milk from Holstein cows
- 1/2 teaspoon unflavored high-vitamin fermented cod liver oil or 1 teaspoon regular cod liver oil[1,2]
- 1 teaspoon expeller-expressed sunflower oil[1]
- 1 teaspoon extra virgin olive oil[1]
- 2 teaspoons Frontier brand nutritional yeast flakes[1]
- 1/4 teaspoon acerola powder[1]

    1.   Available from Radiant Life 888-593-8333, www.radiantlifecatalog.com.
    2.   Use only recommended brands of cod liver oil. See http://westonaprice.org/cod-liver-oil/cod-liver-oil-basics#brands.

INSTRUCTIONS
- Put 2 cups filtered water into a pyrex measuring pitcher and remove 2 tablespoons (which will give you 1 7/8 cups water).
- Pour about half the water into a pan and place on a medium flame.
- Add the gelatin and lactose to the pan and let dissolve, stirring occasionally.
- Stir in the coconut oil and optional high-vitamin butter oil; stir until melted.
- When the gelatin and lactose are dissolved, remove from heat and add the remaining water to cool the mixture.
- Meanwhile, place remaining ingredients into a blender.
- Add the water mixture and blend about three seconds.
- Place in glass bottles or a glass jar and refrigerate. You may also use the formula with a breastfeeding aid (see Sources).
- Before giving to baby, warm bottles by placing in hot water or a bottle warmer. NEVER warm bottles in a microwave oven.

pump is a mother's best friend. Very small babies may not have enough strength to nurse effectively; the breast pump will help keep the milk flowing until baby gets stronger. Many mothers produce more milk in the morning than in the evening, when they are tired. With a breast pump, she can give some of her morning milk to baby in the evening. And for working moms, the breast pump used several times during the day will ensure that mom continues to produce breast milk and baby continues to enjoy its advantages.

There are many brands of breast pumps on the market, and in general the more expensive ones are worth paying for. If you will be using the breast pump every day, purchase a larger, heavier model as the smaller compact models may not be strong enough to maintain your milk supply, nor sturdy enough to last through the months of breastfeeding. For occasional use, however, the smaller breast pumps may be adequate (see Sources).

Often left out of the promotional literature is the fact that the "horns" that fit on the breast come in different sizes. Having a suction horn that fits your breast will make a big difference in how much milk you get. Horns of different sizes are available on the Internet (see Sources).

Milk extracted with a pump can be given with a bottle or with a breastfeeding aid (see Sources). If you use a bottle, be sure to use a nipple that best approximates that shape of the breast—these often come with the breast pump. The breast feeding aid is a plastic bag that you fill with the pumped milk (see Sources). It has a small tube that is placed on the breast so that baby gets the extra milk while nursing. With baby continuing to nurse at the breast, plus the extra milk extracted by the pump, many mothers can get over the hump of low milk supply that may occur during the early weeks, or even later, when baby goes through a growth spurt and is especially hungry.

Most importantly, the breast pump provides an accurate picture of how much milk a mother is producing. If, after pumping consistently, mom still only produces an ounce or two of milk per day, she will know for sure that supplementation is an absolute necessity.

Pumped breast milk should be stored in very clean glass bottles. It will keep up to six hours at room temperature, up to twenty-four hours in a cooler with ice packs and five to eight days in a refrigerator. It may also be frozen for up to several months. If you are freezing the milk, don't fill the bottle too full, but leave some space at the top for air expansion.

To warm the milk, set in a bottle warmer or pan of simmering water. Never, *never* heat baby's bottle in a microwave oven.

GALACTAGOGUES

A galactagogue is a substance that promotes lactation in humans and other animals, usually an herbal preparation such as fenugreek, blessed thistle or alfalfa. Others include anise, astragalus root, burdock, nettle, fennel, flax, soapwort, vervain and red raspberry leaf. These may be formulated with marshmallow root, which increases the absorption rate. The classic European remedy is fenugreek seed

---

GOAT'S MILK FORMULA

Although goat's milk is rich in fat, and in some cases more digestible for the infant, it must be used with caution in infant feeding as it lacks folic acid and is low in vitamin B_{12}, both of which are essential to growth and development. Inclusion of nutritional yeast will provide folic acid. To compensate for low levels of vitamin B_{12}, (as well as folic acid) if preparing the Cow's Milk Formula (page 123) with goat's milk, add 2 teaspoons organic raw chicken liver, frozen for 14 days, finely grated or 1/2 teaspoon desiccated liver (see Sources) to the batch of formula.

Once baby is eating solid foods, which should include liver, the goat's milk formula can be made exactly as the cows milk formula.

and blessed thistle. Formulations of fenugreek and blessed thistle are widely available, both as dried herbs and as a tincture (see Sources).

Pharmaceutical galactagogues, available usually by medical prescription, include domperidone and metoclopramide. Domperidone, a dopamine antagonist, is available in the U.K. but not approved for enhanced lactation in the U.S. Some drugs, primarily atypical antipsychotics such as Risperdal, may cause lactation in both women and men. Most of those discovered have been found to interact with the dopamine system in such a way to increase the production of prolactin. Obviously, such drugs should be used with great care as all drugs have side effects.

Foods reported to increase milk supply include raw milk, bone broths, soaked porridge such as oatmeal, lacto-fermented beverages such as kombucha and unpasteurized beer.

Acupuncture has also proven effective for increasing milk supply.

HOMEMADE FORMULA

"Nature does not always confer upon a woman the important capacity for nursing her baby, but the women who are able should do so. Every pregnant woman should not only be impressed with the importance of this duty on her part, but with the essential preparation for accomplishing it. However, there are women who for some reason cannot perform this natural function—for these, it is necessary to learn to take advantage of the way now available to them to feed the infant artificially. The logical substitute for human milk is cow's milk (or goat's milk)." So wrote F. T. Proudfit in *Nutrition and Diet Therapy*, published 1942. All books on infant feeding published before the Second World War recommended cow or goat milk—usually certified raw cow or goat milk—when mother's milk was not sufficient.

In fact, until the Second World War, part of the preparation for women during pregnancy, aside from a diet enriched by special animal foods, was the scouting out of a cow that would be given the best of pasture and whose milk would be available to the infant throughout his childhood. Today we know that for infants, we should dilute the milk and add other whole foods in order to approximate the nutrient profile of human milk, but even before we knew these things, millions of babies thrived on rich whole milk from a variety of animals. Yet some of the strongest words in the medical literature today are aimed at commercial formula's only competition—homemade formula based on raw cow or goat milk.

HOMEMADE WHEY FOR HOMEMADE INFANT FORMULA

Makes about 5 cups.

Homemade whey is easy to make from good quality plain yogurt, kefir or buttermilk. Ideally, use yogurt, kefir or buttermilk that you have made from whole raw milk. Second choice would be commercial brands of yogurt or kefir listed in the Shopping Guide from the Weston A. Price Foundation.

You will need a large strainer or colander that rests over a bowl and a linen kitchen towel.

Place 2 quarts yogurt or kefir in a strainer or colander lined with a linen kitchen towel set over a bowl. Cover with a plate and leave at room temperature overnight. The whey will drip out into the bowl. Place whey in clean glass jars and store in the refrigerator.

The thick yogurt or kefir that is left is delicious mixed with maple syrup or raw honey—a great food for mom while she is nursing and a good food for baby once he begins solid food. (Note: do not give the thick yogurt or kefir mixed with raw honey to baby until he is at least one year old; use maple syrup instead.)

LIVER-BASED FORMULA

Makes about 36 ounces.

Our liver-based formula also mimics the nutrient profile of mother's milk. It is extremely important to include coconut oil in this formula as it is the only ingredient that provides the special medium-chain saturated fats found in mother's milk. As with the milk-based formula, all oils should be truly expeller-expressed. This formula has been a life saver for babies with severe allergies to milk of all kinds.

INGREDIENTS
- 3-3/4 cups homemade beef or chicken broth (see Recipes)
- 2 ounces chicken, duck or turkey liver, cut into small pieces
- 5 tablespoons lactose[1]
- 1/4 teaspoon *Bifidobacterium infantis*[1]
- 1/4 cup homemade liquid whey (See recipe for whey, page 145)
- 1 tablespoon coconut oil[1]
- 1/2 teaspoon unflavored high-vitamin fermented cod liver oil or 1 teaspoon regular cod liver oil[1,2]
- 1 teaspoon unrefined sunflower oil[1]
- 2 teaspoons extra virgin olive oil[1]
- 1/4 teaspoon acerola powder[1]

1. Available from Radiant Life 888-593-8333, www.radiantlifecatalog.com.
2. Use only recommended brands of cod liver oil, See www.westonaprice.org/cod-liver-oil/cod-liver-oil-basics#brands.

INSTRUCTIONS
- Simmer liver gently in broth until the meat is cooked through.
- Liquefy using a handheld blender or in a standing blender.
- When the liver broth has cooled, stir in remaining ingredients.
- Store in a very clean glass or stainless steel container.
- To serve, stir formula well and pour 6 to 8 ounces in a very clean glass bottle.
- Attach a clean nipple and set in a pan of simmering water until formula is warm but not hot to the touch, shake well and feed to baby. (Never heat formula in a microwave oven!)

Our recipes for homemade baby formula were developed with Mary G. Enig, PhD, nutritionist and expert in lipids. Since first published, in the first edition of *Nourishing Traditions*, 1996, the formula has nourished hundreds if not thousands of infants, almost always with excellent results. In fact, babies who cannot tolerate commercial formula and who seem to be lactose intolerant often thrive on the raw milk formula.

Based on whole, unpasteurized cow or goat milk, the formula provides similar immune-stimulating, health-promoting and antimicrobial components as human breast milk. Some specific human proteins and maternal immune factors will be missing, but these can be obtained with a hybrid formula-breast milk program.

Our first choice is formula based on cow's milk. Although goat milk is easier for some babies to digest, it is low in folic acid and vitamin B_{12}. There are several reports in the scientific literature of problems developing in infants fed goat milk exclusively.[71] If you use goat milk and the formula is baby's only food, then it is imperative to add a little liver to supply folic acid and vitamin B_{12}. Once baby is eating solid foods, which should include liver, then goat milk formula can be made exactly as the cow's milk formula.

BREAST MILK AND HOMEMADE FORMULA NUTRIENT COMPARISON CHART

Based on 36 ounces.

These nutrient tables were derived from standard food nutrient tables and do not take into account the wide variation in nutrient levels that can occur in both human and animal milk, depending on diet and environment.

	BREAST MILK	COW'S MILK FORMULA	GOAT MILK FORMULA	LIVER-BASED FORMULA
Calories	766	856	890	682
Protein	11.3 g	18 g	18 g	15 g
Carbohydrates	76 g	79 g	77 g	69 g
Total Fat	48 g	52 g	54 g	36 g
Saturated Fat	22 g	28 g	30 g	16 g
Mono Fat	18 g	16 g	16 g	12 g
Poly Fat	5.5 g	5.6 g	5.7 g	5.6 g
Omega-3 FA	.58 g	1.3 g	1.2 g	1.0 g
Omega-6 FA	4.4 g	4.2 g	4.4 g	4.5 g
Cholesterol	153 g	137 mg	166 mg	227 mg
Vitamin A*	946 IU	5000 IU	5,000 IU	12,000 IU
Thiamin-B_1	.15 mg	1.05 mg	1.1 mg	19 mg
Riboflavin-B_2	.4 mg	1.2 mg	1.2 mg	1.9 mg
Niacin-B_3	1.9 mg	2.5 mg	4.4 mg	14.2 mg
Vitamin B_6	.12 mg	.51 mg	.6 mg	.65 mg
Vitamin B_{12}	.5 mcg	1.9 mcg	.8 mcg	39 mcg
Folate	57 mcg	236 mcg	284 mcg	159 mcg
Vitamin C	55 mg	57 mg	59 mg	62 mg
Vitamin D	480 IU	450 IU	525 IU	460 IU
Vitamin E***	9.9 mg	6.2 mg	4.7 mg	4.9 mg
Calcium	355 mg	532 mg	548 mg	NA**
Copper	.57 mg	.38 mg	.58 mg	1.9 mg
Iron	.33 mg	1.4 mg	2.2 mg	5.4 mg
Magnesium	37.4 mg	91.3 mg	96.1 mg	34.5 mg
Manganese	.29 mg	.034 mg	.12 mg	.24 mg
Phosphorus	151 mg	616 mg	729 mg	344 mg
Potassium	560 mg	949 mg	1228 mg	750 mg
Selenium	18.8 mcg	15.4 mcg	18.7 mcg	31.1 mcg
Sodium	186 mg	308 mg	320 mg	NA**
Zinc	1.9 mg	2.8 mg	2.7 mg	2.5 mg

* Vitamin A levels in human milk will depend on the diet of the mother. Nursing mothers eating vitamin A-rich foods such as cod liver oil will have much higher levels of vitamin A in their milk. Commercial formulas contain about 2400 IU vitamin A per 800 calories.

** Calcium and sodium values for homemade broth are not available.

*** Vitamin E values are derived from commercial vegetable oils. The vitamin E levels for homemade formulas will be higher if good quality, expeller-expressed oils are used.

FORTIFIED COMMERCIAL FORMULA

Makes about 35 ounces.

This stopgap formula can be used in emergencies, or when the ingredients for homemade formula are unavailable.

INGREDIENTS
- 1 cup milk-based powdered formula[1]
- 29 ounces filtered water (3 5/8 cups) Note: never use fluoridated water for baby formula!
- 1 egg yolk, preferably from a pastured hen
- 1/2 teaspoon unflavored high-vitamin or high-vitamin fermented cod liver oil or 1 teaspoon regular cod liver oil[2]

1. The best choice for commercial formula today seems to be Baby's Only Organic Dairy Formula (see Sources). Unfortunately, it contains iron (mandated by FDA) but otherwise contains higher quality ingredients than any of the other commercial formulas. It is also the only brand on the market at this time without added oils containing industrial ARA and DHA (see page 139). If you are forced to use commercial formula, make sure that baby is getting cod liver oil, either added to the formula or given separately with an eye dropper or syringe. As soon as possible, introduce solid foods like egg yolk, liver, meat and bone broths.
2. Use only recommended brands of cod liver oil. See www.westonaprice.org/cod-liver-oil/cod-liver-oil-basics#brands.

INSTRUCTIONS
- Place all ingredients in a blender or food processor and blend thoroughly.
- Place 6-8 ounces in a very clean glass bottle. (Store the rest in very clean glass bottles or a very clean glass jar in the refrigerator for the next feedings.)
- Attach a clean nipple to the bottle and set in a pan of simmering water until formula is warm but not hot to the touch, shake well and feed to baby. (Never heat formula in a microwave oven!)

A third formula, based on liver and broth, is provided for the rare baby that cannot tolerate the cow or goat milk formula. We have several reports of babies thriving on this formula. In the days before soy-based infant formula, Gerber produced a meat-based formula for babies who could not tolerate milk-based formula.

THE COMBO:
FORMULA AND BREAST MILK

Many moms who have trouble with supply settle into a combo or hybrid solution, both breastfeeding and giving baby homemade formula using a bottle or breastfeeding aid (see Sources). The breast-feeding aid is the better way to give the milk, as it keeps baby stimulating the breast by nursing, and never poses the problem of nipple confusion. Stay-at-home moms can easily use the breastfeeding aid to give formula at the same time as the breast. Sometimes the relief of seeing her baby nourished and content will be enough to increase a mother's supply to the point where she no longer needs to supplement.

Breastfeeding advocates warn against giving baby the breast and a bottle alternately because baby may prefer the bottle to the breast and refuse to nurse. Some lactation consultants recommend giving pumped breast milk or formula with a syringe or even from a cup. However, many babies easily adjust to both bottle and breast.

Working moms will need to have someone give either formula or pumped milk—or a combination—using a bottle during the day, and many have succeeded in getting baby to accept both breast and bottle. Use a nipple with a small hole so baby has to work at getting the formula, preferably one with a shape comparable to a human nipple. One trick is to always have someone other than mom give the bottle, with mom giving the breast only.

Sometimes babies will go on a nursing strike, refusing the breast in an obvious play for the bottle. But if you are firm, you can get over this hump. Babies may fuss and even scream but don't give up. Try expressing milk directly into baby's mouth, or even putting a little bit of formula on your nipple to get him started. You might try giving the bottle to get baby started, then switch craftily to the breast. Pumping for a few minutes will get milk flowing so nursing is easier. Baby may even cry himself to sleep, but then be ready to nurse when he wakes up. The important thing is not to get upset—watch TV, zone out, take your focus off the baby, and he may start nursing. Most babies soon learn to switch hit without any problem.Conversely, some babies refuse the bottle. Try different nipples, different people, different angles of the bottle. Have someone else feed baby while you leave the house. One trick is to warm the nipple in your bra before putting it on the bottle!

WORKING MOTHERS

A large portion of mothers work today, with many of them continuing to breastfeed for many months. Baby will need to get bottles during the day, either of pumped breast milk, homemade formula, or a combination.

The important thing is to prepare for your return to work well in advance, pumping and storing milk. Baby needs to get used to taking a bottle from someone else—and mom needs to get used to leaving someone else in charge. Mom will return to work in a more relaxed frame of mind if she has prepared herself and baby in advance, and has a supply of breast milk in the fridge and freezer. If she is supplementing her breast milk with homemade formula, she needs to get the formula-making routine down pat, and be assured that baby is doing well on it.

Most states require workplaces to provide breaks for pumping and a place to do so that is not a bathroom. In practice this means that lawyers, editors and other white collar workers, who know their rights, can manage the breastfeeding-pumping in a flexible, supportive environment. For teachers, bus drivers and other service workers, it might be much more difficult to juggle the pumping with the job. (For help and encouragement, visit www.workandpump.com.)

CONSTIPATION IN BABY

One problem occasionally reported with the homemade formula is constipation—indeed, even breastfed babies can become constipated. The following are suggestions for relieving this uncomfortable condition.

- Constipation is more frequent with the goat milk formula than the cow's milk formula. If baby is constipated on the goat milk formula, switch to cow's milk if you can.
- Use homemade kefir or yogurt made from raw milk in place of the sweet milk in the formula.
- Use 1/2 cup fresh whey and reduce the amount of water by 1/4 cup.
- Increase the *Bifidobacterium infantis* from 1/4 teaspoon to 1/2 teaspoon.
- Add 1 teaspoon molasses to the formula; add to the hot water-gelatin mixture.
- Replace regular cream in the formula with cultured or sour cream.
- Give baby Digestive Tea (see Recipes) in a bottle.
- Give baby a little diluted prune juice in a bottle.
- Homemade chicken broth in a bottle can soothe the digestive tract and help relieve constipation.

If none of these work, use an infant suppository on your baby as a last resort. Bear in mind that babies vary in how often they move their bowels; however once every two days should be considered a minimum.

If you are at the weaning stage, don't be tempted to give baby rice cereal, Cheerios, teething biscuits or bread rolls, as these can be a recipe for constipation. See Chapter 9 for appropriate weaning foods.

A typical schedule for a working mother goes like this:

- Wake up, immediately nurse baby.

- Shower, dress, breakfast.

- Nurse baby again before you leave for work or when you drop her off at daycare.

- Pump at work midmorning, just after lunch and in the afternoon—this might take about one hour in all—keeping the milk in a small refrigerator or a freezer bag with a cold pack.

- Nurse immediately when you get home.

- Nurse before baby's bedtime.

Pumped milk should be stored in bottles for baby's feeding the next day. If you do not produce enough milk for three to four daily feedings, you can supplement with homemade formula. (And it might be a good idea to have the formula ingredients on hand for emergencies.)

Although the formula is ideally made fresh every day, you can make it every other day or even just twice a week, storing it in the coldest part of the refrigerator.

Be sure to bring enough bottles and parts with you so you don't have to do any washing of bits and pieces at work. Breastfeeding while working sounds complicated and requires you to be organized, but lots of dedicated moms have made it work.

PROBLEMS WITH HOMEMADE FORMULA

Overall, mothers who have used our homemade formula have reported excellent success, but sometimes there are problems.

If baby cries, seems to be suffering from indigestion, or vomits, you can eliminate some of the ingredients that might be problematic, such as nutritional yeast or gelatin. Cod liver oil can be given separately, with an eye dropper. Some mothers have reported excellent results replacing cream with melted ghee or even raw colostrum. If baby becomes constipated, follow the suggestions on page 149.

If the cow's milk formula is not working, the second choice is formula made with goat milk. If the formula is baby's only food, the baby must get an additional source of folic acid and vitamin B_{12}. This can be achieved by adding liver to the formula. If you are using the breastfeeding aid, the powdered liver is probably a better choice as it is difficult to blend the grated liver fine enough to pass through the plastic tube.

Once baby begins eating solid food, which should include puréed liver, then the goat milk formula can be made exactly as the cow's milk formula.

Making the formula may seem like a lot of trouble, but you will soon get into the routine. It takes about twenty minutes to make a fresh batch every morning.

Heat gently by setting the bottle into simmering water or a bottle warmer—never in a microwave. Test the temperature of the milk by shaking a few drops on your wrist.

Please note that you should only use fresh whey in the formula—this is easily made using whole yogurt or kefir. Powdered whey is an industrial product—it will not contain good bacteria and the whey proteins are damaged by the powdering process. Cheese whey will cause the formula to curdle. If the baby is getting only formula, you will need to make fresh whey from one quart yogurt or kefir about once a week. The by-product is a delicious quark cheese, a wonderful food for mom and the rest of the family, as well as a good weaning food for baby.

FOR FURTHER INFORMATION

The Nursing Mother's Companion by Kathleen Huggins.

Breastfeeding Answer Book by Nancy Mohrbacher.

Wise Woman Herbal for the Childbearing Year by Susun Weed.

www.westonaprice.org/childrens-health/recipes-for-homemade-baby-formula, includes frequently asked question, testimonials and a video on making the homemade baby formula.

Chapter 8
Bringing Up Baby

Of all mammalian species, only humans require long-term care and assistance from birth with every facet of life—clothing and warmth, protection from danger, cleanup of waste products, feeding of special foods, training and structure, even an environment that is both safe and interesting—parents of human children must supply all of these or their offspring will perish. Fortunately, the hormones that course through the bloodstream of both father and mother as they look upon their tiny darling make them well disposed to devotion and care.

But hormones alone cannot help modern parents navigate between the conflicting recommendations they hear and read on how to bring up their babies—and almost every subject is rife with controversy, from where he sleeps, to the way he is cuddled, to how he is disciplined. As you navigate these difficult waters, remember that the most fruitful course can usually be found in the middle of the channel, avoiding the rocky extreme of hardline disciplinarianism and the treacherous sands of indulgent overparenting. Above all, enlist your sense of humor and sense of wonder during the brief but fascinating period of babyhood, remembering that no one is a perfect parent. Fortunately babies are very resilient, especially well-fed babies; they will survive their parents' mistakes and, in the vast majority of cases, emerge from childhood ready for the challenge of life.

CUDDLING, STROKING and HOLDING

Just as mammalian mothers lick their babies, human parents instinctually cuddle and stroke their infants. Babies left alone in their cribs in orphanages suffer from extreme emotional trauma and even death.

The skin of the infant serves as a kind of external brain—indeed skin and brain develop from the same embryonic tissue. Recent studies show that when we stimulate baby's skin through touch, we stimulate brain development.[1] Touching and stroking also enhance immune function; antibody production is increased. Touching also increases the production of growth hormone, the master hormone that regulates all endocrine functions of the body.

Truly, tactile and loving human contact is necessary for normal emotional and even physical life. Yet, just a few decades ago, child care books cautioned parents against kissing and cuddling their offspring. John B. Watson, author of *Psychological Care of Infant and Child* (1928) warned that cuddling a child was a "sex-seeking response" on the part of frustrated mothers, which could ruin a child's "vocational future and. . . . chances of marital happiness."

A reaction to this harsh attitude can be found in the extreme application of what is called attachment parenting, which stipulates that parents hold and cuddle their infants at all times, never leaving them

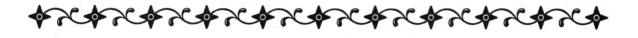

alone, not even to sleep. The right course of action lies somewhere between these two extremes, providing affection and comfort along with freedom to develop as an independent human being.

The most important place to stroke a baby is her soft, fuzzy head. Move your hand gently back and forth with a light touch—a motion that calms baby outwardly but stimulates the growth of nerve cells inwardly. Mothers do this instinctually while they are nursing.

From the very first weeks, babies will differ in the amount of cuddling they want and need. Some babies are happy to nestle in a parent's arms; others will wiggle and squirm to get free.

Baby's transition from womb to outside world

CAN BABIES BE OVERSTIMULATED?

In the early 1900s, Luther Emmett Holt, president of the American Pediatric Society, warned against the "overstimulation" of babies. Raised on a quiet farm, Holt believed that the noise and distractions of the city, "factory and locomotive whistles, trolley cars and automobiles. . . door bells and telephones in the house," disrupted the neurocognitive development of babies. Rattle-waving by doting mothers only added to the onslaught, he warned. Modern babies growing up in quiet suburbs are often subjected to stimulation of another sort in the form of picture books, constant classical music and Baby Einstein DVDs thrust in front of them at three months old—compared to which city noises and the occasional rattle-waving mother seem downright bucolic.

The Baby Einstein movement grew out of research on brain plasticity in the 1990s, which posits the brain as "plastic," able to be molded by experience, especially during the first three years of life. The more stimulation in early life, so goes the theory, the greater the brain development. In the hands of anxious parents and clever marketers, the brain plasticity theory morphed into a whole philosophy of child rearing, wherein babies were subjected to foreign languages via DVDs and toddlers were exposed to flash cards of famous paintings and taken on numerous trips to museums.

In 2007, researchers at the University of Washington published a paper on the effects of television and DVD/video viewing on language development in children under two years of age. The study concluded that among infants aged eight to sixteen months, exposure to "baby DVDs/videos"—such as Baby Einstein and Brainy Baby—was strongly associated with *lower* scores on a standard language development test. This result was specific to baby-oriented educational videos and did not hold for other types of media, and was not related to shared parental viewing. Among toddlers aged seventeen to twenty-four months, the study found no significant effects, either negative or positive, for any of the forms of media that were viewed. Daily reading and storytelling, however, were found to be associated with somewhat higher language scores, especially for toddlers.[2]

The fact is that intelligent, creative individuals have emerged from childhood over hundreds, even thousands of years without the aid of educational DVDs for babies. Newborns learn about their world predominantly through the senses of touch and taste, and through trial and error in movement; flat images on a screen have no meaning for them and can distract them from their important work of learning about their world—the real world. Instead of exposing their babies to fine paintings and foreign words, parents could use their time more productively in the kitchen preparing choline-rich custards and liver paté to support the production and connection of glial cells going on in baby's brain.

It is interesting to watch a baby at work-play. She grabs an object, puts it in her mouth, looks at it, holds it, lets go, perhaps repeating the exercise several times. Then she becomes quiet, as if assimilating the experience. Or, she interacts with mom, smiling and cooing, perhaps for half a minute, then turns her head to stare at the wall, again as a kind of repose. To interrupt this process with constant stimulation is to interrupt the natural way that babies learn about their world.

should be a gradual one. During the first month or two after birth, babies like to be swaddled—wrapped tightly in a blanket—as having arms and legs free often triggers a startle reflex. But as the weeks go by, baby will want to move more and have arms and legs free.

The idea that baby, especially an older baby, should be held and carried for hours does a disservice to both mother and baby. Very few mothers have the strength to carry baby throughout the day, especially as baby grows. And mom has work to do, even if she is a stay-at-home mom—food preparation, laundry, care for other children and at-home work.

It also does a disservice to baby. Baby needs to spend some time on a blanket on the floor (or in a playpen if the household is a busy one) kicking and learning to use his hands, learning to roll over, exercising by lifting his head, and eventually sitting up, getting on his knees and crawling. He can't do this if he is always held in a backpack or sling.

Many traditional cultures swaddled their babies in a cradle board, which kept arms and legs rigid, a practice that seems abhorrent to westerners. Children were swaddled to keep them safe, often until the second birthday. Swaddling did, however, provide one advantage—it allowed parents to put their infants in an upright position so baby could observe the goings on around him. Babies do get bored if left on the floor too long.

A modern solution, one that keeps baby safe but allows freedom of movement in the arms and legs, is an infant seat that keeps baby at a forty-five degree angle. Baby is strapped in but can move his arms and legs; more importantly, he can observe what is going on around him.

The seat can be placed on a counter while mom or dad is preparing meals, on the floor while someone is doing housework or siblings are playing, and on the dining room table while the family shares a meal. Just remember that if the infant seat is on the counter or table, baby must be watched at all times.

Alternating between holding baby, putting him on the floor or in a playpen, and allowing him to be in a semi-upright position in a baby seat will help alleviate boredom and fussiness; mom or dad are right there to keep watch, interact and observe, but still free to carry out household chores.

DIAPERS

Human babies in indoor civilized settings need diapers—your baby will generate more than two thousand wet or messy diapers in the first year alone. One of the first choices parents make is the type of diaper to use—cloth or disposable. Either way, baby needs to be changed often and the diapers and their contents disposed of in a responsible way. Cloth diapers should be rinsed out in the toilet and washed with soap and very hot water, then rinsed with an extra rinse cycle (or sent out to a diaper service); disposables should be wrapped up and placed in a receptacle reserved for the diapers alone. Once your baby is excreting well-formed feces, the responsible course of action is to transfer as much of the waste as possible into the toilet.

Diaper changing provides a good gauge on how baby is doing. As a newborn, she should have six to eight wet diapers per day, and several soiled with feces. Learning your child's patterns will help you interpret what's normal and what's not.

Most babies have their first bowel movement within the first two days of life. These stools, called meconium, tend to be thick, sticky and tarlike. They consist of skin cells the baby shed and then swallowed while he was in the womb. After the meconium is passed, stools will vary depending on whether your newborn is breastfed or formula-fed. Breast-milk stools tend to be soft, seedy and mustard colored, and babies will pass many small stools each day. It's normal for a breastfed two-week-old to have eight to ten stools a day, often runny at first, but gradually becoming firm.

A formula-fed baby's stools are yellow to brown in color and firmer than the stools of a breastfed baby. Formula-fed newborns also pass fewer—but larger and smellier—stools. Stools of babies fed our raw milk formula are much more like those of a breastfed baby.

Without your becoming obsessive about it, monitoring the frequency and quantity of bowel motions is one of the best ways of knowing whether the baby is getting enough milk.

After the first three or four weeks of life, some breastfed babies may suddenly change their stool pattern from many each day, to one every three days or even less. Some babies have gone as long as fifteen days or more without a bowel movement. As long as the baby is otherwise well, and the stool is the usual pasty or soft yellow movement, this is not constipation and is of no concern. However any baby between five and twenty-one days of age who does not pass at least one substantial bowel movement within a twenty-four-hour period should be seen by a pediatrician. Generally, small, infrequent bowel movements during this time period mean insufficient intake.

By one month of age, your baby will defecate less, regardless of how he's fed. The number of stools for breastfed babies drops to about four per day; formula-fed babies may pass a stool two times a day or as infrequently as once every other day. If baby goes more than two days without a bowel movement, follow our suggestions for constipation (page 149).

When your baby starts solid food, stools will turn brown, although they may occasionally reflect the color of foods eaten. Solid food tends to make the stools of breastfed infants firmer and the stools of formula-fed infants softer, but in either case the stools will probably smell worse.

DIAPER CHANGING OPPORTUNITY

You will probably want to set up a diaper changing station somewhere in your home, ideally a long counter or changing table in a warm bathroom. From the very start, even before baby can turn over, make it a habit to have a hand on your baby at all times during diapering. If you have to turn around,

CLOTH VERSUS DISPOSABLE DIAPERS

The argument for cloth diapers is persuasive.

ENVIRONMENT: Over ninety percent of disposable diapers end up in landfills, where they represent four percent of solid waste. Disposable diapers generate sixty times more solid waste, and they use twenty times more raw materials—such as crude oil and wood pulp—than cloth diapers. To produce one year's supply of disposable diapers for one baby requires more than three hundred pounds of wood, twenty pounds of chlorine, and fifty pounds of petroleum.[3] Of course, cloth diapers need to be washed, which uses up energy and clean water. However, the outcome, dirty water, is more easily recycled than a diaper in a landfill, which by some estimates takes two hundred fifty to five hundred years to degrade, even though today's conventional diapers are about forty percent biodegradable.

COST: If you wash baby's diapers at home, cloth diapers are a clear winner, costing about one thousand dollars less over three years than disposables. If you use a diaper laundering service, you will pay about the same amount as disposables—two thousand dollars or more over three years.

HEALTH AND COMFORT: Cloth diapers are more comfortable and less likely to cause diaper rash. Disposable diapers are more breathable, but their moisturizing, absorbent chemicals can be irritating. If you use disposables, be sure they are chlorine-free.

CONVENIENCE: Cloth diapers no longer require complicated folds and menacing pins; they now come with Velcro or snap closures, shapes fitted to baby, waterproof bands around the waist and legs, and removable linings, making the cloth change almost as quick and easy as the disposable (see Sources). Cloth diapers aren't as absorbent, though, so you'll have to change them more often.

On the downside, many day care centers don't allow cloth, and cloth diapers are not convenient for traveling. Even in the home setting, disposable diapers are easier to change and dispose of, and they tend to keep babies drier at night. Many a dedicated mom, having sworn to use cloth diapers, ends up using disposables instead. Fortunately, there are at least two nontoxic, biodegradable brands to choose from (see Sources).

keep your hand on baby's tummy to ensure he is safe. Some diaper changing tables have a strap to keep baby secure—by all means use this!

Set up your changing area to have clean diapers, changes of clothes, waste bucket, clothes hamper and a damp cloth or baby wipes handy. Premoistened wipes are very convenient, but the chemicals in them can cause or exacerbate diaper rash, so do opt for the non-chlorinated, gentle kind, or just use a moistened cloth to clean baby's bottom.

With everything in place and convenient, you can use diaper changing time as an opportunity to interact with your baby—cooing, smiling and stroking. As baby grows, he will use the diaper changing time to smile, gurgle and kick. Often baby's first smile occurs on the changing table.

BATHING BABY

Bathing baby for the first time can be a nerve-wracking experience. Fortunately, bathing isn't necessary for the first couple of weeks. Baby is born with a protective coating called vernix case-osa, which is best left on (see page 101). Baby can be dried after birth, and his bottom kept clean after diaper changings, but otherwise the first bath can

wait. The American Academy of Pediatrics recommends sponge baths until the umbilical cord stump falls off—which might take up to three weeks. But even sponge baths are not necessary.

Many babies get their first bath in the kitchen sink, but if that makes you nervous, you can use a plastic baby bathing tub set on a towel on the floor. The plastic tub can also be set in the bathtub—some are molded to support baby's back in a semi-upright position.

The important thing is to get everything ready before you start. The room and water should be warm, the towel ready and a mild shampoo on hand (see Sources). Have baby's next diaper and clean clothes nearby.

Your baby may not like his first bath very much, but with familiarity, will come to enjoy it. Once baby can sit up in the bath tub, he will enjoy his bath very much. Just remember, even if baby can sit up in the bath, he needs to be watched every minute.

There's no need to give your newborn a bath every day. In fact, bathing your baby more than several times a week can dry out his skin. Soap on baby's delicate skin is counterproductive. Just warm water

---

DIAPER RASH

Baby comes into the world with a beautiful, smooth bottom, but it seldom stays that way. Diaper rash is extremely common, in most cases mild and nothing to be concerned about. A good nutrient-dense diet will help baby build strong, resilient skin, and there are many things that parents can do to minimize the risk of diaper rash.

1. Change diapers frequently—at least every two hours in newborns. You can space this out as baby starts to urinate less often. You'd get diaper rash too if you had to wear a wet diaper!
2. Change poopy diapers right away—this is a lot of trouble at first since newborns often have small, frequent stools. Changings will become less frequent as baby grows.
3. Use "natural," scent-free brands of diapers and wipes, with as few chemicals as possible.
4. Wipe well and dry well. Be sure to wipe all the stool and urine away and then dry well with a soft cloth.
5. If using disposables, another brand or size may fit a little better and cause less friction.
6. Rinse cloth diapers by adding one-half cup of vinegar to the rinse cycle. This helps remove alkaline irritants. Your diaper service can also do this.
7. Apply coconut oil at every diaper changing. Coconut oil will heal and protect. Another choice is Weleda Diaper Cream (see Sources).
8. If you see a rash coming on, mix some cod liver oil with the coconut oil. Vitamins A and D in cod liver oil will help protect and heal the skin.
9. If weather permits, allow baby to play naked in the back yard to allow his bottom to "air out."

and a little scrub in the folds of his bottom, arms and knees is enough. Wash hair with a gentle shampoo and rinse by holding baby's head back. One of the advantages of the kitchen sink is the sprayer, which can be used to rinse baby's head. Just be sure to check the temperature of the water coming out of the sprayer before you use it.

After his bath, baby should be wrapped in a large, absorbent towel and thoroughly dried—including between the toes and in the creases.

BABY'S SLEEPING ARRANGEMENTS: CRIB OR BED?

A recent focus in child care involves baby's sleeping arrangements. Should baby sleep in the same room as his parents (called co-sleeping) or in the same bed (called bed-sharing) or in a separate room? The debate between those who advocate co-sleeping or bed-sharing and those who urge a separate room and crib for a newborn is often acrimonious, each side accusing the other of long-term damage to baby's psyche; in fact, one satirist called the dis-

ATTACHMENT PARENTING

Attachment parenting, a phrase coined by well-known pediatrician William Sears, is a parenting philosophy based on the principles of attachment theory in developmental psychology. According to attachment theory, the child forms a strong emotional bond with caregivers during childhood, with lifelong consequences. Sensitive and emotionally available parenting helps the child form a secure attachment style, which fosters a child's socio-emotional development and well-being.

While based on psychological theory, attachment parenting manifests in practice in three ways: co-sleeping, often to an advanced age; carrying baby in a sling until he is of an advanced age, usually until he can walk; and spending a large amount of time with the growing child, talking and interacting, described as "consistent, attentive responsivemess."

Critics of attachment parenting note that it can be very strenuous and demanding on parents—many mothers develop back and shoulder problems carrying a heavy baby in a sling. Writer Judith Warner contends that a "culture of total motherhood," which she blames in part on attachment parenting, has led to an "age of anxiety" for mothers in modern American society.[4] Sociologist Sharon Hays argues that the "ideology of intensive mothering" imposes unrealistic obligations and perpetuates a "double shift" life for working women.[5]

One can also criticize the effects of attachment parenting on the child. Does the developing baby and infant really want to be held all the time, or subjected to a barrage of "consistent, attentive responsiveness?" Are children so psychologically fragile that they need constant reassurance that their parents are right there? Children naturally want to accomplish milestones due to their own efforts, and they need to learn to be alone at times; they especially need to learn to play alone (see Chapter 10). Attachment parenting can interfere with a child's need to learn about the world on his own, and his gradual emergence into his sense of an independent self.

As with so many other controversies in the field of child development, most parents wisely choose a happy medium between constant parenting and cruel neglect. During the first few months of life, baby will do best with lots of contact, including co-sleeping and frequent carrying in a baby sling. But as baby gets older, he will benefit from *not* being carried. After all, he has important work to accomplish, learning to roll over, crawl, walk and explore his fascinating world. And baby will not suffer psychological harm from parental silence or even from being alone for a while. We all want time to ourselves, and that includes our infants. One very important milestone occurs when baby wakes up in his crib alone and spends time talking to himself. When he is ready for your company, he will let you know!

cussion "parenthood's all-out war" in a humorous essay, "Cribs vs. Beds."[6]

Proponents for co-sleeping and bed-sharing note that these were standard practices in many parts of the world, often for the very practical reason of keeping baby warm at night. Certainly, in many traditional cultures, bed-sharing is the only way to keep a baby safe. Proponents argue in addition that bed-sharing promotes bonding, facilitates breastfeeding and can even save babies' lives by preventing sudden infant death syndrome (SIDS). They also make the claim that co-sleeping allows parents to get more sleep.

Opponents of bed-sharing (including the American Academy of Pediatrics) cite the danger of baby being smothered or falling out of bed. Critics claim that it promotes an unhealthy dependence of the child on the parents and interferes with sexual relations of the parents.

The most well-known proponent of bed-sharing—or "shared sleep" as he calls it—is Dr. William Sears, author of *The Baby Book: Everything You Need to Know About Your Baby from Birth to Age Two*. He and his wife began the practice of bed-sharing with their fourth baby, who cried persistently when left alone in her crib. Bringing the baby into the bed was an act of desperation, one that allowed both baby and parents to get some sleep. The arrangement proved workable and harmonious; Dr. Sears observed that mother and baby slept on their sides, facing each other, with their breathing in sync.

On the other side of the debate, parenting experts such as Dr. Spock and Gary Ezzo, author of *Baby Wise*, claim that bed-sharing children will become manipulative, clingy and needy. And according to Ezzo, "The most serious sleep problems we've encountered are associated with parents who sleep with their babies."

The sleep advice given by *Baby Wise* is similar to Richard Ferber's advice given in his popular book *Solve Your Child's Sleep Problems*. The Ferber method of getting a baby to sleep starts with putting the baby to bed when awake. Baby is expected to learn how to fall asleep alone. Both authors warn parents against using aids such as pacifiers to ease the baby into sleep, and both methods describe putting the infant to sleep without prior rocking, cuddling or nursing applied for the sole purpose of calming the child into sleep. "Crying it out" is expected from the infant during the early training periods, until about eight weeks of age—advice that goes against all maternal instincts and could only come from men.

Between these extremes—bed-sharing for several years and letting a tiny baby cry it out in her crib—there has to be some middle ground, and in fact, there are many middle grounds, depending on the personality of the baby, the family dynamics and the sleep patterns of the parents.

Generally, during the first weeks mom will want to sleep with her newborn in the bed or nearby in a basinet or small crib. This allows her to breastfeed

SLEEPING SCHEDULES

Sleep is as important as food for a growing baby!

- At two months old, babies average 14.5 hours of sleep over a 24-hour period, 9.5 at night and 5 during naps.
- At six months of age, babies still average 14.5 hours , with 11 at night and 3.5 during naps.
- At one year, babies average 14 hours of sleep, 11.5 at night and 2.5 during naps.
- After about four months, the night time sleep should include one long period of "sleeping through the night," either from bedtime at 7-7:30 to 4-4:30 in the morning; or from about midnight (after a five-hour sleep) to about 7:30 in the morning.
- A good rule of thumb is for baby to sleep through the night before he can pull himself up in the crib. Babies have a hard time going back to sleep when they are standing up!

several times in the night without getting up; she will know when baby needs to nurse and can even snooze while baby is breastfeeding. In the early stages, her every instinct and hormone make separation painful. Dad may want to sleep in a different room during this early period. If all three share the bed, care must be taken to avoid crushing baby. Indeed, baby cots with crib bars on three sides, the fourth side open against the bed, can be purchased to allow safe bed-sharing.

This period may be a short one. As baby matures and mom's hormones wane, she may prefer to have baby in another room. Again, this need not be an all-

or-nothing decision. Mom can nurse baby to sleep in the family bed and then transfer the sleeping baby to a crib in the adjacent room; or, she may bring baby into the bed in the morning for nursing and snuggling.

Sarabenet Sequeira, a California holistic pediatrician, feels that the greatest danger of prolonged bed-sharing is lack of time for intimacy between mom and dad. Mom proudly announces at the one-year checkup that she is still bed-sharing and at the two-year checkup, confesses that she is divorced. Sequeira urges mothers to put baby in a crib in another room around the age of four months, about

PREVENTING SUDDEN INFANT DEATH SYNDROME

Sudden Infant Death Syndrome (SIDS), also referred to as cot death or crib death, is defined as the sudden death of an infant that is unexpected by medical history and remains unexplained even after autopsy. It is more common in male babies, babies of teenage mothers, babies born to mothers with lower rates of education and babies exposed to maternal smoking in utero. It is more common in premature babies and in formula-fed babies than in breastfed babies. The incidence increases with subsequent children—if a first child dies of SIDS, a SIDS death is more likely in a subsequent child.

SIDS occurs most frequently between the ages of two and four months, the age when babies begin receiving vaccinations. The medical establishment denies any connection between vaccinations and SIDS, but in a scientific study of SIDS, episodes of apnea (cessation of breathing) and hypopnea (abnormally shallow breathing) were measured before and after DPT vaccinations. "Cotwatch" (a precise breathing monitor) was used, and the computer printouts it generated (in integrals of the weighted apnea-hypopnea density—WAHD) were analyzed. The data clearly showed that vaccination caused an extraordinary increase in episodes where breathing either nearly ceased or stopped completely. These episodes continued for months following vaccinations. Dr. Viera Scheibner, the author of the study, concluded that "vaccination is the single most prevalent and most preventable cause of infant deaths."[7] As an epidemiological confirmation, when Japan changed the start time for vaccinating from three months to two years, their SIDS rate plummeted.

Another theory holds that SIDS is caused by normally harmless fungi and other microorganisms that consume the phosphorus, arsenic and antimony added as fire retardants and plastic softeners in baby mattresses and bedding. Before World War II, unexplained infant deaths were unusual. But after 1950, the governments of nearly all the rich industrialized countries required treatment of baby and child mattresses with flame retardant chemicals. Phosphorus and antimony were most commonly used; arsenic was sometimes added later as a preservative. After that, American SIDS deaths ballooned four hundred-fold; the toll has since declined. The presumed mechanism of death is the generation of extremely poisonous gases from the chemicals added to the mattresses. In consuming the chemicals, the fungi emit heavier-than-air neurotoxic gases based on phosphine (PH_3), arsine (AsH_3)[4] and stibine (SbH_3). These gases are about one thousand times more poisonous than carbon monoxide. They are about as toxic as Sarin, used in the 1980s Iran-Iraq war and in a Tokyo terrorist subway poisoning in 1995. The longer a fungi-infested mattress sits in a house, the more toxic gases it is likely to produce—an explanation for the increased rates of SIDS in children whose older siblings died of SIDS.

the time that mom wants to return to a more normal life. It certainly is normal for baby to be the center of attention during his first few months; but it is not normal for baby to be the center of attention for the longterm. Rest assured, sleeping in a room alone will not turn your child into an axe murderer—much more important is your loving attention and a nutritious diet during his waking hours.

What ultimately determines how long baby shares a bed with mom is how well mom—not baby—sleeps with this arrangement. Contrary to assumptions, baby is not quiet during sleep. He moves, sighs and fidgets, making sweet noises to which his mother is exquisitely sensitive. Many mothers simply cannot sleep a wink with their babies beside them, in which case baby should go into a crib in an adjoining room so that his cries, but not small noises, can be heard. A good night's sleep is of paramount importance for a new and nursing mother. If she is lucky, dad will get baby when he wakes during the night, change him and then bring him in to nurse so that mom doesn't have to get out of bed.

And while Dr. Sears and his wife, in desperation for sleep, brought their baby into the bed, sometimes the reverse is necessary and parents will indeed need to let baby "cry it out,"—although certainly not when baby is a tiny infant.

PREVENTING SUDDEN INFANT DEATH SYNDROME

In some cases, fungal growth in polyvinyl chloride (PVC), a soft plastic commonly used as the mattress covering, was associated with development of a pink stain in the shape of the sleeping infant. Such mattresses were always found to be generating one or more of the gases. Pink stain often results from, and demonstrates presence of, this type of fungal growth. There is even a reference and health warning in the Bible to pinkish mildew (*Leviticus* 14).

To prevent crib death, an appropriate gas-impermeable barrier is needed between mattress and baby. An inexpensive slip-on mattress cover called BabeSafe®—invented by New Zealander T. J. Sprott, PhD—came to market in New Zealand in 1996. Among one hundred thousand or so babies sleeping on this and similar products there and elsewhere, not one crib death has been reported.

If possible, use an organic mattress for baby, one that has not been treated with fire retardants. If using a conventional mattress, be sure to cover it with the BabeSafe mattress cover (see Sources). The mattress should be fitted with an organic mattress pad and a tightly fitted organic sheet. There should be no covering sheets or blankets, no pillow, no soft toys and no bumpers in the crib with baby. Keep him warm by dressing him in a sleep sack—made of organic cotton, of course (see Sources).

The American Academy of Pediatrics recommends putting baby to sleep on his back, which reduces the chance of suffocation or of breathing in toxic fumes from the mattress. Some practitioners have argued that putting baby on his back will limit the development of neck muscles, or cause baby to have flat spot on the back of the head. But Anat Baniel, author of *Kids Beyond Limits*, explains clearly that neck muscles will develop normally without giving baby "tummy time."[8] In any event, well nourished, strong babies will quickly learn to turn onto their stomachs, and these babies are also strong enough to move their heads from side to side as they sleep.

Having a fan in the room has been shown to reduce the incidence of SIDS. And while we often focus on keeping baby warm, it's important that baby be protected from overheating. SIDS deaths have occurred when sunlight coming through the window overheated a sleeping baby. Pull the shades down when baby sleeps and always make sure there is fresh air circulating in his room.

Source: *The Infant Survival Guide: Protecting Your Baby From the Dangers of Crib Death, Vaccines and Other Environmental Hazards* by Lendon Smith, MD and Joseph Hattersley, MA; *The Cot Death Coverup* by Jim Sprott.

SLEEPING THROUGH THE NIGHT

Entire parenting philosophies are built around the cause of getting baby to sleep through the night. *On Becoming Baby Wise: Giving Your Infant the Gift of Nighttime Sleep* is a controversial book by the aforementioned Gary Ezzo and conservative Christian pediatrician Robert Bucknam; the book presents an infant care program which the authors say will cause babies to sleep through the night beginning between seven and nine weeks of age. A reaction to "attachment parenting," in which a primary caregiver, usually mom, is constantly present to satisfy baby's every need, it emphasizes parental control of the infant's sleep, play and feeding schedule rather than allowing the baby to decide when to eat, play and sleep.

As can be expected, the *Baby Wise* program has come under criticism from a number of pediatricians and parents who are concerned that an infant reared using the book's advice will be at higher risk of failure to thrive, malnutrition and emotional disorders.

Certainly, sleeping through the night is an important milestone—not as much for baby as for her sleep-deprived parents. Absent from the whole discussion is the observation that all babies eventually sleep through the night, and they generally do so when their digestive systems are mature enough to make a midnight feeding unnecessary. Babies whose pregnant and nursing mothers eat according to our dietary principles tend to be excellent sleepers, usually sleeping through the night by the end of their second month.

Babies wake up in the night for many reasons, but a

BABY STUFF

Having a baby these days seems like a recipe for buying lots of equipment; in fact, if you are not careful, the equipment along with toys can take over your house, yard and car. It's hard to keep simple with so much high tech stuff on the market. Fortunately, the Internet allows you to carefully weigh your choices and shop judiciously.

CRIB: Baby will need a crib. If you are planning to co-sleep or bed-share, a crib that allows one side to go down, sometimes called a "side car cot," can be placed next to your bed. The crib can be moved to another room and used with the side put up when baby (or rather Mom) is ready to sleep alone. Most important is an organic mattress that has not been treated with flame retardants. If you are purchasing a used crib with a regular mattress, do obtain an organic cotton mattress pad and sheets if at all possible.

BABY SLING: These are great for carrying small babies. There are many designs available, some easier to use than others. Make sure that whatever you purchase has a good buckle or clasp that will not slip out. The important thing is a design that places baby sideways against your body or facing you with legs folded up or straight down, not facing you with his legs spread open.

CHANGING TABLE: You will need a safe place to change baby. Many moms have successfully used a kitchen or bathroom counter covered with a towel, but if you can afford a changing table with a strap to hold baby in, by all means purchase one. Changing tables are usually equipped with shelves to hold diapers, washcloth or wipes and baby clothes, thus helping prevent the invasion of baby stuff into the household's general living area.

PLAY PEN: Not an absolute necessity—you may be able to keep baby safe in a confined area using baby gates. Tiny babies can be set on a clean blanket or quilt on the floor. However, if your household is a busy one, you will need a playpen to protect baby from being stepped on. One model, called Pack and Play, doubles as a crib for babies up to about six months. It packs up into a neat package for traveling and use in non–child friendly environments. Also available are panels that make up an enclosed play area; they can be easily dismantled and are totally portable.

major one is when their blood sugar drops and they need nourishment; high-fat breast milk or high-fat homemade formula will keep baby's blood sugar stable so he can sleep longer.

Rather than suffer from sleep deprivation, or let their baby cry it out, parents of babies who are not sleeping through the night by three months of age should reexamine their diets. Is mom getting enough fat in her diet? Is she letting baby nurse long enough to get the high-fat hind milk from her breast? If baby is getting our homemade formula, try adding more cream to the bottle. By four months, even breastfed babies should be on cod liver oil, which supports maturation of the digestive and nervous systems, and will help turn baby into a good sleeper. If a fully breastfed baby is still waking up after four months, it's time to introduce solid food, with a feeding of egg yolk, puréed liver or even a teaspoon or more

of cream (preferably raw, but not ultrapasteurized) along with breastmilk or homemade formula right before bedtime. Baby can then go longer before needing food and presto! He sleeps through the night.

Be sure to lower the shades during naptimes and make sure that baby has fresh air in the room, ideally with an open window—he'll have trouble sleeping if the air in the room is hot and stuffy. When the weather is cold, dress baby in warm organic cotton pajamas or sleeping bag, but keep the window open just a crack; baby will be warm but will breathe cool fresh air.

It's a very good sign when baby plays and coos alone before going to sleep or upon waking—an indication of a well-nourished, contented baby. Baby needs time alone just as much as adults do!

BABY STUFF

INFANT SEAT: You will find an infant seat an extremely valuable piece of equipment for babies up to about six months old. They allow baby to observe household activities from a sitting up position and are great for feeding baby when solid food is introduced. Some models double as car seats. Baby should never be left alone in an infant seat.

CAR SEAT: These are required by law—all babies need to be in an approved car seat facing backwards when transported in a car. One important caveat: Never, never leave baby alone in a car in his car seat, not even for a few minutes. Cars heat up rapidly, especially when the windows are closed, and many babies have died due to overheating in a car seat.

STROLLER: You can spend hundreds of dollars on a stroller but it is not necessary. An inexpensive collapsible "umbroller" serves just as well. And you don't even need a design with a sunshade—sunlight is good for baby, and when the sun is very bright, baby can wear a hat. Many fancy strollers keep baby enclosed in protective plastic sheets—not a good idea when the whole point of taking baby for a stroll is to give him fresh air.

BABY GATES: As soon as baby begins to crawl, you will need these to keep baby in childproofed areas of the house. If you have stairs, baby gates may be necessary at the top and bottom.

CHILDPROOF LATCHES: You'll need these for lower cupboards in the kitchen and bathrooms, as soon as baby can sit up and scoot across the floor. Even with latches, it's a good idea to clear lower cupboards of anything poisonous or dangerous, as many toddlers soon learn to open them. This includes household cleaning items, especially dishwasher powder, and anything breakable.

BATHING TUB: Plastic baby-friendly tubs for bathing can be used in the kitchen sink, on the floor or in the bath tub. They make bathing time less nerve-wracking; but remember, even with these shallow tubs, baby should never be left alone in the bath.

BABY POTTY: An inexpensive baby potty is very helpful for toilet training.

If baby has trouble sleeping, wakes up frequently or sleeps fretfully, look first to the diet. Is breastfeeding mom eating processed food, full of MSG and related flavoring agents, refined sweeteners, caffeine and industrial fats and oils? Components that cause insomnia can come through the breastmilk, affecting your baby's sleep patterns. Or, is baby getting commercial baby foods including canned food containing hydrolyzed vegetable protein (which contains MSG) or commercial baby formula, another source of MSG? In sensitive people, even small amounts of MSG can disrupt sleep patterns, so why not also in infants?

Above all, make sure your baby is getting enough fat, from your rich breastmilk or from a cream-rich homemade formula. Nothing ensures restful sleep like a diet containing plentiful healthy fats.

Another consideration to baby's successful sleep is chemical-free sleepwear and bed linens. They should be pure organic cotton, free of chemicals such as flame retardants (see Sources).

PACIFIERS AND TEETHING

Pacifier use is seen worldwide as as a soothing and calming device for infants. Many parents have strong opinions about whether or not infants should use pacifiers at all.

The main objection to pacifier use is "nipple confusion" in breastfed infants. The concern is that these infants may wean earlier from the breast, though the evidence for this is not conclusive. It is generally recommended to withhold pacifiers from breastfed infants until one month of life, at which time the

NOT GOOD FOR BABY

While parents have many choices of fine baby equipment these days, from strollers to carseats, there are some items they need to avoid.

BABY MONITOR: Better not to use one as wireless baby monitors in North America constantly emit microwave radiation. The base station of the baby monitor is kept near the crib while the parent takes the receiver and either wears it in a hip pocket or on a belt, or places it nearby. Ideally a baby monitor base station should be voice-activated, meaning that it transmits sound only when it senses a sound from the baby. This would reduce the microwave exposure of both infant and parent. Unfortunately, most baby monitors emit microwave radiation all the time that they are on.[9]

Low EMF monitors from Europe, called Babyfon, are available on Amazon in the U.K., but they are not sold in the U.S.! If you import one, you would need to purchase the right voltage converter.

Try to organize your house so that you can hear baby from his crib, rather than having to resort to a baby monitor. This might mean a second crib, basinet or bed in the main part of the house.

BABY WALKERS: It's very tempting to put baby in a baby walker—babies love them and parents like the fact that when baby is in his walker, they are free to get things done. But parents should know that walker use typically delays motor development—and that it may delay mental development even more.

As they grow, healthy babies develop a strong urge to move across the floor. At first, this is a struggle for them as they work their arms and legs, stretching, rolling, scooting or crawling. They find delight in accomplishment as they achieve their goal of grabbing an object out of reach. Later, the focus of their work will turn to pulling themselves upright.

Babies who use a walker skip some of this magnificent developmental journey. With their toes in an unnatural position, they glide across the floor with ease, moving upright before they are physically ready to do so.

infant-mother "mechanics" of breastfeeding as well as maternal milk supply should be well established.

Pacifier use has also been associated with a slight increase in ear infections[12] as well as oral yeast (thrush),[13] presumably from contamination of the pacifier with these organisms. And some recalled models have caused cases of choking on the devices, and strangulation on pacifier cords.

Lastly, vigorous sucking of pacifiers is said to alter the structure of the roof of the mouth and teeth over time, resulting in malocclusion, although as we have shown, the shape of the jaw is largely determined by nutrition (see page 124). In any event, manufacturers claim that newer varieties are configured so as to minimize inpact on palate shape.

The most compelling benefit for pacifier use is a decrease in the incidence of SIDS by about 50 percent.[14] The exact mechanism for this finding is unknown but the result has been reported in several studies from different countries.

The objection to the pacifier is that it is a prop, and a plastic one at that. It is sometimes difficult to wean older children off the pacifier—and while it may seem normal for babies to suck on a pacifier, most of us balk at the sight of an older child still sucking away.

Hopefully, with our dietary guidelines, the pacifier will never be needed to calm fussiness.

Take care when choosing a pacifier that it is made

NOT GOOD FOR BABY

Babies who use walkers learn to stand and walk later than they would have otherwise, and continue to show delayed motor development for months after they have learned to walk. The delay is about two to three weeks in learning to walk.[10] Worse, with walkers, babies often skip the crawling stage, and some child development experts theorize that children who skip crawling are likely to have reading difficulties later on. This may help explain delays in mental development and lower scores on mental developmental testing, still present ten months after initial walker use.

In addition, walkers are dangerous. In 1994, the Consumer Products Safety Commission declared that baby walkers were responsible for more injuries than any other children's product. The types of injuries included head injuries, broken bones, broken teeth, burns, entrapment of fingers and even amputations or death. Walkers allow mobility beyond a baby's natural capability, and faster than a parent's reaction time. Most of the injuries involve falls down stairs, but injuries can also come, for instance, from allowing baby to reach hot, heavy or poisonous objects. Today's walkers are safer, but they are still hazardous— and of no benefit to the baby.[11] Stationary activity centers for babies can provide many of the benefits parents are looking for from walkers, without the serious problems.

BABY JUMPERS: Not only are walkers bad for development, but baby jumpers are too. Infants in jumpers will push as if they are wanting to push and jump, but what's really happening is that the devices are exploiting a reflex (the homologous push reflex) at the expense of others. There are a handful of healthy and basic reflexes that all infants have and these reflexes are the beginnings of developing neurological motor patterns necessary for conscious and healthy movement.

When a single reflex is exploited over and over, like the push reflex in the jumpers, its balancing reflex is left behind and the baby will, if left in this device too long, develop neurological movement patterns that may seem harmless at first, but over time can create vulnerabilities in movement. A baby in the Johnny jumper will have excessive development in extensor tone and will be more likely to be a toe walker, a problem that is very difficult to overcome later in life.

Furthermore, the jumpers can be dangerous—baby can hit his head, and the jumpers can break.

pure, natural rubber (see Sources). Newer plastic ones are free of bisphenol-A, but there are plenty of other endocrine-disrupting chemicals in plastics.

As for soothing the teething baby, the best remedy is a teething ring, again of pure rubber, free of the many toxic additives found in plastic (see Sources).

SCHEDULES

Until Dr. Spock came along, most baby rearing manuals advocated strict feeding and sleeping schedules for babies; feeding at three-hour intervals was the usual recommendation for infants and toilet training beginning at three months! (John B. Watson, author of the *Psychological Care of Infant and Child*, 1928, recommended toilet training starting at three weeks.) Dr. Spock wisely advised mothers to relax and not worry about strict schedules; toilet training was mercifully put off until an age when the child could walk to the toilet and understand its use.

The success of a feeding schedule depends first and foremost on mom's breastmilk supply. If she has plenty of milk, and the milk is of good quality, her newborn will go at least two hours between feedings just after birth and settle into a three-hour schedule within a matter of days. This translates into about six feedings per day and one during the night. Babies who cry and need to be fed more often are probably not getting enough with the feeding. If she has the time to feed baby on demand many times per day, mom may be able to wait until the introduction of solid food and then settle into a schedule; but if she has many demands on her time, she will need to supplement with our homemade baby formula so that baby can settle into a reasonable sort of routine.

While you do not need to worry about strict feeding and sleeping schedules for an infant, the goal as baby grows is a structured day of feedings and sleep times. Feedings at early morning, and mid morning followed by a short morning nap, then at noon, followed by nap time, then afternoon, evening and

---

TOYS

As with baby equipment, the motto is, keep it simple, and keep it safe. Stuffed animals should be made with chemical-free materials; nothing should have sharp edges; painted toys should be nontoxic; and no toy should be smaller than anything that can be put into a film canister.

Remember that almost anything can serve as a toy to an infant—wooden spoons, stainless steel bowls, a set of measuring spoons and wooden slotted clothes pins can all serve as play things. The key is providing objects that are safe for baby to put into his mouth—because that is what baby will do.

Old magazines make great distractions for babies—they love to rip the pages out!

As baby grows, toys that allow him to imitate adults have great appeal. A small broom and dust bin can keep a toddler occupied for long stretches of time. With a small rag he can "dust" the furniture.

Crayons and a large pad of paper on an easel provide a much more appropriate artistic outlet for your child than flash cards of famous paintings.

Toys that last and that exercise your child's creative abilities are a good investment. These include wooden blocks, Duplos and wooden train sets. When your child outgrows these, they can be put away and brought out again for grandchildren!

There's no getting around gender preferences when it comes to toys. Girls are likely to be attracted to dolls and horses, boys to trucks, airplanes and trains.

Above all, don't let a huge collection of toys overrun your house. Large baskets or boxes to store toys in will prevent clutter. As baby gets older, do let her help with putting toys away.

bed time feedings, provide a comforting pattern for baby and allow a well-rested mom to plan and accomplish her chores.

As baby grows, he will soon settle into a schedule of breakfast, lunch, nap and early dinner, with a snack after nap time if dinner is late. Sticking more or less to this schedule will prevent low-blood sugar meltdowns and bouts of exhausted crying. The key is nourishing, satisfying food at each feeding and withholding snacks between the expected feeding times.

Much more important than strict schedules for infants is a reliable meal pattern for toddlers and growing children. Children should not be fed on demand or given whatever they want to eat. Rather, parents should institute a workable meal schedule and provide meals that are nutritious, satisfying and tasty. Children should expect as normal that they eat what their parents prepare for them, and eat at regular meal times. Obviously, this means that parents should keep snack foods out of sight, and follow a regular meal pattern themselves.

CLOTHING

Keep it simple, and keep it pure. Purchase clothing that is as chemical-free as possible, and wash with a mild detergent. Never use fabric softener or detergents with artificial scents added. Above all, avoid sleepwear treated with flame retardant.

Flame retardants pose a real danger to all of us, but especially to the infant. One of them, polybrominated diphenylether or PBDE, can adversely affect your baby's developing brain and developing reproductive system. There is limited evidence to indicate that PBDE can cause cancer.[15]

The bromine in PBDE and similar products can replace iodine in the thyroid gland, thus seriously jeopardizing the normal development of your baby.[16] Unlike many other industrial chemicals, brominated flame retardants build up inside the human body and are very difficult to detoxify.

PBDEs are found in mattresses, upholstered furniture, carpets, baby seats and blankets; but the worst offender is children's sleepwear, which exposes baby to these chemicals constantly during sleep.

Choose your baby's clothing carefully. Currently, all sleepwear for babies sized twelve months and up that is not snug-fitting nor 100 percent cotton is treated with flame retardants. Instead of loose fitting pajamas, use a cotton tee shirt and loose cotton pants for sleepwear. Above all, check with the manufacturer about whether their baby clothes are treated.

Tiny babies need cotton undershirts and pajamas, preferably one-piece pajamas with feet. Older children do well in overalls that close with snaps on the inside legs.

For natural, chemical-free baby clothes as well as chemical-free sheets, mattress pads and baby blankets, see Sources.

SUNLIGHT

It's good for baby! Older books on baby care universally advised putting baby in the sun to sunbathe whenever possible. Today in our solarphobic society, moms get dire warnings about letting their children play in the sunlight; even the naturalistic Dr. Sears advises slathering babies with sun screen from the age of six months.

Of course, we should protect our children against sunburn. If baby is going to be out in the bright sun for any length of time, cover his torso with a tee shirt and head with a hat. But ten to thirty minutes of sun per day on baby's bare body helps him produce vitamin D and may have many other benefits. Start when baby has reached twelve pounds or so. Coconut oil on his skin will protect against dryness. In fact, the natives studied by Dr. Price believed that sunlight shining on coconut oil actually nourished the skin.[17]

For his sunbath, place baby face down on a clean blanket, wearing nothing but his diaper—if he has diaper rash, omit the diaper and let the sunlight do its magic healing work. For very fair babies, the sunbath should occur before ten in the morning or after four in the afternoon. Begin with five minutes to a side, gradually working up to ten minutes. After five to ten minutes, turn baby over, When baby is on his back, make sure that his eyes are shaded.

Baby can spend even longer naked in the fresh air

if he is in the shade. Such sun and fresh air therapy may do wonders for fussiness and fretful sleep patterns.

The recommendation to slather children with sunscreen—many parents apply sunscreen daily under baby's clothes, "just in case" he might get exposed to sunlight—is highly irresponsible. Dermatologists and pediatricians have insisted that such sunscreen use would prevent skin cancer and protect our health. However, over the past decade, many scientists studying cancer have come to the opposite conclusion; that is, the use of sunscreen chemicals may be increasing the incidence of cancer while sunlight exposure can decrease human cancer rates and improve our health.

Sunscreens increase cancer rates by virtue of their free radical-generating properties. And more insidiously, many commonly used sunscreen chemicals have strong estrogenic actions that may cause serious problems in sexual development and adult sexual function. The body has difficulty removing these chemicals; they can accumulate in the tissues for serious longterm effects.

Most chemical sunscreens contain, as UVA and UVB blockers, from 2 to 5 percent of compounds such avobenzone, benzophenone, ethylhexyl p-methoxycinnimate, 2-ethylhexyl salicylate, homosalate, octyl methoxycinnamate and oxybenzone (benzophenone-3) as the active ingredients.[18] Benzophenone (and similar compounds) is one of the most powerful free radical generators known. It is used in industrial processes as a free radical generator to initiate chemical reactions. Benzophenone is activated by ultraviolet light energy, which breaks benzophenone's double bond to produce two free radical sites. The free radicals then react with other molecules and produce damage to the fats, proteins and DNA of the cells—the types of damage that produce skin aging and the development of cancer.

Adding to the problem is the fact that large amounts of applied sunscreens can enter the bloodstream though the skin. This may be a factor in the large increases in cancer (breast, uterine, colon, prostate) observed in Northern Australia, where the use of sunscreen chemicals has been heavily promoted by medical groups and the local governments.

These free radical-generating sunscreen chemicals also have estrogen-like effects. Such effects can increase cancers, cause birth defects in children, lower sperm counts and penis size in men, plus contribute to a plethora of other medical problems. These effects are similar to those of many banned chemicals such as DDT, dioxin, PCBs.

Estrogenic chemicals can mimic hormonal estrogen, the key female sex hormone. When the body's hormone receptors recognize the estrogenic chemical as estrogen, the result is feminization of the tissue.[19]

Conventional sunscreen is not something you want to put on your precious child! However, for intense sun exposure, use a natural zinc oxide on baby's nose, shoulders and other vulnerable spots (see Sources).

Strange as it may seem, you may be able protect your child from sunburn to a certain extent with his diet. Many have reported that babies who consume mostly saturated fats, found in butter, cream, meat fats and coconut oil, are more likely to tan, while a diet of polyunsaturated vegetable oils is a recipe for skin that sunburns.

GERMS

The sun is our friend, not our enemy, and so are germs. The goal is not to prevent contact with germs by using antibacterial wipes and soaps, but to develop an immunity to the harmful ones and a symbiotic relationship with the friendly ones. Your child's diet, based on breastmilk or raw milk, rich in vitamins A and D, as well as lacto-fermented foods, is a key factor for building immunity for life.

But to build this immunity, baby also needs to be exposed to germs! Don't worry about baby being on the floor, playing in the dirt, snuggling pets or generally getting exposed to life. As long as his diet supports the immune system, the contact with microbial life will be beneficial. One study even showed that exposure to germs made mice smarter![20]

Of course, you will want to prevent contact with rotten food, animal feces, infected or stagnant water, dead animals and other potential sources of bacteria and parasites that might create a toxic overload, but otherwise well-nourished babies are perfectly capable of handling the myriad species of bacteria with which they come in contact.

CHILDPROOFING

As baby begins to crawl, you will need to childproof your house. In the kitchen and bathroom, that means putting all household cleaners and toiletries up on high shelves. Childproof latches will keep babies out of cupboards for a while, but most toddlers will learn to open them by watching you.

In the rest of the house, you will need to put all objects that are breakable, that have sharp edges, or that present a swallowing danger away until your child is older and no longer tempted by every object that meets his eye. Baby will be safer and you will be a much more relaxed mother if you put your valuable and cherished objects out of sight for a few years.

Gates that keep your child away from the stairs and corralled in an area (usually a room) where baby will be safe without your having to keep a constant eye on him are a must in today's open plan houses.

It goes without saying that if you have a swimming pool, it needs to be enclosed with a childproof fence that is kept securely locked at all times.

Be careful to turn pot handles away from you on the stove to avoid spills of scalding liquids; in any case, baby should be kept well away from the stove area.

Cords for curtains and shades present the danger of strangulation. Make sure these are out of reach. Never place baby's crib within arm's length of curtain or shade cords.

If you have a garden area where your child can play, that should be childproofed also. Obviously, you should not use any pesticides or herbicides in your garden. Gate latches and locks should be placed well above your child's head and all sharp garden implements should be safely stored away. Children can spend many happy hours in a garden with large balls, a tricycle and plastic child-sized gardening implements.

TOILET TRAINING

Starting in 1914, the U.S. Department of Labor Children's Bureau put out a series of publications called *Infant Care*, which provides us with an interesting history of toilet training philosophies over the years. The 1914 edition recommended toilet training to begin by the third month "with the utmost gentleness." The 1929 and 1935 editions recommended a method that used suppositories to put the baby on a strict schedule of bowel movements. In 1938, parents were advised to start bowel training "as early as the sixth month."

However, by 1951, fears of psychological ramifications from early training emerged, and parents were advised to wait "between one and a half to two years" to commence training. In 1957, the average age of starting toilet training was still under one year, at eleven months, and 90 percent of children were dry during the day by two years.

Today, toilet training takes place much later. In 2002, the average age that parents recognized their child "showing an interest in using the potty" was about twenty-four months, and daytime dryness was achieved on average at almost three years of age. Nighttime accidents are now considered normal until five or six years of age.[21]

It's easy to speculate on the reasons for the increasing age of successful toilet training. Is it because children are getting harder to train, or are parents more concerned about the psychological effects of early training? Or, do parents simply have less incentive to toilet train with modern diapers, washing machines and indoor plumbing? Whatever the reason, most books on baby and child care advise parents not to be concerned if their child is not toilet trained until the age of three or even four—it's comforting to realize that all normal children, and even most developmentally challenged children, eventually learn to use the toilet.

Some children, usually girls, become potty trained very early, simply by sitting on a baby potty in the bathroom and imitating mommy. Others—most often boys—seem to actively resist training, even though they are obviously aware of the need to eliminate and sufficiently verbal to understand a parent's explanations.

Pediatrician Lindy Woodard believes that a child can and should be trained by thirty months; in her professional experience, children who are trained at an older age have more problems learning to use the toilet.

Numerous books and manuals address the subject of toilet training the modern child. Most agree that it is fruitless to begin training until your child is ready. Signs of readiness include:

- Your child signals that his diaper is wet or soiled.
- Your child seems interested in the potty chair or toilet.
- Your child says that he would like to go to the potty.
- Your child understands and follows basic instructions.
- Your child feels uncomfortable if his diaper is wet or soiled.

- Your child stays dry for periods of two hours or longer during the day.
- Your child wakes up from naps with a dry diaper.
- Your child can pull his pants down and then up again.

Actual training involves discipline in the true sense of the word—a learning process in which the teacher provides instruction through example, explanation, watchfulness and praise.

Start by allowing your child to be present when you go to the bathroom and make him feel comfortable in the bathroom. Allow him to see urine and bowel movements in the toilet. Let him practice flushing the toilet—he will love doing this! Have your child become familiar with the potty chair by placing it in the normal living and play area. You can also install a potty seat on the toilet and let him sit there if he wants to.

ELIMINATION COMMUNICATION

Elimination Ccommunication (EC) is a process that involves observing baby's signs and signals, providing cue sounds and elimination-place associations so that baby can go diaper free (at least during the day) from a very early age. The theory is that the natural age at which babies can signal their elimination needs is much earlier than the age currently acknowledged in our society.

The practice assumes a lot of time on the part of the mother, engaged in co-sleeping, nursing freely and promptly responding to baby's needs. With such closeness, mom might notice, for example, that baby pees five minutes after nursing, or grunts just before he poops.

If you think your baby is ready to urinate or defecate, the next step involves sitting on the toilet holding baby's back to your stomach and making a specific cueing sound to "invite" your baby to pee or poop. In most places where EC is practiced culturally, caregivers use a watery sound such as "psss." This sound, along with a particular position, is used to signal or stimulate the baby's elimination. When you are starting out, make your cueing sound every time you notice your baby peeing. Within a few days, your baby will associate the sound with the act of eliminating. By practicing EC consistently, your baby will learn to release her bladder at will upon hearing the cueing sound when being held in the potty position. A grunt sound will cue your baby to defecate. For further information, visit www.diaperfreebaby.org/.

Critics contend that the training involves "attachment parenting" in spades, and is simply off limits for mothers who work or have large families. It involves constant attention to the baby, looking for "signs," when modern diapers—whether disposable or not—are a blessing that allows mom to have time of her own, even with an infant in the house.

Nevertheless, many mothers and caregivers enthusiastically report good results with EC. Pediatrician Lindy Woodard notes that many babies who suffer from colic stop crying when their mothers "EC" them. While not for everyone, she reports that caregivers and babies practicing EC seem attached, confident and contented. The process is most easy and natural around the age of eighteen months.

Allow your child to observe, touch and become familiar with the potty chair. Tell him that the potty chair is his own chair; he can sit fully clothed on the potty chair, as if it were a regular chair if he wants to. After your child has become used to the potty chair and sits on it regularly with his clothes on, try having him sit on the potty without wearing pants and a diaper. The next step is to show your child how the potty chair is used. Place stool from a dirty diaper into the potty chair. Allow him to observe the transfer of the stool from the potty chair into the toilet. Let him flush the toilet and watch the stool disappear down the toilet.

After your child has become comfortable with flushing the toilet and sitting on the potty chair, you may begin teaching him to go to the bathroom. Keep him in loose, easily removable pants—you can call them

SHAKEN BABY SYNDROME

Shaken baby syndrome (SBS) is a triad of medical symptoms—subdural hematoma (blood on the surface of the brain), retinal hemorrhage and cerebral edema (water in the brain)—from which doctors infer child abuse caused by intentional shaking. In a majority of cases there is no visible sign of external trauma. SBS is often fatal or causes severe brain damage, resulting in lifelong disability. Estimated death rates among infants with SBS range from 15 to 38 percent. Parents accused of SBS often face charges of child abuse or even murder, and have their children taken into foster care.

The theory that shaking babies could cause intracranial hemorrhages was introduced in a 1972 paper by Dr. John Caffey, "On the Theory and Practice of Shaking Infants: Its Potential Residual Effects of Permanent Brain Damage and Mental Retardation."[22] Caffey based his theories on whiplash studies inducing intracranial hemorrhaging in rhesus monkeys in rear-end collisions, even though the author of the study advised Caffey that no information could substantiate such injuries in humans from shaking.[23] Unfortunately, Caffey's theory has prevailed in medicine and law ever since. In a later paper, Caffey claimed that subdural and retinal hemorrhaging without signs of external physical abuse would be sufficient to diagnose child abuse.[24] Many parents have suffered the anguish of finding their baby unresponsive, only to be followed by the further anguish of losing their child to foster care. Sometimes they are charged with child abuse when a doctor finds a bruise with a follow-up x-ray showing multiple bone fractures.

A new theory, delineated in a 2011 paper by attorney Matthew B. Seeley, JD, argues that SBS is actually a manifestation of vitamin D deficiency and rickets. In cases of SBS, he suggests that children be given a single-photon absorptiometry test, which has been used for years to measure bone density in children. That type of test could exonerate or prove SBS charges, especially if an infant were born prematurely, or when there are no signs of physical abuse presenting on the child's body.[25] Additionally, Seeley argues that a blood serum Vitamin D test should be mandated and taken of both the supposedly abused infant *and* his postpartum mother. The mother's test results could indicate the proclivity to *in utero* rickets, depending upon how long after the birth the SBS tragedy occurred, while the infant's test results would confirm insufficient Vitamin D levels, which allowed the child to have bone fractures either during the birthing process or even from normal daily baby care, since no one knew of the child's fragile bones.

Deficiency of vitamin C is another potential cause of SBS. Infantile scurvy still occurs today and can be mistakenly diagnosed as nonaccidental injury.

Another possible culprit is vaccinations, especially vaccinations given to tiny babies. Many incidences of SBS occur after an inoculation, to which a vitamin D- ot vitamin C-deficient baby may be especially vulnerable.[26]

The tragic consequences of shaken baby syndrome should give parents extra incentive to follow a nutrient-dense diet, rich in vitamin D and other fat-soluble vitamins as well as calcium and vitamin C, throughout pregnancy and lactation, and to feed their babies nourishing traditional foods.

"big girl" or "big boy" pants to motivate your child.

Place your child on the potty chair whenever he signals the need to go to the bathroom. Your child's facial expression may change when he feels the need to urinate or to have a bowel movement. He may stop any activity he is engaged in when he feels the need to go to the bathroom.

Most children have a bowel movement shortly after eating, and they urinate within an hour after having a large drink. So in the early stages of toilet training, parents need to be watchful.

In addition to watching for signals that your child needs to urinate or have a bowel movement, place him on the potty at regular intervals.

ALBION'S SEED: FOUR PHILOSOPHIES OF CHILD REARING

Childrearing philosophies are a contentious issue in America, perhaps because the different immigrant groups coming to this country had different views on the nature of childhood and the type of upbringing that children need. *Albion's Seed: Four British Folkways in America* is a 1989 book by David Hackett Fischer that examines the the folkways of four groups of settlers from the United Kingdom to the American colonies. According to Fischer, the foundation of American culture was formed from four mass emigrations from four different regions of the British Isles by four different socio-religious groups.

New England's constitutional period occurred between 1629 and 1640 when Puritans, most from East Anglia, settled there. The next mass migration was of southern English cavaliers and their Irish and Scottish servants to the Chesapeake Bay region between 1640 and 1675. Then, between 1675 and 1725 thousands of Irish, English and Welsh Quakers led by William Penn, along with large numbers of Germans who strongly sympathized with the Quakers, settled the Delaware Valley. Finally, Irish, Scottish and English settlers from the borderlands of Britain and Ireland migrated to Appalachia between 1717 and 1775. Each of these migrations produced a distinct regional culture that can still be seen in America today. Each of these distinct cultures had its own child rearing practices.

The Puritans of New England subscribed to the doctrine of original sin and believed in the natural depravity of the child; small children were disposed to do evil, and so their wills must be broken at an early age. New England autobiographies of that era remember childhood not with nostalgia but with persistent feelings of pain and guilt. The "breaking of the will" constituted a determined effort to destroy the spirit of autonomy in a small child. Any manifestations of willfulness were restrained and repressed. This process was usually achieved by strict and rigorous supervision rather than corporal punishment, although most Puritans subscribed to the epigram "better whipped than damned." Children were trained to regard their elders with a mixture of love and fear; they were required, for example, to stand and bow when their parents approached, and forbidden to show fondness and familiarity. In addition, the Puritans subscribed to the custom of "sending out," usually at the age of puberty. Children were sent to be raised in other homes, for practical purposes, such as to place a child close to a school, to prepare for a profession, or to put a child in an intact family after the loss of a parent. In addition, the Puritans believed that children would learn better manners and behavior in a setting outside the home.

Among the Virginian aristocrats, as well as their servants, growing up was a process full of pain and difficulty. Virginians appeared to be exceptionally indulgent toward their children, and children were not considered inherently evil. But growing up involved a process of "bending the will," of adherence to two different and contradictory demands. Youngsters were expected and compelled to develop strong and autonomous wills; but also expected to yield willingly to the requirements of an hierarchical culture. These psychic tensions took a heavy toll. Parents took pride in "childish acts of autonomy," and boys were expected to be willful and wild. Boys, but not girls, were expected to develop strong wills and boisterous emotions—if not they were thought unmanly; in fact, boys were usually booted out of the manor house at puberty to live elsewhere on the plantation, in a *garconière*, where they could be as wild as they wanted to be, without parental supervision. The "bending of the will" to strict demands of comportment and etiquette by adulthood was accomplished by requiring children to observe elaborate

Stay with your child when he is on the potty chair. Reading or talking to him when he is sitting on the potty may help him relax. Praise your child when he goes to the bathroom in the potty chair, but do not express disappointment if he does not urinate or have a bowel movement in the potty. Patience is key!

Once your child has learned to use the potty chair, he can begin using an over-the-toilet seat and a step-up stool.

Experts disagree about whether to use disposable training pants. Some think that training pants may confuse children and make them think it is okay to use them like diapers. This may slow the toilet

---

ALBION'S SEED: FOUR PHILOSOPHIES OF CHILD REARING

rituals of self-restraint and rules of conduct, all epitomized in formal dancing instruction. All children of every level of society were compelled to learn these rules of conduct. George Washington's list of "Rules of Civility and Decent Behavior in Company and Conversation" serve as an example of the expectations imposed on children from an early age. The social creed was fundamentally a form of stoicism to which all children and young adults were expected to adhere. A gentleman of Virginia was expected to have boisterous feelings, manly passions and a formidable will; in addition, he was expected to achieve a stoic mastery of self. These expectations put considerable stress on growing children and resulted in a society with a patina of politeness that harbored a fair number of sexual predators.

Quakers generally rejected the idea that children were evil, believing that small children were "harmless, righteous and innocent creatures." The Society of Friends believed that children were incapable of sin until old enough to understand their acts. Quaker society held a special intensity and interest in the young—it was much more child-centered than the other cultures. Settlers in Pennsylvania and nearby regions believed that small childen should be sheltered from the world and raised within a carefully controlled environment—"trained up" by control of their surroundings. As the child grew, parents preferred "bracing the will" of their children through appeal to their reason. The Quakers made heavy use of rewards rather than punishment, promises rather than threats. Corporal punishment was used in moderation. But the culture was not permissive. Children were trained to silence and subjection, not so much to parents or elders but to the larger family of the meeting. Individuality was subordinated to the entire community. Training up children was a communal process that involved lots of socializing with other children. The culture was fairly egalitarian, with the same standards expected of both sexes and a big emphasis on treating all siblings fairly. Quaker parents imposed much more restraint than the other three groups when their children reached puberty—the Quakers had strict rules against dancing and drinking—and children lived at home longer than in other cultures.

The backwoods culture of Appalachia aimed at "building the will." The rearing of male children was meant to foster fierce pride, stubborn independence and a warrior's courage. The effect was a society of autonomous individuals "who were unable to endure external control and incapable of restraining their rage against anyone who stood in their way." Stories told to children celebrated courage, pride and independence, and sports celebrated one-on-one contests such as wrestling, running and fighting. Recklessness and fearless courage were highly admired traits in backwoods boys. Infants of both sexes received indulgent attention, attention that dwindled as the child grew. The culture was not egalitarian; female children were expected to exhibit the virtues of obedience, patience, sacrifice and devotion, to be self-denying, while male chilfdren were expected to be self-asserting. Corporal punishment was frowned on, but in practice many children received terrific beatings. Thus the process of child rearing was highly volatile, permissive most of the time but punctuated by acts of angry violence, often compounded by alcohol.

Even today we can recognize these differing attitudes in various child-rearing books and manuals; and parental child-rearing methods often reflect the cultural attitudes of their ancestors.

training process. Others think training pants may be a helpful step when you are training your child. Sometimes, training pants are used at nighttime, when it is more difficult for a child to control his bladder.

It is normal for a child to have an occasional accident even after he learns how to use the toilet. Sometimes, children get too involved in activities and forget that they need to use the bathroom. Suggesting regular trips to the bathroom may help prevent some accidents.

If your child does have an accident, stay calm. Do not punish him. Simply change him and continue to encourage him to use the potty chair.

Some children learn to use the toilet with just a few weeks of training; others take as long as three to six months. If your child resists, discontinue training for a while and then take it up again.

What if your child reaches preschool age, has normal communication skills and still resists toilet training? You may need to take your child out of diapers and just hope for the best—usually the embarassment of wet or soiled pants will quickly con-

vince your child that using the toilet is best. Some parents, in desperation, have used reverse psychology and forbidden their recalcitrant five-year-old to use the toilet! In defiance, the child becomes toilet trained.

DISCIPLINE

The debate about whether and how to discipline children has been ongoing for decades, hardliners arguing for strict discipline starting in infancy, with spankings and corporal punishment if necessary for toddlers and older; "softliners" are adverse to any kind of corrective action other than patient explanations of why a child should not engage in certain behaviors.

The word for discipline comes from the Latin *disciplina*, meaning teaching or learning, not punishing. The word "disciple" has the same root as "discipline." All cultures have ways of teaching children how to avoid danger and engage in acceptable social behavior—and all children need this kind of molding.

Unfortunately, much of what we call discipline is simply bad parental behavior. Being a parent is hard

TV FOR TODDLERS?

Many idealistic parents swear that they are not going to allow their children to watch TV—a noble sentiment, but be careful! As your child grows, you may find him wanting to spend most of his time at the neighbor's, where the TV is on all the time. And while you may not have a TV in your living area, you may have an au pair or relative who has a TV in her room. Don't be surprised if your child wants to spend his time there instead of with you.

Most parents at least try to limit TV watching, which can only be a good idea. Some experts suggest waiting until age two to introduce the television. But whenever your child is allowed to watch, the beauty of modern electronics allows parents to organize TV so that their children never have to watch an advertisement for sugary cereal or cheap toys. Appropriate cartoons, *Sesame Street*, *Mister Rogers' Neighborhood*, classic Disney movies, nature films, even films about trucks, trains and airplanes are available through DVD services like Netflix and through streaming services like Amazon Instant and Hulu. You can also download these shows to an iPad for entertainment while traveling.

And that's what TV is, entertainment, not education. And there's nothing wrong with entertainment. Some people bristle at the notion of using TV as a babysitter, but that is a perfect use for television. Used judiciously, TV can be a special treat, for example on Saturday mornings, to keep children entertained while mom and dad do chores. TV should never take the place of reading to your child, or of letting your child play, both indoors and out. But there is no harm in limited amounts of exposure to the better quality children's programs.

work, a realization that often comes as a terrible shock to new parents. Impatience, anger, scoldings, shouting, confinement and physical violence to children can occur without any teaching motive whatsoever, but simply because the parent is impatient, angry, under stress or lacking self-discipline. By the same token, a hands-off approach to discipline, whereby a child is rarely corrected, may simply reflect laziness or fatigue on the part of the parent. Some, in fact, much of such parental behavior may stem from poor nutrition, leading to low blood sugar, adrenal malfunction and neurological deficits. Truly, our diet for pregnant women and growing children applies to every family member if the family life is to be truly harmonious.

But just because some parents set a bad example and impose excessive punishment on their children does not mean that children don't need discipline. Children need to learn that it is dangerous to go into the street and unacceptable to hit others or engage in destructive actions. As they grow, they need to learn to be helpful, to assist in chores, to refrain from anti-social behavior—and not because we are trying to force them into an arbitrary mold but because we want to give them the gifts of self-discipline, goal-oriented behavior and successful integration into human society.

The type of discipline needed will change as your child grows. Discipline in the early months is completely inappropriate. Those who advocate "disciplining" an infant into a strict feeding schedule or toilet training, letting a tiny baby "cry it out" and similar behaviors simply don't understand that these measures can only harm the noncomprehending infant, or perhaps they harbor a grudge against children or humanity in general.

Likewise, the type of discipline a parent engages in may be predicated on the nature of the child. Some children are docile and compliant, easily molded, and also easily injured by any sort of correction that isn't sensitive and gentle. Other children may be more independent, even openly defiant, and require a stricter approach.

THE TIME-OUT TECHNIQUE

Time-out is one of the most widely researched techniques for dealing with inapproproate behavior in children. It involves having a child sit on a stool or face the corner of a room—in other words removed from all activity—for a short period of time. The child should not be sent to his room, where he can continue to play, but instead exposed for a brief period to a very boring, unrewarding environment.

Set an oven timer or small mechanical timer to buzz when the time is up. The child learns to control himself for a short period of time, and also understands when the time-out is over.

While the child should know that his parent means business, time-out spares the parent from haranguing or preaching to the child. In fact, the whole point is that the parent becomes quiet and refuses to engage with the child, refuses, in other words, to reward bad behavior with attention. Instead, the child is simply put in the corner and forced to think about why he is there. For the first few times, a parent may have to stand behind the child with a hand on his shoulder to keep him there. But eventually, the child will stay without any parental supervision. Parents should ignore any questions or requests to go to the bathroom. The time-out should be a period of complete silence.

The time-out technique can begin with a child as young as eighteen months and will work well even until the seventh year—although when instituted early, it will probably not be necessary past the age of three or four. Start with a three-minute time-out for a toddler, increasing to ten minutes for the recalcitrant older child.

The child should be told why he is put in the corner with a simple statement, "We do not bite," or "We do not throw things in the house." But when the time-out is over, parents should not say anything about it. There is no need to discuss the behavior or the fairness of the punishment. The child will get the message without any further comment.

Most likely the first things that require discipline are destructive behaviors like throwing, hitting and hair pulling. A stern look and a sharp "No!" may be all the correction that baby needs.

Distraction is a parent's best tool. Is baby throwing objects? Let him scrunch up pieces of newspaper or magazine pages and throw those. Or move him outside where throwing is allowed. Has he colored on a wall? Explain that he can color on paper at an easel, not on the wall. You may need to use a stern voice and look for this one. (Some enlightened parents let their children color on just one wall, say in a hall, which can be easily repainted when your child grows out of the wall-coloring stage. In fact, there are indoor paints that take chalk drawings which can be wiped off.)

If some kind of punishment is needed, it should be immediate, appropriate, gentle. . . and even fun. Your toddler hits? He gets a three-minute "time out" on the kitchen stool—you can even have an egg timer for this that he can watch. Your two-year-old pulls your hair? Five minutes standing in the corner facing the wall. Your child will understand what the punishment is for, will experience it as a teaching procedure, and rejoice that it is over quickly. Sometimes children will even climb on the stool or go to

MILESTONES FOR THREE MONTHS

MOVEMENT MILESTONES
- Raises head and chest when lying on stomach
- Supports upper body with arms when lying on stomach
- Stretches legs out and kicks when lying on stomach or back
- Opens and shuts hands
- Pushes down on legs when feet are placed on a firm surface
- Brings hand to mouth
- Takes swipes at dangling objects with hands
- Grasps and shakes hand toys

VISUAL AND HEARING MILESTONES
- Watches faces intently
- Follows moving objects
- Recognizes familiar objects and people at a distance
- Starts using hands and eyes in coordination
- Smiles at the sound of your voice
- Begins to babble
- Begins to imitate some sounds
- Turns head toward direction of sound

SOCIAL AND EMOTIONAL MILESTONES
- Begins to develop a social smile
- Enjoys playing with other people and may cry when playing stops
- Becomes more communicative and expressive with face and body
- Imitates some movements and facial expressions

DEVELOPMENTAL HEALTH WATCH
If you notice any of the following warning signs in your infant at this age, discuss them with your pediatrician.

- Doesn't seem to respond to loud sounds
- Doesn't notice her hands by two months
- Doesn't smile at the sound of your voice by two months
- Doesn't follow moving objects with her eyes by two to three months
- Doesn't grasp and hold objects by three months
- Doesn't smile at people by three months
- Cannot support her head well at three months
- Doesn't reach for and grasp toys by three to four months
- Doesn't babble by three to four months
- Doesn't bring objects to her mouth by four months
- Begins babbling, but doesn't try to imitate any of your sounds by four months
- Doesn't push down with her legs when her feet are placed on a firm surface by four months
- Has trouble moving one or both eyes in all directions
- Crosses her eyes most of the time (occasional crossing of the eyes is normal in these first month.
- Doesn't pay attention to new faces, or seems very frightened by new faces or surroundings
- Still has the tonic neck or "fencing" reflex at four to five months

the corner on their own, stay there, and come away smiling. Gentle discipline is actually a joy for the child, a sign that the world imposes limits but in a mild and loving way.

Above all, avoid the temptation to frighten the child with lies such as "If you don't go to bed a lion will come and eat you." Children soon learn to lose all respect for parents who lie to them. But they will respect a parent who refuses to negotiate and simply states, "It's time to go to bed now."

Good nutrition plays a definite role here—children who are well nourished seldom misbehave, are easy to correct and take directions easily. A child who is malnourished, who lacks good fats in the diet, who consumes pasteurized milk, or a lot of fruit juice and sugar misbehaves because he has low blood sugar or feels awful. He may whine constantly, cry frequently, engage in destructive behavior—discipline in these cases only adds to the child's misery. The remedy for the child who constantly whines and misbehaves is a nourishing traditional diet, not punishment for the parents' unwise dietary decisions.

Sometimes even well nourished children can be

MILESTONES FOR SEVEN MONTHS

MOVEMENT MILESTONES
- Rolls both ways (front to back, back to front)
- Sits with, and then without, support of her hands
- Supports her whole weight on her legs
- Reaches with one hand
- Transfers object from hand to hand
- Uses raking grasp (not pincer)

VISUAL MILESTONES
- Develops full color vision
- Distance vision matures
- Ability to track moving objects improves

LANGUAGE MILESTONES
- Responds to own name
- Begins to respond to "no"
- Distinguishes emotions by tone of voice
- Responds to sound by making sounds
- Uses voice to express joy and displeasure
- Babbles chains of consonants

COGNITIVE MILESTONES
- Finds partially hidden object
- Explores with hands and mouth
- Struggles to get objects that are out of reach

SOCIAL AND EMOTIONAL MILESTONES
- Enjoys social play
- Interested in mirror images
- Responds to other people's expressions of emotion and appears joyful often

DEVELOPMENTAL HEALTH WATCH
- Seems very stiff, with tight muscles
- Seems very floppy, like a rag doll
- Head still flops back when body is pulled up to a sitting position
- Reaches with one hand only
- Refuses to cuddle
- Shows no affection for the person who cares for him
- Doesn't seem to enjoy being around people
- One or both eyes consistently turn in or out
- Persistent tearing, eye drainage or sensitivity to light
- Does not respond to sounds around him
- Has difficulty getting objects to his mouth
- Does not turn his head to locate sounds by four months
- Doesn't roll over in either direction (front to back or back to front) by five months
- Seems inconsolable at night after five months
- Doesn't smile spontaneously by five months
- Cannot sit with help by six months
- Does not laugh or make squealing sounds by six months
- Does not actively reach for objects by six to seven months
- Doesn't follow objects with both eyes at near (1 foot) and far (6 feet) ranges by seven months
- Does not bear some weight on legs by seven months
- Does not try to attract attention through actions by seven months
- Does not babble by eight months
- Shows no interest in games of peekaboo by eight months

very naughty indeed—these are times when scoldings are appropriate. Your child should know that you are displeased. If you react to bad behavior with a swift spank on the bottom, don't be hard on yourself. Most important is following up with an explanation and a hug, then even a story or time doing something together.

Along with good nourishment, the key to raising a happy, independent, well-behaved child is consistency, gentleness and patience—something that no parent can achieve one hundred percent of the time. But not to worry: children are resilient and for the most part forgiving of our mistakes. Whatever style of parenting you adopt, your children are likely to grow up fine.

MILESTONES FOR TWELVE MONTHS

MOVEMENT MILESTONES
- Gets to sitting position without assistance
- Crawls forward on belly by pulling with arms and pushing with legs
- Assumes hands-and-knees position
- Creeps (crawls) on hands and knees supporting trunk on hands and knees
- Gets from sitting to crawling or prone (lying on stomach) position
- Pulls self up to stand
- Walks holding on to furniture
- Stands momentarily without support
- May walk two or three steps without support

MILESTONES IN HAND AND FINGER SKILLS
- Uses pincer grasp
- Bangs two cubes together
- Puts objects into container
- Takes objects out of container
- Lets objects go voluntarily
- Pokes with index finger
- Tries to imitate scribbling

LANGUAGE MILESTONES
- Pays increasing attention to speech
- Responds to simple verbal requests
- Responds to "no"
- Uses simple gestures, such as shaking head, for "no"
- Babbles with inflection
- Says "Dada" and "Mama"
- Uses exclamations, such as "oh-oh!"
- Tries to imitate words

COGNITIVE MILESTONES
- Explores objects in many different ways (shaking, banging, throwing, dropping)
- Finds hidden objects easily
- Looks at correct picture when the image is named
- Imitates gestures
- Begins to use objects correctly (drinking from cup, brushing hair, dialing phone, listening to receiver)

SOCIAL AND EMOTIONAL MILESTONES
- Shy or anxious with strangers
- Cries when mother or father leaves
- Enjoys imitating people in play
- Shows specific preferences for certain people and toys
- Tests parental responses to his actions during feedings (What do you do when he refuses a food?)
- Tests parental responses to his behavior (What do you do if he cries after you leave the room?)
- May be fearful in some situations
- Prefers mother and/or regular caregiver over all others
- Repeats sounds or gestures for attention
- Finger-feeds himself
- Extends arm or leg to help when being dressed

DEVELOPMENTAL HEALTH WATCH
- Does not crawl
- Drags one side of body while crawling (for over one month)
- Cannot stand when supported
- Does not search for objects that are hidden while he watches
- Says no single words ("mama" or "dada")
- Does not learn to use gestures, such as waving or shaking head
- Does not point to objects or pictures

MILESTONES

The observation that most babies tend to achieve the same developmental accomplishments at certain ages began in the 1920s with the work of Arnold Gesell, a psychologist and pediatrician who launched the field of child development. Gesell's main finding was that development takes place in distinct stages. Adults can influence this development only in minor ways.

Gesell's classic study involved twin girls, both given training for motor skills but one given training for longer than the other. There was no measurable difference in the age at which either child acquired the skills, indicating that development happens in a genetically programmed way, irrespective of the training given. Thus, given a normal environment, a child learns basic movement, social and language skills without parental interference, suggesting that physical development is largely pre-programmed.

By studying thousands of children over many years, Gesell came up with "milestones of development" —stages by which normal children can accomplish different tasks. With certain variations and additions, these guidelines are still used today.

Gesell's successor was Jean Piaget who was involved in the administration of intelligence tests to

MILESTONES FOR TWO YEARS

MOVEMENT MILESTONES
- Walks alone
- Pulls toys behind her while walking
- Carries large toy or several toys while walking
- Begins to run
- Stands on tiptoe
- Kicks a ball
- Climbs onto and down from furniture unassisted
- Walks up and down stairs holding on to support

MILESTONES IN HAND AND FINGER SKILLS
- Scribbles spontaneously
- Turns over container to pour out contents
- Builds tower of four blocks or more
- Might use one hand more frequently than the other

LANGUAGE MILESTONES
- Points to object or picture when it's named for him
- Recognizes names of familiar people, objects, and body parts
- Says several single words (by fifteen to eighteen months)
- Uses simple phrases (by eighteen to twenty-four months)
- Uses two- to four-word sentences
- Follows simple instructions
- Repeats words overheard in conversation

COGNITIVE MILESTONES
- Finds objects even when hidden under two or three covers
- Begins to sort by shapes and colors
- Begins make-believe play

SOCIAL AND EMOTIONAL MILESTONES
- Imitates behavior of others, especially adults and older children
- Increasingly aware of herself as separate from others
- Increasingly enthusiastic about company of other children
- Demonstrates increasing independence, the "terrible twos"
- Begins to show defiant behavior
- Increasing episodes of separation anxiety toward midyear, then they fade

DEVELOPMENTAL HEALTH WATCH
- Cannot walk by eighteen months
- Fails to develop a mature heel-toe walking pattern after several months of walking, or walks exclusively on his toes
- Does not speak at least fifteen words by eighteen months
- Does not use two-word sentences by age two
- Does not seem to know the function of common household objects (brush, telephone, bell, fork, spoon) by fifteen months
- Does not imitate actions or words by the end of this period
- Does not follow simple instructions by age two
- Cannot push a wheeled toy by age two

MILESTONES FOR THREE TO FOUR YEARS

With your child's third birthday, the "terrible twos" are officially over and the "magic years" of three and four begin—a time when your child's world will be dominated by fantasy and vivid imagination. During the next two years, he'll mature in many areas.

MOVEMENT MILESTONES
- Hops and stands on one foot up to five seconds
- Goes upstairs and downstairs without support
- Kicks ball forward
- Throws ball overhand
- Catches bounced ball most of the time
- Moves forward and backward with agility

MILESTONES IN HAND AND FINGER SKILLS
- Copies square shapes
- Draws a person with two to four body parts
- Uses scissors
- Draws circles and squares
- Begins to copy some capital letters

LANGUAGE MILESTONES
- Understands the concepts of "same" and "different"
- Has mastered some basic rules of grammar
- Speaks in sentences of five to six words
- Speaks clearly enough for strangers to understand
- Tells stories

COGNITIVE MILESTONES
- Correctly names some colors
- Understands the concept of counting and may know a few numbers
- Approaches problems from a single point of view
- Begins to have a clearer sense of time
- Follows three-part commands
- Recalls parts of a story
- Understands the concept of same/different
- Engages in fantasy play

SOCIAL AND EMOTIONAL MILESTONES
- Interested in new experiences
- Cooperates with other children
- Plays "Mom" or "Dad"
- Increasingly inventive in fantasy play
- Dresses and undresses
- Negotiates solutions to conflicts
- More independent
- Imagines that many unfamiliar images may be "monsters"
- Views self as a whole person involving body, mind, and feelings
- Often cannot distinguish between fantasy and reality

DEVELOPMENTAL HEALTH WATCH
- Cannot throw a ball overhand
- Cannot jump in place
- Cannot ride a tricycle
- Cannot grasp a crayon between thumb and fingers
- Has difficulty scribbling
- Cannot stack four blocks
- Still clings or cries whenever his parents leave him
- Shows no interest in interactive games
- Ignores other children
- Doesn't respond to people outside the family
- Doesn't engage in fantasy play
- Resists dressing, sleeping, using the toilet
- Lashes out without any self-control when angry or upset
- Cannot copy a circle
- Doesn't use sentences of more than three words
- Doesn't use "me" and "you" appropriately

MILESTONES FOR FOUR TO FIVE YEARS

By age four or five, the somewhat calm child of three becomes a dynamo of energy, drive, bossiness, belligerence and even out-of-bounds behavior. During this time there is a tremendous spurt of imaginative ideas that spring from children's minds and mouths.

MOVEMENT MILESTONES
- Stands on one foot for ten seconds or longer
- Hops, somersaults
- Swings, climbs
- May be able to skip

MILESTONES IN HAND AND FINGER SKILLS
- Copies triangle and other geometric patterns
- Draws person with body
- Prints some letters
- Dresses and undresses without assistance
- Uses fork, spoon, and (sometimes) a table knife
- Usually cares for own toilet needs

LANGUAGE MILESTONES
- Recalls part of a story
- Speaks sentences of more than five words
- Uses future tense
- Tells longer stories
- Says name and address

COGNITIVE MILESTONES
- Can count ten or more objects
- Correctly names at least four colors
- Better understands the concept of time
- Knows about things used every day in the home (money, food, appliances)

SOCIAL AND EMOTIONAL MILESTONES
- Wants to please friends
- Wants to be like her friends
- More likely to agree to rules
- Likes to sing, dance, and act
- Shows more independence and may even visit a next-door neighbor by herself
- Able to distinguish fantasy from reality
- Sometimes demanding, sometimes eagerly cooperative
- Aware of sexuality

DEVELOPMENTAL HEALTH WATCH
- Exhibits extremely fearful or timid behavior
- Exhibits extremely aggressive behavior
- Is unable to separate from parents without major protest
- Is easily distracted and unable to concentrate on any single activity for more than five minutes
- Shows little interest in playing with other children
- Refuses to respond to people in general, or responds only superficially
- Rarely uses fantasy or imitation in play
- Seems unhappy or sad much of the time
- Doesn't engage in a variety of activities
- Avoids or seems aloof with other children and adults
- Doesn't express a wide range of emotions
- Has trouble eating, sleeping, or using the toilet
- Can't differentiate between fantasy and reality
- Seems unusually passive
- Cannot understand two-part commands using prepositions ("Put the cup on the table;" "Get the ball under the couch.")
- Can't correctly give her first and last name
- Doesn't use plurals or past tense properly when speaking
- Doesn't talk about her daily activities and experiences
- Cannot build a tower of six to eight blocks
- Seems uncomfortable holding a crayon
- Has trouble taking off her clothing
- Cannot brush her teeth efficiently
- Cannot wash and dry her hands

SOURCE: University of Michigan Health System, http://www.med.umich.edu/yourchild/topics/devmile.htm.

children and became interested in the types of mistakes children of various ages were likely to make. Piaget began to study the reasoning processes of children at various ages. He theorized that cognitive development proceeds in genetically determined stages that always follow the same sequential order.

Another important developmental theorist was Erik Erikson, who also proposed a stage theory of development, but his theory encompassed development throughout the human lifespan. Erikson believed that each stage of development is focused on overcoming a conflict. Success or failure in dealing with conflicts can impact overall functioning. Erikson's findings are echoed in hands-off child-rearing philosophies, which recommend parents allow children to make their own mistakes—from learning to walk to developing social skills—and not make life too easy for them as they grow.

Developmental milestones can be a two-edged sword. They can provide assurance that baby is developing normally; and they can be a source of anxiety to parents when baby lags behind. When parents are following the principles of good nutrition outlined in this book, babies almost always meet their milestones; if they do not, then parents are alerted to the fact that something needs to be addressed with therapy or even medical intervention.

Sometimes babies meet their milestones to a certain point and then regress. The most commonly reported cause of such regression is a vaccination, but exposure to pesticides and other toxins, changes in diet (such as use of pasteurized or ultrapasteurized milk, consumption of school lunches or introduction to junk food) or even a psychological upset such as a frightening experience, loss of a parent or sexual molestation may also cause regression. Thus, the milestones, albeit preprogrammed, can provide important clues to a child's overall environment.

When gauging a child's development according to accepted milestones, remember that each child is different and may learn and grow at a different rate. However, if your child cannot do many of the skills listed for his or her age group, you should consult a health practitioner.

If your child was born early, be sure to deduct the number of months early from his age. A five-month-old born two months early would be expected to show the same skills as a three-month-old who was born on his due date.

Chapter 9
Nourishing a Growing Child

As we have stated many times in this book, the feeding of your child ideally begins long before she is born; good nutrition continues with mom's diet during breastfeeding, or with our homemade infant formula. Then, starting at four to six months, solid food is carefully introduced, food specific to baby's needs.

We realize that many parents reading this book may not have instituted the ideal diet until after their baby was born; rest assured, it is never too late to start. A nutrient-dense diet during the early years can help your child recover from earlier deficiencies and give her the best chance for a full and healthy life.

WHEN TO START

Somewhere between the fourth and sixth month, baby should be started on solid food. The exact moment depends on the size and maturity of your infant. Babies who have reached twelve pounds and who are achieving their milestones (see pages 174-179) are probably ready for solid food at age four months. Infants ready for solid food will stop pushing their tongue out when a spoon or bit of food is placed in their mouth—a reflex common in infants that disappears at around four months of age. For less mature babies, wait until five or six months. But by the halfway mark to baby's first year, he will need solid food in addition to breast milk or formula.

The reason is that it is at this time of life when baby runs out of iron, and neither breast milk nor raw milk from another species is likely to provide adequate iron for baby's needs. One study found that babies exclusively breastfed even for six months were more likely to develop anemia than those introduced to solid foods at four to six months.[1]

Exclusive breastfeeding, that is, breastfeeding without any other food for up to a year, is a recent fad. The result is pale, anemic babies who tend to be timid and clingy. In virtually all traditional cultures, baby gets his first solid food by six months, usually liver or other organ meat which the mother has pre-chewed. Liver is the best source of usable iron for baby, along with vitamin B_{12} and a host of other nutrients, all of which will put color in baby's cheeks and liveliness in her behavior. The other recommended weaning food is grass-fed egg yolk, loaded with choline, vitamin D and cholesterol, as well as iron, all necessary for baby's developing brain.

The consequences of iron deficiency in children are serious. According to a study published in the *Journal of Nutrition*, "Infants with chronic, severe iron deficiency have been observed to display increased fearfulness, unhappiness, fatigue, low activity, wariness, solemnity and proximity to the mother during free play, development testing and at home." Anemic infants who did not receive iron supplementation, "never smiled, never interacted socially, and never showed social referencing."[2] Fortunately such unhappy consequences are easily prevented with the feeding of iron-rich foods to your baby, starting by the sixth month of age.

WHAT'S WRONG WITH COMMERCIAL BABY FOOD

The time to prepare baby's food begins with the first feeding—get in the habit of preparing baby's food from the very first meal, and it will soon become second nature. Baby's foods are easy to fix and can be frozen and stored for later use. Working moms find that with just a couple hours devoted to food preparation on the weekend, baby can be well nourished all week long. Time spent in the kitchen can mean far less time spent at the doctor, dentist, learning specialist or therapist as your child grows.

Why not commercial baby food? For one reason, the really nutritious foods like egg yolk and liver are not available as baby food in jars. Even baby food meat is hard to find. Most baby foods consist of puréed vegetables and fruit where water is a major ingredient. How would you feel if you only got puréed vegetables and fruit for a meal? You'd soon be whiny and cranky from low blood sugar and crying for food—which might be a high-carbohydrate snack from your perplexed and hassled mother.

TAKE IT SLOWLY

As you introduce baby foods, it is important to go slowly and be observant; every baby will have an individual response to different foods. Introduce new foods one at a time and continue to feed that

BABY FOOD INGREDIENTS

Heeding concerns about additives in baby food, the two major baby food companies, Gerber and Earth's Best, provide additive-free baby foods, the latter company using all organic ingredients. But the foods baby needs most—liver and egg yolks—are not available as baby food in jars.

Commercial baby foods are either extremely simple—just one ingredient plus water—or strangely complex. If you must use commercial baby food, opt for the simple choices; heat them gently and add butter or cream and a pinch of salt. The concoctions containing a number of ingredients are not appropriate for babies; they usually contain grains and improperly prepared legumes. If baby reacts, it's difficult to know which ingredient is causing the problem. When baby reaches the age when he can handle grains like rice or wheat, he will be too big for baby food anyway.

Hopefully, the ingredient lists of typical factory-produced baby foods will inspire you to make baby's food in your own kitchen.

- Gerber Squash: Squash, Water

- Gerber Peas: Peas, Water

- Gerber Apple Blueberry: Apples, Blueberries, Water, Ascorbic Acid

- Gerber Chicken: Ground Chicken, Water, Cornstarch

- Earth's Best Chicken Mango Risotto: Water, Organic Carrots, Organic Mango Purée, Organic Finely Ground Chicken, Organic Whole Grain Brown Rice, Organic Yellow Split Pea Flakes, Calcium Carbonate.

- Earth's Best Chicken & Brown Rice: Water, Organic Butternut Squash, Organic Ground Chicken, Organic Corn, Organic Whole Grain Brown Rice.

- Earth's Best Spaghetti with Cheese: Water, Organic Carrots, Organic Tomato Paste, Organic Cheddar Cheese (Pasteurized Organic Whole Milk, Cheese Culture, Enzymes), Organic Spaghetti (Organic Whole Wheat Durum Flour), Organic Whole Wheat Flour, Organic Onions, Organic Garbanzo Beans.

same food for at least four days, without introducing any other food, to rule out the possibility of a negative reaction. Signs of intolerance include redness around the mouth; abdominal bloating, gas and distention; irritability, fussiness, overactivity and awaking throughout the night; vomiting; constipation and diarrhea; frequent regurgitation of foods; nasal or chest congestion; and red, chapped or inflamed eczema-like skin rash.[3] If a newly introduced food causes any one of these reactions, hold off from serving it to baby for a few months, then try again.

In addition, be sure to respect the tiny, still-developing digestive system of your infant. Babies have limited production of enzymes necessary for the digestion of foods. In fact, it takes at least sixteen months for the carbohydrate enzymes (namely amylase) to come on line.[4] Foods like cereals, grains and breads are very challenging for little ones to digest. Thus, these foods should be some of the last to be given to baby. (One carbohydrate enzyme that

baby's small intestine does produce is lactase, for the digestion of lactose in milk.)

Foods introduced too early can cause digestive troubles and increase the likelihood of allergies (particularly allergies to those foods introduced). If baby's digestive tract is not well developed, large particles of food may be absorbed. If these particles reach the bloodstream, the immune system mounts a response that leads to an allergic reaction.

Babies do produce functional enzymes (pepsin and proteolytic enzymes) and digestive juices (hydrochloric acid in the stomach) that work on proteins and lipase enzymes that work on fats.[5] This makes perfect sense since the milk from a healthy mother has 50-60 percent of its energy as fat, which is critical for growth, energy and development.[6] In addition, the cholesterol in human milk supplies an infant with close to six times the amount most adults consume from food.[7] In China, a new mother is encouraged to eat six to ten eggs a day and almost ten

CHEERIOS: A BAD STRATEGY FOR BABY

CHEERIOS: "Whole Grain Corn, Whole Grain Oats, Sugar, Whole Grain Barley, Whole Grain Wheat, Whole Grain Rice, Corn Starch, Brown Sugar Syrup, Corn Bran, Salt, Canola and/or Rice Bran Oil, Tripotassium Phosphate, Color Added. Vitamin E added to preserve freshness. VITAMINS AND MINERALS: Calcium Carbonate, Zinc, Iron, Vitamin C, Vitamin B3, Vitamin B6, Vitamin B2, Vitamin B1, Folic Acid, Vitamin B12, Vitamin D3."

It's a common sight these days: a baby in a stroller with a small plastic bag containing Cheerios. Baby fusses, mom plunks a Cheerio in baby's mouth. The rationale for giving Cheerios is that they ensure "complete nutrition" with all the added vitamins and minerals, and that the hole in Cheerios will keep baby from choking! Only a high-priced advertising agency could have thought that one up.

What's wrong with Cheerios? Cheerios (and all dry breakfast cereals) are made by a process called extrusion, which damages the delicate proteins in grains; unpublished research indicates that when extruded, the proteins in grains become toxic to the nervous system.[9] The levels of these proteins will be higher in whole grains compared to refined. Furthermore whole grains that are not properly prepared are very difficult to digest. Finally, it's likely that refined sweeteners are the major ingredient in Cheerios—if you add the brown sugar syrup (eighth ingredient) to the sugar (third ingredient) it's possible that total sugars are number one on the list.

Cheerios given to babies is a recipe for blood sugar highs and lows with ensuing crankiness, whining and tantrums. Digestive disorders and later learning problems are a distinct possibility—all very inconvenient effects from the convenience of giving Cheerios.

Much better traveling food for babies: small cubes of cheese, naturally made salami and crispy nuts like pecans (see Recipes). These are convenient, nourishing foods with plenty of fat to keep blood sugar stable and the nerves calm.

ounces of chicken and pork for at least one month after birth.[8] This fat-rich diet ensures her breast milk will contain adequate healthy fats.

Thus, a baby's earliest solid foods should be mostly animal foods since his digestive system, although immature, is better equipped to supply enzymes for digestion of fats and proteins than carbohydrates, especially grains.[9]

MEAT VERSUS CEREAL

Remember that the amount of breast milk or formula decreases when solid foods are introduced. This decrease may open the door for insufficiencies in a number of nutrients critical for baby's normal growth and development. The nutrients that are often in short supply when weaning begins include protein, zinc, iron and B vitamins. One food group that has these nutrients in ample amounts is meat.

Unfortunately, cereal is the most often recommended early weaning food. A Swedish study suggests that when infants are given substantial amounts of cereal, they may suffer from low concentrations of zinc and reduced calcium absorption.[10]

In the U.S., Dr. Nancy Krebs headed up a large infant growth study which found that breastfed infants who received puréed or strained meat as a primary weaning food beginning at four to five months grew at a slightly faster rate than infants given cereal. Kreb's study suggests that inadequate protein or zinc from common first foods may limit the growth of some breastfed infants during the weaning period. More importantly, both protein and zinc levels were consistently higher in the diets of the infants who received meat.[11] Thus, the custom of providing large amounts of cereals and excluding meats in the weaning period may short-change the nutritional requirements of the infant.[12]

HAPPY BABY OR ADDICTED BABY?

One of the most fascinating fields of biochemistry today involves the body's production and use of feel-good chemicals called endorphins. The well nourished body will make compounds that are chemically identical to the addictive molecules in marijuana, opium, heroin and other drugs, but in tiny amounts that the body can clear without adverse effects. Mammalian milk also contains these compounds. The fat-soluble activators A and D, plus cholesterol and choline, support the proper function of receptors for these feel-good chemicals and then help get rid of them without addictions or side effects.

We all know the devastating effects of these drugs when introduced to the body from the outside—addictions and side effects such as rapid aging. And it has become increasingly clear that large amounts of these substances can be produced in the gut when we eat the wrong foods and when the gut flora is damaged. Poorly digested grains and pasteurized milk create dietary opiates, excitotoxins and cannabinoids that mimic morphine, heroin and marijuana.[13] Sugar produces dopamine and endorphins that mimic cocaine, morphine, opium and heroin: sugar stimulates the production of adrenaline and norepinephrine, which mimic methamphetamine; and sugar feeds yeasts that can produce ethanol and acetyladehyde, resulting in symptoms of inebriation and hangover.[14] Finally, artificial sweeteners such as aspartame, artificial flavors such as MSG and hydrolyzed protein, and emulsifiers such as carrageenan produce glutamate, a powerful brain stimulant that can be toxic in large amounts.[15] When children are fed these foods, can we blame them for fussiness, whining, crying, crabbiness, sullenness, tantrums, insomnia and general bad behavior?

When parents put their efforts into preparing super nutritious foods for baby, and dedicate themselves to keeping harmful foods out of baby's diet, the rewards are great: happy, curious, intelligent, well-behaved children. These children produce their own feel-good chemicals in just the right amounts and without side effects. The national angst about bringing up baby fades into a pleasant partnership when attention is focused on the diet rather than on the child's psychology. Truly diet can do more to support good behavior than any particular child-rearing philosophy.

Meat is also an excellent source of iron. Heme iron (the form of iron found in meat) is better absorbed than iron from plant sources (non-heme). Additionally, the protein in meat helps the baby more easily absorb iron from other foods.[16] Two important studies[17] have examined iron status in breastfed infants who received meat earlier in the weaning period. While researchers found no measurable change in breastfed babies' iron stores when they received an increased amount of meat, the levels of hemoglobin (iron-containing cells) circulating in the bloodstream did increase. Meat also contains a much greater amount of zinc than cereals, which means more is absorbed.[18] These studies confirm the practices of traditional peoples, who gave meat—usually liver—as the first weaning food. Furthermore, the incidence of allergic reactions to meat is minimal and lower still when puréed varieties are used.[19]

THE IMPORTANCE OF FATS

While dietitians and government officials blithely assure the public that the lowfat, low-cholesterol diet they recommend for growing children carries no risk, the scientific literature on the subject, although sparse, indeed indicates that such diets shortchange the growing child. One report details growth failure in children put on lowfat, low-cholesterol diets.[20] Studies on European children brought up on lowfat, low-cholesterol macrobiotic diets showed poor growth, poor psychomotor development and numerous nutrient deficiencies.[21]

The majority of energy in mother's milk comes from fat, much of it saturated fat, which is needed throughout growth and development, and that means right up to young adulthood. Milk fats and animal fats give energy and also help children build muscle and bone. In addition, the animal fats provide vitamins A, D_3 and K_2 necessary for protein and mineral assimilation, normal growth and hormone production.

Choose a variety of fats and oils to provide your child with a range of fat-soluble nutrients, but emphasize stable saturated fats found in butter, meat, lard, and coconut oil, and monounsaturated fats, found in chicken, duck and goose fat, avocados and olive oil.

COD LIVER OIL

Many books on feeding babies written before the Second World War recommended cod liver oil for babies, sometimes starting at three weeks—even baby photo albums had a place to note baby's age when first given cod liver oil. Advertising for cod liver oil stressed its vitamin A and D content as critical for normal growth, and even normal behavior. The generation of babies born just before the Second World War that was given cod liver oil, in both America and Europe, grew up healthy, strong and intelligent, in spite of the privations of the Depression and the war years.

If you are breastfeeding, you can give your baby cod liver oil through your breast milk by taking cod liver oil yourself; if you are giving the homemade formula, you can add the cod liver oil to the formula. But sometime around four months, you should start giving it separately to baby, using a syringe or eye dropper.

Unfortunately, most brands of cod liver oil today come from Europe where they are highly processed, with a large portion of the critical vitamins A and D removed, often replaced by synthetic vitamins. In addition, the oil is heated to high temperatures,

LITTLE FISHES

A common food for babies in Asia and Africa is tiny dried whole fishes. Japanese children often carry these morsels to school in a special little case. They are salty and crunchy—a super nutrition replacement for junk food snack chips. As the fish are whole, baby gets the nutrition from head and organs. These little fish are rich in vitamins A and D, iron, calcium, protein, iodine and a host of minerals (available from Radiant Life, see Sources).

Instead of this nutritious super snack, Western parents give their children "goldfish" made of white flour, sweeteners and vegetable shortening—a very poor substitute!

which damages the fragile omega-3 fatty acids EPA and DHA. Fortunately, we now have an American-made brand of cod liver oil that is low temperature-processed and filtered in such a way as to leave the valuable natural vitamins in the oil. The oil is fermented, which is how it was traditionally processed, a process that creates vitamin K_2 in the oil, an important complement to vitamins A and D. We refer to this product as fermented high-vitamin cod liver oil (see Sources).

Start with a 1/4 teaspoon of high-vitamin cod liver oil doubling the amount at six to eight months. Use an eye dropper or syringe at first; later baby can take cod liver oil mixed with a little water or fresh orange juice. If you start young enough, you will have no trouble getting your child to take cod liver oil.

INTRODUCTORY FOODS

Egg yolks, rich in choline, cholesterol and other brain-nourishing substances, can be added to your baby's diet sometime between four and six months. Prepare by boiling three minutes, or until the white is congealed but the yolk still slightly soft. Discard the white and add a little sea salt to the yolk.

Most babies love their egg yolk but occasionally a baby reacts badly by vomiting. This is why we recommend introducing egg yolk very slowly, with just one-half to one teaspoon for the first time, gradually increasing to the whole yolk. One tip is to start by giving baby just a tiny bit of the egg yolk from the fried or poached egg you have made for your own breakfast.

SUPERFOODS FOR BABY

Baby should have plenty of superfoods in his diet every day, even every meal.

RAW MILK: Designed for the developing baby to build the gut wall, create the immune system and ensure the assimilation of 100 percent of the nutrients; and, raw milk contains an ideal blend of protein, fat and carbohydrates. Raw milk from humans and from other mammals all have these health-promoting properties.

EGG YOLK: A superlative source of choline, cholesterol and arachidonic acid for baby's developing brain. Grass-fed yolks will also be rich sources of vitamins A, D, iron and folic acid.

LIVER: Not only supplies choline, cholesterol and arachidonic acid, but a powerhouse of minerals (including all-important iron) and vitamins (including crucial and hard-to-obtain vitamins B_6 and B_{12}). Poultry liver (chicken, turkey, duck and goose) are the best choices because they contain a good balance of vitamins A, D_3 and K_2.

BONE MARROW: A rich, high-fat food bursting with factors that nourish the blood.

BRAIN: In Elizabethan times, babies were fed a dish of jellied brains. Perhaps that's why these people had such a great facility with language. If you have access to brains, by all means prepare them for baby.

FISH EGGS: Not all babies take to fish eggs, but some will pick up colorful salmon eggs and eat them with relish. Small fish eggs can be mixed with cream or yogurt.

WHOLE FISHES: As described on page 185, these crunchy whole fishes rival liver in the range of nutrients they contain.

COD LIVER OIL: An insurance policy for Western children, who may be unlikely to eat many organ meats; cod liver oil provides all important fat-soluble activators A and D.

GRASS-FED BUTTER: The perfect fat for developing babies, with an ideal fatty acid profile and balance of fat-soluble vitamins. Butter is also a great source of iodine and other minerals.

FEEDING BABY BY AGES

4-6 MONTHS
- Minimal solid foods as tolerated by baby.
- Egg yolk if tolerated, preferably from pastured chickens, lightly boiled and salted.
- Organic liver, frozen for fourteen days, then grated and added to egg yolk.
- Banana or avocado, mashed, for babies who are very mature and seem hungry.
- Cod liver oil, 1/4 teaspoon high vitamin or 1/2 teaspoon regular, doubling by six months, given with an eye dropper.

6-8 MONTHS
- Organic chicken or duck liver, cooked and puréed.
- Salmon eggs—baby may enjoy picking these up with his fingers!
- Puréed meat, lamb, turkey, beef, chicken, liver and fish.
- Bone broth (chicken, beef, lamb, fish) added to puréed meats and vegetables, or offered as a drink.
- Fermented foods: small amounts of yogurt, kefir, lacto-fermented sweet potato or taro, if desired.
- Raw mashed fruits such as banana, melon, mangoes, papaya, avocado.
- Cooked, puréed fruits such as organic apricots, peaches, pears, apples and berries with cream.
- Cooked vegetables such as zucchini, squash, sweet potato, carrots, beets, with butter or coconut oil.
- Cod liver oil: 1/2 teaspoon high-vitamin or 1 teaspooon regular cod liver oil.

8-12 MONTHS
- Continue to add variety and increase thickness and lumpiness of the foods.
- Creamed vegetable soups.
- Homemade braised meats or stews, all ingredients cut small or mashed.
- Dairy such as yogurt cheese, cottage cheese, mild harder raw cheese, cream, custards.
- Finger foods, when baby can grab and adequately chew, such as lightly steamed veggie sticks, mild cheese, avocado chunks, salmon eggs, pieces of banana and peeled tropical fruit.
- Lacto-fermented sauerkraut and pickles.
- Cod liver oil: 1/2 teaspoon high-vitamin or 1 teaspooon regular cod liver oil.

OVER ONE YEAR
- Grains and legumes, properly soaked and cooked. Babies especially love oatmeal.
- Crispy nut butters (see Recipes).
- Leafy green vegetables, well cooked, with butter.
- Raw salad vegetables such as cucumbers, tomatoes, etc.
- Citrus fruit, fresh and organic.
- Whole egg, cooked.
- Meats such as additive-free bacon, natural salami, smoked salmon, smoked oysters.
- Cod liver oil: Increase to 1 teaspoon high-vitamin or 2 teaspooon regular cod liver oil by age two.

FOODS TO AVOID
- Up to six months: Raw and even cooked vegetables, which are hard for baby to digest.
- Up to nine months: Citrus and tomato, which are common allergens.
- Up to one year: Because infants do not produce strong enough stomach acid to deactivate potential spores, infants should not be given honey. Use blackstrap molasses, which is high in iron and calcium, or maple syrup. Egg whites should also be avoided up to one year due to their high allergenic potential. All grains should be withheld until baby reaches one year, and then introduced slowly, and carefully prepared.
- Always avoid commercial dairy products (especially ultra-pasteurized), modern soy foods, margarines and shortening, fruit juices, reduced-fat or low-fat foods, extruded grains, all processed foods.

BABY FOOD RECIPES

EGG YOLK FOR BABY (4 months +)
Use the best quality eggs you can find, ideally from chickens kept on pasture and fed a soy-free mix. Boil an egg for three to four minutes (longer at higher altitudes), peel away the shell, discard the white and mash up yolk with a pinch of unrefined sea salt. (The yolk should be soft and warm, not runny.) Small amounts of grated, raw organic liver (which has been frozen 14 days) may be added to the egg yolk. Some mothers report their babies tolerate the yolk better with the liver. For a demonstration of egg yolk preparation, see http://www.thehealthyhomeeconomist.com/video-first-food-for-baby/.

PUREED MEATS (6 months +)
Cook meat gently in filtered water or homemade stock until completely tender, or use meat from stews, etc., that you have made for your family. Make sure the cooked meat is cold and is cut into chunks no bigger than 1 inch. In a blender, food processor or baby mill, grind up the meat until it becomes a clumpy powder. Then add water, formula or breast milk, or the natural cooking juices as the liquid. Grind again until well blended and add a small amount of unrefined sea salt. Place into small dishes for individual servings. These will keep about 2 days in the refrigerator. If you are making a lot of meat at one time, you can put portions into an ice cube tray, cover and freeze. Remove one frozen cube at a time and gently heat in a dish placed in simmering water until soft to serve to baby. When warm and just before serving, you may mix in a little softened butter.

BABY PATE (6 months +)
Place 1/4 pound organic chicken livers and 1/4 cup broth or filtered water in a saucepan, bring to a boil and reduce heat. Simmer for eight minutes. Pour liver with liquid into a food processor, blender or baby mill with 1-2 teaspoons butter and a 1/4 teaspoon unrefined sea salt and blend to desired consistency. Place individual servings in small containers and refrigerate or freeze.

VEGETABLE PUREE (6 months +)
Use squash, sweet potatoes, parsnips, rutabagas, carrots or beets. Cut vegetables in half, scoop out seeds from squash and bake in a 400 degree oven for about an hour, or steam them (in the case of carrots and beets) for 20 to 25 minutes. Purée in a blender, food processor or baby mill, mixing in some butter and a little unrefined sea salt at the end. You can cook these vegetables for your own dinner and purée a small portion in a baby mill for your baby.

STEWED FRUIT (6 months +)
Use fresh or frozen peaches, nectarines, apples, blueberries, pitted cherries, pears, berries or a combination. Note: Whenever possible, use organic fruit, and peel the fruit if it is not organic. Cut fruit and put in a saucepan with 1 cup filtered water for every 1/2 cup of fruit. Bring to a boil; reduce to a simmer for about 15 minutes or until the fruit is cooked. Purée the mixture in a blender or food mill and strain if necessary. You may add a pinch of allspice or nutmeg, as well as a small amount of unrefined sea salt. To serve, heat gently and stir in a little butter or cream. From *Natural Baby Care* by Mindy Pennybacker.

DRIED APRICOT PUREE (6 months +)
Bring 2 cups filtered water to a boil with 1 pound unsulphured dried apricots and simmer for 15 minutes. Reserve any leftover liquid to use for the puée. Purée, adding the reserved liquid as necessary to achieve a smooth, thin paste. Blend with butter or cream.

FERMENTED SWEET POTATO OR TARO (6 months +)
Poke a few holes in 2 pounds sweet potatoes or taro root and bake in an oven at 300 degrees for about 2 hours or until soft. Peel and mash with 1 teaspoon seasalt and 4 tablespoons fresh whey. Place in a bowl, cover, and leave at room temperature for 24 hours. Place in an airtight container and store in the refrigerator.

BABY FOOD RECIPES

BABY CUSTARD (6 months +)
Mix 1 cup whole coconut milk (see Sources for coconut milk in BPA-free cans), 1 cup raw cream, 6 beaten egg yolks, 1/2 teaspoon vanilla and 1 tablespoon maple syrup. Pour into buttered ramekin dishes placed in a Pyrex dish filled part-way with water. Preheat oven to 300 degrees and cook for about 1 hour. For an extra treat, add 1 cup cooked and mashed sweet potatoes.

MARROW CUSTARD FOR BABY (6 months +)
Soak 4 marrow bones (cut 2-3 inches in length) in cold water, changing water several times, for 12-24 hours. Cover the bones with cold water, bring slowly to a boil and barely simmer for about 20 minutes. Scoop the cylinder of marrow out with the handle of a small spoon. Mix with 1 cup raw cream, 3 egg yolks and a little sea salt. Pour into four small buttered ramekins, place in hot water and bake at 300 degrees for about 20 minutes or until the custard is set.

SMOOTHIE FOR BABY (8 months +)
Blend 1 cup whole yogurt with 1/2 banana or 1/2 cup puréed fruit, 1 raw egg yolk (from an organic or pastured chicken) and 1 teaspoon of maple syrup. Wash egg in warm, soapy water before cracking.

COCONUT FISH PATE (8 months +)
Place 1 cup leftover cooked fish, 1/4 teaspoon seasalt, 1/4 teaspoon fresh lime juice in a food processor and process with a few pulses. Add 1/2-1 cup whole coconut milk to obtain desired consistency.

YOGURT FOR BABY (8 months +)
Mix 1/2 cup whole yogurt, preferably homemade from raw milk, with 1-2 teaspoons maple syrup or molasses (warmed up for easier mixing). Can be mixed with 1 tablespoon mashed fruit.

BABY CAVIAR (8 months +)
Mix 1 teaspoon caviar with 1 tablespoon thick cream or yogurt cheese and 1/4 teaspoon grated onion.

CEREAL GRUEL FOR BABY (1 year +)
Mix 1/2 cup freshly ground organic flour of spelt, Kamut® , rye, barley or oats with 2 cups warm filtered water plus 2 tablespoons yogurt, kefir or buttermilk. Cover and leave at room temperature for 12 to 24 hours. Bring to a boil, stirring frequently. Add 1/4 teaspoon salt, reduce heat and simmer, stirring occasionally, about 10 minutes. Let cool slightly and serve with cream or butter and small amount of a natural sweetener, such as raw honey.

SALMON AND RICE MOUSSE (1 year +)
Heat 2 cups chicken broth to a slow boil and add 1/4 cup soaked brown rice. Lower the heat, cover tightly, and let cook for 30 minutes or until almost tender. Wash 3 ounces salmon thoroughly and remove all bones carefully. Add the salmon to the rice, cover, and let it poach for 10 minutes or until done all the way through. Allow the salmon and rice to cool enough that it can be puréed safely in the blender or food processor. If it is too thick, add just enough water to obtain the consistency you want. Season with a little seasalt and add 1-2 tablespoons butter. Serve with a puréed vegetable. From *The Crazy Makers* by Carol Simontacchi.

CRISPY NUT BUTTER (1 year +)
Purée equal amounts of crispy nuts, raw honey and coconut oil. Add salt to taste. Serve at room temperature.

NOTE: See Recipe appendix for recipes for stock, whey, yogurt, yogurt cheese and crispy nuts.

If baby has a bad reaction, discontinue and try again one month later. Some mothers have reported that adding a little grated frozen liver to the yolk prevents baby from reacting to the egg yolk.

Cholesterol is vital for the insulation of the nerves in the brain and the entire central nervous system. It helps with fat digestion by increasing the formation of bile acids and is necessary for the production of many hormones. Since the brain is so dependent on cholesterol, it is especially vital during this time when brain growth and neural connections are taking place.

Choline is another critical nutrient for brain development. The traditional practice of feeding egg yolks early is confirmed by current research. A study published in the June 2002 issue of the *American Journal of Clinical Nutrition* compared the nutritional effects of feeding weaning infants six to twelve months of age regular egg yolks, enriched egg yolks, and an otherwise normal diet. The researchers found that both breastfed and formula-fed infants who consumed the egg yolks had improved iron levels when compared with the infants who did not. In addition, those infants who got the egg yolks enriched with extra fatty acids (the equivalent of grass-fed egg yolks) had 30-40 percent greater DHA levels than those fed regular egg yolks.[22]

Thus, the best choice for baby is yolks from pasture-fed hens since they will contain higher levels of DHA. If at all possible, try to obtain egg that are not only pasture-fed, but not fed soy.

Why just the yolk? The white is the portion that is most difficult to digest and most often causes allergic reactions, so wait to give egg whites until after your child turns one year old.

TIPS FOR FEEDING BABY

- Keep in mind, all babies are different and will not enjoy or tolerate the same foods or textures. Experiment by offering different foods with various textures. Remember, just because your baby doesn't like a food the first time it is introduced does not mean he will not like it the second time. Continue to offer the food, but never force.

- Baby's food should be lightly seasoned with unrefined salt, but in the beginning there is no need to add additional seasonings, such as herbs and spices. However by ten to twelve months, your baby may enjoy a variety of natural seasonings.

- To increase variety, take a small portion of the same food you are preparing for the rest of the grown-up family or leftovers, and purée it for baby (thin as necessary with homemade stock or water).

- To gradually make food lumpier, purée half of the food, roughly mash the other half and combine the two.

- Frozen finger foods are a great way to soothe a baby's teething discomfort.

- Keep a selection of plain whole yogurt, yogurt cheese, eggs, fresh fruit (especially ripe bananas) and ripe avocados handy to prepare almost instant natural baby food any time, even when vacationing or traveling.

- Organic foods have minimal toxicity, thus placing a smaller chemical burden on the body. This is particularly a benefit for our youngsters. They are more vulnerable to pesticide exposure because their organs and body systems are not fully developed and, in relation to body weight, they eat and drink more than adults. Remember that most of these pesticides are estrogenic, which means they cause hormonal disruption. Furthermore, the presence of these chemicals in the environment leads to further contamination of our air, waterways and fields.

- Let baby eat with a silver spoon—the small amount of silver he will get from the spoon really does help fight foodborne illness!

The other introductory food is liver. You can add a little grated frozen chicken, turkey or duck liver to the egg yolk, or make a separate liver purée (see Recipes).

Why add salt? Salt provides chloride, needed for the production of hydrochloric acid and the digestion of meats; and sodium activates an enzyme critical for neurological development. Use unrefined salt to supply a variety of trace minerals.

If baby is very mature and seems hungry, he may be given very ripe mashed banana during this period. Ripe banana is a great food for babies because it contains amylase enzymes to digest carbohydrates. It's also a wonderful source of vitamin B_6. Mashed ripe avocado is another great food for baby. It can be mixed with cream or yogurt.

AT SIX MONTHS

Puréed meats, including puréed chicken, goose or duck liver, can be given at six months (or even earlier if baby is very mature). Poultry liver provides a good balance of vitamins A, D_3 and K_2, and all meat helps ensure adequate intake of iron, zinc and protein with the decrease in breastmilk and formula.[23]

A variety of fruits can be introduced at this time. Avocado is a wonderful food for baby, mashed with a little salt or mixed with yogurt or cream. Melon, mangoes and papaya can be mashed and given raw. They also can be mixed with a fat source, such as cream or egg yolk.

High-pectin fruits such as peaches, apricots, apples, pears, cherries and berries should be cooked to break down the pectin, which can be very irritat-

---

BABY-LED WEANING?

The influential book *Baby-Led Weaning* by Gill Rapley and Tracey Murkett builds on the theory that eating problems such as pickiness are caused by babies starting "their journey to grown-up eating by being spoon-fed their first mouthfuls of puréed food on a date decided by their parents." The authors propose letting baby "show you when he's ready to start" and sharing "your meals from the very beginning."

The problem with this theory is that babies *do* need solid food long before they are old enough to know what to eat, let alone have the coordination to pick it up and eat it themselves. And the early foods that babies need should be puréed—remember, babies don't have teeth! By six months, baby needs egg yolk and puréed liver, foods he has no capability of eating on his own except for small amounts that might be transferred from his fingers to his mouth. And getting fed puréed food on a spoon is not an unpleasant experience for babies. While the first few feedings might be difficult and messy, once baby gets used to being fed, he will kick joyfully with every bite. What *is* unpleasant is cleaning up the mess that a small baby will make trying to feed himself. No one should have to do this several times per day.

Of course, as baby gets older, he will want to use his hands to put food into his mouth and eventually will learn to use a spoon. During this transition period you can start his meal by feeding him puréed food with a spoon, and then giving him some chunks of fruit for dessert, to eat by himself. As for sharing meals with a baby, mom and dad may very well wish to enjoy meals by themselves or with older children, after baby has been fed, cleaned up and put to bed.

The main premise of baby-led weaning—that babies and children should make their own choices about what they eat—is one to be resisted. Baby's parents should be squarely in charge of what baby eats from the beginning, and vigilant about ensuring that baby eats only what is good for him, especially during the early years when such control is possible. Of course, the food they feed baby should taste good, and they should not force feed a food that baby clearly does not like. But pickiness is rare in a well-nourished child, and exposure to foods of various tastes and textures during the early years is the ticket to adventurousness in eating as baby grows.

ing to the immature digestive tract. Again, cooked fruits should be mixed with cream, yogurt, melted coconut oil or butter.

As baby matures, you can increase the complexity and textures of the foods you give him. At about six to eight months, vegetables may be introduced, one at a time so that any adverse reactions can be observed. Carrots, sweet potatoes and beets are excellent first choices. All vegetables should be cooked (steamed preferably), mashed and mixed with a liberal amount of fat, such as butter or coconut oil, to provide nutrients to aid in digestion.

 If you want to have some fun, try giving baby some salmon eggs—fish eggs are held in high esteem in Asia as a food that makes babies smart! Babies enjoy picking up the beautful orange eggs with their fingers. Smaller fish eggs (caviar or roe) can be mixed with cream or yogurt cream.

Early introduction to different tastes is always a good plan to prevent finickiness. Feed your little one a touch of buttermilk, yogurt or kefir from time to time to familiarize him with the sour taste. Lacto-fermented root vegetables, like sweet potato or taro, are another excellent food for babies to add at this time (see Recipes).

AT EIGHT MONTHS

Baby can now consume a variety of foods including creamed vegetable soups, homemade stews and dairy foods such as cottage cheese, mild harder raw cheese and custards.

This is a good time to introduce lacto-fermented foods like sauerkraut or pickles.

Hold off on grains until one year, with the possible exception of soaked and thoroughly cooked brown rice, which can be served earlier to babies who are very mature.

HOW MUCH AT EACH MEAL?

With the rough outline below, one food portion is equal to approximately one tablespoon, depending on the type of ice cube or other food trays you may be using for freezing baby food. Start out slowly. Prepare a teaspoon-sized portion of whatever food you have chosen to begin with. Your baby will most likely only eat half of that small portion for the first few attempts with solids. Ultimately, baby will signal when he has had enough. Your main concern should be making what he does eat as nutritious as possible. As your baby becomes accustomed to eating solids, you can gradually increase the portion size. Once you have ruled out sensitivities and allergies to different foods, be sure to rotate the acceptable foods in the diet; that is, try to avoid having the same food day in and day out.

6-8 MONTHS:
- Breakfast: Breast milk or formula; 1 egg yolk; 1 cube meat; 1-2 tablespoons yogurt; yogurt cheese or smoothie.
- Lunch: Breast milk or formula; 1 cube meat; mashed banana or 1 cube fruit or vegetable.
- Dinner: Breast milk or formula; 1 cube of meat; 1-2 tablespoons fermented taro or sweet potato.

PORTIONS INCREASE FOR 8-10 MONTHS:
- Breakfast: Breast milk or formula; 1 egg yolk; 1-2 cubes fruit or vegetable; 1 cube meat.
- Lunch: Breast milk or formula; 1-2 cubes meat; 1-3 cubes vegetable; optional dairy such as yogurt or cheese.
- Dinner: Breast milk or formula; 2 cubes meat; 1-3 cubes fruit and vegetables; yogurt or cheese.
- Snacks: Finger foods or smoothie.

Remember, not all babies will be eating the same amounts of foods. This portion outline is just an example. Some infants are not ready to eat three "meals" per day until well into the nine-to-ten month range. You should use the above information as a general guideline only, being observant of baby's cues, weight gain and general process of development.

AT ONE YEAR

Grains, nuts and seeds should be the last foods introduced to babies. This food category has the most potential for causing digestive disturbances or allergies. Babies do not produce the needed enzymes to handle cereals, especially gluten-containing grains like wheat, before the age of one year. Even then, it is a common traditional practice to pre-digest grains by soaking them in water and a little yogurt or buttermilk overnight or for up to twenty-four hours (see Recipes). This process jump-starts the enzymatic activity in the food and begins breaking down some of the harder-to-digest components.

The easiest grains to digest are those without gluten, like brown rice. When grains are introduced, they should be soaked in an acidic medium and cooked with plenty of water for a long time. This will make a slightly sour, very thin porridge that can be mixed with other foods.

After one year, babies can be given nut butters made with crispy nuts (see Recipes), cooked leafy green vegetables, raw salad vegetables, citrus fruit and whole egg. Scrambled egg with an extra yolk is a great breakfast food for baby, starting at one year of age.

If baby is still nursing at one year of age—wonderful! If she is on our formula, you can switch over to raw whole milk. Whenever baby is weaned or even before, she can consume milk from a mug or sippy cup. The quantity of milk often decreases at this age to about sixteen to twenty ounces per day.

WATER

Opinions vary as to when to offer babies water. Many resources suggest giving water about the same time solids are introduced. This is often in combination with cup drinking or sippy-cup training. Keep in mind, breast milk and formula are providing the majority of nutrients in the first six to nine months, so it is important for baby not to get full on water.

When do you offer water, make sure it is filtered or spring water in glass (not plastic) containers, and never give your child fluoridated water (see sidebar, page 198).

Water with a squeeze of lemon and a pinch of salt will hydrate baby better than plain water.

When solids become a larger part of the diet, more liquid may be needed for hydration and digestion.

BABIES DO NEED SALT!

Between 1984 and 1991, several lawsuits took place involving two brands of chloride-deficient formula, produced by a company called Syntex. The plaintiffs argued that by removing chloride (in the form of sodium chloride) from the formula, their children did not achieve their full intellectual potential. Experts testified that chloride (from sodium chloride, salt) was essential for the growth and development of the brain. Syntex went out of the infant formula business because of adverse publicity about their products. Today all baby formula has added salt.

Salt to provide chloride is essential for the developing brain, particularly for the glial cells, those structures that make us capable of higher, creative thinking. Sodium is also critical for neurological development. Yet today, so-called "experts" urge us to restrict salt in children's diets.

Restricting salt in the early months of life can result in poor neurodevelopment in later years. In fact, pre-term babies need even more salt than those who go to term.[24] In the womb, babies get sodium and chloride from the mother, who should be consuming plenty of salt. A wonderful Jewish custom puts a pinch of salt on the tongue of a newborn baby.

Mammalian milk concentrates salt because growing mammals need salt. Human mothers need plenty of salt while they are nursing, to ensure that their breast milk is of high quality; and babies should have salt added to their weaning foods—baby's food should taste slightly, not overly, salty.

Also, extreme heat, dehydration, vomiting and fever may also indicate a need for extra water. Bottom line: follow your baby's cues. In cases of dehydraton, that pinch of salt added to water is a must.

JUST SAY NO!

One important warning: do not give your child juice, which contains too much simple sugar and may ruin a child's appetite for the more nourishing food choices. A 1994 study found that children who drank lots of juice were at risk for failure to thrive.[25] The sorbitol in apple juice is especially difficult for children to digest and the fructose in all juices puts a real strain on the liver.

Soy foods, margarine and shortening, vegetable oils, dry breakfast cereals, soy foods (including tofu) and commercial dairy products (especially ultrapasteurized) should also be avoided, as well as any products that are reduced-fat or lowfat.

CHUBBY BABIES ARE HAPPY BABIES

The current thrust of dietitians and the medical establishment is to restrict food for babies to avoid obesity. But baby fat is a good thing; babies need those extra folds for growth and development. Babies have a lot of what is called brown fat, which helps keep them warm and gives them plenty of energy. Because it increases metabolism, brown fat helps *prevent* excessive weight gain.

It is easier for baby to make muscle from fat than from nothing. And baby fat produces important immune-supporting compounds.

If you are concerned about weight gain, just make sure to withhold high-carbohydrate foods and all empty processed foods. Even if these foods don't cause weight gain right away, they will dispose your baby to overweight later on.

NOT A GOOD IDEA FOR BABIES!

The proliferation of beverages—often called "milk"—based on soy, almonds, rice and even hemp poses a temptation to parents wanting to feed their children right; parents often turn to these beverages in an attempt to avoid milk allergies, perhaps not knowing about raw milk, or not having any access to it. But these alternative beverages are not good foods for your baby; they are highly processed, often containing refined sweeteners and industrial oils, plus inappropriate additives such as carrageenan (very difficult for babies to digest) and the synthetic form of vitamin D (vitamin D_2, which can have the opposite effect of the animal form, vitamin D_3). Soy milk with its high levels of plant-based estrogens (called isoflavones) is out of the question; the other milks may not contain isoflavones, but they are low in nutritive factors and not good foods for baby—nor for their brothers and sisters!

Almond Breeze Vanilla (Almond Milk): Purified water, evaporated cane juice, almonds, tricalcium phosphate, natural vanilla flavor and other natural flavors, sea salt, potassium citrate, carrageenan, soy lecithin, d-alpha tocopherol (natural vitamin E), vitamin A palmitate, vitamin D_2.

Rice Dream "Heartwise" Rice Drink Original: Filtered water, brown rice (partially milled) gum arabic, expeller pressed high oleic safflower oil, tricalcium phosphate, CorowiseTM phytosterol esters, sea salt, vitamin A palmitate, vitamin D_2, vitamin B_{12}.

365 Organic Rice Milk Vanilla: Filtered water, partially milled organic rice, organic expeller pressed canola oil, tricalcium phosphate, natural vanilla flavor with other natural flavors, sea salt, carrageenan, vitamin A palmitate, vitamin D.

365 Organic Soymilk, Plain: Filtered Water, Whole Organic Soybeans, Organic Evaporated Cane juice, Calcium Carbonate, Sea Salt, Natural Flavors, Carrageenan, Vitamin A Palmitate, Vitamin D_2, Riboflavin (Vitamin B_2), Vitamin B_{12}.

DOESN'T LIKE VEGETABLES?

Don't sweat it, mom! Most of baby's nutrition should come from animal foods at this early age. Baby doesn't have the enzymes online yet to obtain much nourishment from vegetables; he can't convert the carotenes in vegetables to vitamin A, for example. In addition, many of the minerals in vegetables are blocked by antinutrients like oxalic acid. When you do feed vegetables, they should be well cooked and served with butter or other healthy fat. Hopefully your child will learn to like vegetables as he grows older.

PRINCIPLES OF HOMEMADE BABY FOOD

Making homemade baby food may not be as easy as opening a jar, but once you have organized a cook-and-freeze routine, it becomes second nature. Making your own baby food gives you control over food choices and cooking methods, and allows you to avoid synthetic preservatives. With careful preparation, you will maximize the nutrient and enzyme content of your baby's food. This will make for easier digestion and better overall nutrition.

One timesaving method is to cook and purée a selection of fruits, vegetables and meats in adult quantities, then freeze them in glass custard dishes or porcelain ramekins, or just clumps on a baking sheet. You can also freeze them in ice cube trays. These cubes can then be placed in freezer bags, labeled and sealed, available for quick thawing and reheating.

Thawing in the refrigerator is the most nutrient-saving method. Simply place a covered dish containing food cubes in the fridge; they will thaw in three to four hours. It only takes one to two hours at room temperature. Frozen meats can be warmed up by placing them in a container set in simmering water. When on the go, put the cubes in a glass container and add hot water or place the container in hot water to thaw. Most importantly, avoid the temptation of thawing the nutritious baby food you have made in the microwave!

Little attention is necessary to seasoning baby foods except to add adequate salt—baby's food should taste slightly salty, not overly so. But texture is important. Besides the basic taste, the smoothness or thickness of a food is what concerns baby most. To thin purées, use breast milk, homemade formula or homemade bone broth.

The only special equipment you need is a food processor, blender or a baby food mill and a simple metal collapsible steamer basket. Don't forget the

---

WHEN RAW MILK IS NOT AVAILABLE

Raw milk is an important part of our dietary protocol for babies and children. But what if you have no access to raw milk? Not to worry. Although raw milk is a wonderful food for growing children, you can still raise healthy children without it. The important thing is not to give pasteurized milk, which is highly allergenic and can cause digestive disorders, asthma and chronic ear infections. Here are some tips if you don't have access to raw milk:

- If you need to use a homemade formula, use the liver-based formula, with added whey made from a good quality store-bought yogurt.

- Use lots and lots of bone broth throughout the growing years, added to baby food and used in soups, sauces and stews. When making the bone broth, you can add egg shells for extra calcium.

- As soon as baby is old enough, add raw cheese to his diet. Raw cheese is legal everywhere, and can be ordered on the Internet if not available in your town.

- If you can obtain raw or pasteurized (but not ultra-pasteurized) cream, serve it frequently. Check the Shopping Guide of the Weston A. Price Foundation for sources of frozen raw cream. This can be diluted with water and consumed as a raw dairy beverage.

unbreakable serving bowls, baby spoons and bibs. Two-handed weighted cups for drinking lessons are also helpful.

Never hesitate to add fat to baby food, fat such as butter, cream or coconut milk. A breastfeeding mother naturally produces the needed nutrition when she consumes the necessary nutrients. The composition of healthy breast milk gives us a blueprint for an infant's needs from birth to maturity. That means a diet should contain at least 50 percent of calories as healthy animal fat.

As baby learns to feed himself, stainless steel or silver baby spoons are best as baby will chew on the plastic ones.

INTRODUCING GRAINS

Today we are facing an epidemic of grain allergies, often manifesting as serious illnesses like celiac disease. The treatment for gluten and grain intolerance is to take the child off all grains, often for an extended period of time.

This is a difficult strategy for families in our grain-centered society. It is very hard to avoid grains one hundred percent of the time while also leading a normal life; and, after all, grains are a key factor in making our diet tasty and interesting.

The secret to avoiding problems with grains, as we have stated, is to introduce them slowly and carefully. No grains at all during the first year is the first rule; then in the second year, baby can have certain carefully prepared grain dishes, such as soaked cereal gruel and properly prepared brown rice. If there is a history of celiac disease and gluten intolerance in the family, you might want to wait until the third year before introducing any grains.

Key to avoiding problems with grains are foods rich in cholesterol and the fat-soluble vitamins A and D, which are needed for building a healthy gut wall; equally important is arachidonic acid, a fat found in egg yolks and liver, which the body uses to build tight cell-to-cell junctures, needed for gut integrity.[26]

AVOIDING REFINED SWEETENERS

Keeping refined sweeteners, such as sugar, high fructose corn syrup and agave "nectar," away from your children is a most difficult challenge for parents in modern life, one that requires discipline, planning, creative alternatives and cunning strategy. The following tips may prove useful:

- Don't keep sweets around the house, even if you as parents have the will power to resist temptation. Children will find their way to candies, cookies and other sweet snacks if they are available.

- Never shop when you are hungry.

- Have plenty of nutritious snacks, such as crispy nuts, cheese, salami and raw milk, available for snack times.

- Never send a child to a birthday party or a sleepover on an empty stomach; but fortify her beforehand with a large and nutritious meal or snack.

- Allow occasional desserts sweetened with natural sweeteners, such as maple syrup, maple sugar, unrefined honey, dehydrated cane sugar juice and coconut nectar.

- Be resigned to the fact that you cannot keep refined sweeteners away from your children entirely. Don't make a fuss when they eat sweets and junk foods occasionally while they are with friends or you might give them good reason to rebel. You can protect them from the occasional use of sugar with a diet at home that is consistently nutritious. When they are old enough, be sure to explain just why sugar is so bad for them. Remember that your example is your child's best guide to his adult eating habits.

IRON-FORTIFIED FOODS FOR BABY: NOT SUCH A GOOD IDEA

Iron is very important for the neurological development of children, and the scientific literature is rife with reports of lowered IQ in children with low iron status. For this reason, the U.S. Food and Drug Administration (FDA) mandates the inclusion of a form of iron in infant formula and in infant cereals; indeed iron is added to flour and cereal products for all ages. Unfortunately, such "fortification" has been shown to produce *lower* IQ levels, the very result the inclusion of iron is meant to prevent.

For example, when researchers studied the long-term effects of iron-fortified formula, they found that those on the fortified formula had lower indications of intelligence ten years later compared to those given unfortified formula.[27] The researchers measured IQ, spatial memory, arithmetic achievement, visual-motor integration, visual perception and motor functioning, and those given unfortified formula scored better in every category.

It seems that the iron used in fortification is not processed the same way as iron in food. For example, added iron encourages the growth of iron-loving bacteria in the intestinal tract—and iron-loving bacteria are largely pathogenic. One study found that oral iron supplementation in the tropics in children of all ages was associated with increased risk of clinical malaria and other infections including pneumonia.[28]

One reason to avoid prenatal vitamins is their content of inorganic iron. One study found a correlation between maternal iron supplementation in pregnancy and the most common childhood cancers: leukemia and lymphoma.[29]

Iron supplementation may also cause stunted growth. According to an extensive review of the effects of iron on skeletal developments in early life "iron supplementation in young children without iron deficiency may jeopardize optimal height and weight gains."[30]

Looking forward to adulthood, a Finnish study found that excess iron stores were a stronger risk for heart attack than hypertension or cholesterol levels.[31]

Clearly, pregnant and nursing mothers, and growing babies, need to get their iron—a vital nutrient—from foods, as they have done for centuries, and not the isolated, synthetic type of iron added to formula, vitamin pills and baby foods.

As baby reaches the third year, more grain products can be introduced, such as sourdough bread, soaked pancakes and soaked grain casseroles. Avoid the grain extremes—completely refined grocery store breads and very rough, nonsourdough breads containing bran and added gluten. Above all take care that baby eats his grains with plenty of fat—the butter on his bread should be thick enough to show teeth marks!

AS BABY GROWS

As baby grows, you will be able to add more and more variety to his diet. Before long he will be eating at the table with the rest of the family—which means that the rest of the family should be eating nutrient-dense home-cooked meals as well.

Sometimes pickiness sets in around eighteen months to three years, even if your child was a great eater prior to this period. If a child really reacts negatively to a food, just stop serving it for a while. If your child refuses important foods like eggs, you can hide them in dishes like smoothies and custards. Children who are well nourished from birth usually come back to loving all kinds of foods later in life. (For more on overcoming pickiness, see Chapter 17.)

And one word of caution: don't be overly strict! At the age of two, your baby can share in an occasional homecooked dessert. An outing to a restaurant every now and then is a good experience for the whole family—just make sure that restaurant is at least one notch above a fast food outlet.

And, without a doubt, the child that you have raised so carefully on nutrient-dense food will want to have a social life. You cannot lock your child in a closet. She will want to go to friends' houses where she will invariably be exposed to food that you wouldn't serve at home.

Hopefully, with the good start you have given her, sweets and junk food won't appeal to her. But even if she eats such substandard fare from time to time, you will have given her ample protection with the diet that she eats most of the time at home.

Think of the body as a house. If your child starts out on a nutrient-dense diet, that body will be like a magnificently constructed mansion, requiring very little maintenance and standing impervious to occasional destructive elements for many years. But if a child begins life on substandard foods, the poorly constructed body-house she ends up with may need constant maintenance and be immediately vulnerable to the destructive elements in junk food.

Maintaining the right attitude about diet is a challenging exercise for parents—you will want to provide nutrient-dense food in a loving positive way, without being overly restrictive or critical. Your children should know that it does them no good to ask for junk food, that you won't buy it for them, and they should understand that you are in charge where meals are concerned. At the same time, parents should not make a fuss at the occasional exposure to junk food at sporting events, birthday parties or visits to grandma. If baby has a good start nutritionally, she will be able to handle these occasions.

And as baby grows, she should be gently taught the principles of good nutrition. After all, the goal is not only healthy children, but healthy grandchildren as well.

FOR FURTHER INFORMATION:

Super Nutrition for Babies: The Right Way to Feed Your Baby for Optimal Health by Katherine Erlich, MD and Kelly Genzlinger, CNC, CMTA

FLUORIDE DANGERS

Dental and medical organizations all promote the use of fluoridated water, fluoride drops and fluoridated toothpaste as a way to prevent tooth decay. Yet the healthy natives studied by Weston Price were virtually free of cavities, and they never drank fluoridated water or used fluoridated toothpaste; indeed they never used toothpaste at all!

There is a real downside to exposing your child to fluoride. Fluoride is an enzyme inhibitor and thyroid supressor, which can cause a range of problems, from mottled teeth, weak bones, and sluggish metabolism to behavioral problems.[32]

Even the U.S. government warns parents not to let their children get too much fluoridated toothpaste, for fear of adverse effects.[33] And warnings are also now appearing about using fluoridated water for baby formula.[34]

The latest nail in the coffin for fluoride comes from the journal *Environmental Health Perspectives,* which has recently published a thorough and systematic review by Harvard researchers of eligible studies through the end of 2011 in order to examine the possible adverse effects of exposure to fluoride and the potential of delayed neurobehavioral development in children.[35]

The researchers found that children in high fluoride areas had significantly lower IQ scores than those who lived in low fluoride areas. As a result of their analysis, the researchers concluded that "The results support the possibility of an adverse effect of high fluoride exposure on children's neurodevelopment."

For information on dental health for your child, see Chapter 17.

Chapter 10
From Birth to Adulthood

We have described the accepted physical, behavioral and intellectual milestones for growing children in Chapter Nine. These were developed by Dr. Arnold Gesell and other behavioralists starting in the early twentieth century.

This chapter will look at this subject from a different angle, one described by Rudolf Steiner and other esoteric thinkers who have pondered the wondrous unfolding of the child.

We start by assuming that the child has a soul, an inner life, and that soul changes correspond with changes in the physical body. In addition, the development of the child into an adult in many respects mirrors the changes that all humanity has gone through in its still-evolving process. Let us follow these parallel lines of development and see how they can help us guide our children on their voyage to adulthood.

As we describe these stages, we will see the great danger in rushing your child's development. In virtually every instance where children experience developmental problems, they arise because the child was thwarted from experiencing these stages in their entirety and at the appropriate time. There is never any justification for hurrying a child in his or her development. In fact, the strategy we outline here will encourage you to allow your children to linger back

in these stages, to allow these stages to work deeply into their physical and soul beings. If you rush things, expect problems—poor health, lack of vitality, lack of willpower, depression, the boomerang child who never really grows up. If you allow your child to completely experience each stage of development in its entirety, the vitality and self-mastery that your child attains will literally amaze you.

In the beginning, both humanity and the newborn child experience the world in an "undifferentiated" way. The child comes into the world "trailing clouds of glory," as the poet Wordsworth said. His or her soul has descended from the supersensible worlds into a physical body, and the transition from spiritual to physical world is a gradual one.

As we observe the newborn, it seems reasonable to say that he experiences the world as a unity, or even, we might say, as pure feeling. Nothing is yet named or even considered as a separate object. This correlates with the non-dualistic origin of humanity that is referred to in all native and spiritual traditions, a sort of Garden of Eden where nothing yet has a name or an individual identity.

Imagine living in this stage, where we do not experience a chair or table, nor any other person, nor even oneself. Instead, there is only pure experience. Sometimes the experience is joy, at other times it is hunger, sometimes peace, sometimes it is wetness,

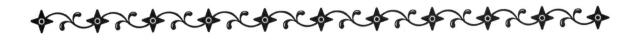

sometimes tummy pain. All this is experienced without judgment, without naming, and completely outside of time.

Amazingly, this is what we try to attain in our endless meditation and yoga classes, this is the state that has been written about by so many gurus and self-help authors and about which we have countless unread books on our shelves. This is the complete non-dualistic, non-judgmental state, the very thing we will want to learn about when we are in our fifties, with nonviolent communication workshops and meditation classes—there it is for the newborn, right off the bat! Why would you want to rush someone out of this stage with alphabet books and learning DVDs?

Unfortunately, most parents do so deliberately or, more often, unconsciously. We have even seen parents put flashcards with the names of all the objects in their house so the baby can more quickly learn these names! Even pointing out objects in a child's world and saying the names has the effect of rushing the child out of the precious, undifferentiated infant period. Much better for a child to glean the names of things through his own effort as he soaks in normal conversation, or to wait until the child asks you, "What's that?"

By the same token, it's important to resist with everything you can muster in helping the child do anything, except in the context of directly answering the child's question. You do not help your baby by putting an object into his hands when he is struggling to do this himself, or by rolling him over when he is working hard towards this accomplishment.

The importance of this first purely experiential stage is that it will imprint deeply in the child's memory the place that adults so ardently seek later in life. That is, in accord with all the profound spiritual teachings, adults long to return to a non-dualistic state in which we become conscious of supersensible worlds, except that as an adult we want to do this having thoroughly developed our mental body, our sense of individuality. Such an accomplishment will be greatly facilitated in your child the more you let the child live into and truly experience this state of being in the first years of life.

It follows therefore that the life of the child in this

first year or so, a process that ends approximately when the child gets his first teeth, should be as minimalist as possible. No museums, no over-stimulation, no flash cards, no DVDs, no gaudy toys, the fewer objects in their lives the better. The child's life is best lived in the warm embrace of the parents and left in quiet to explore her own sensations and the sensations that naturally occur in the world, such as cold, wind and even rain.

The child has a lot to accomplish in that first year—hand-eye coordination, head lifting, rolling over, sitting up, scooting across the floor, crawling and standing.

No "toys" or plastic objects of any kind need be in the child's life; after all, for an undifferentiated being there is no difference between "toy" and anything else. Instead give them household objects to play with—wooden spoons, colored scarfs, measuring cups and unbreakable kitchen ware. "Play" is not even the right word yet, because before the teeth erupt, the child doesn't really play, he just experiences the world and himself. After the teeth come in, however, the child does play, and that is very serious business indeed.

The eruption of the teeth signifies a "hardening," an emergence from this watery, undifferentiated state towards the hardened state of adult life in the physical world. This, like all "falls" and transitions, is often accompanied by some pain and occasional sickness, such as colds and fevers. We call this pain "teething," and the preventative measure is simply at all costs to resist rushing the child's development. If you surround him with toys, place flash cards on the chairs, name the objects in their world, you can expect teething pain—the child is warning you, "It's too soon for this."

As the teeth emerge the child starts to bear down on the first major milestone, when he first refers to himself as "I." In the ideal world, this happens at the age of three and marks the end of non-dualism. In saying the word "I," the child's consciousness shifts squarely to the self as opposed to the non-self world.

Many illnesses emerge as a consequence of immune system dysfunction, in which the body confuses self with non-self. These are the auto-immune diseases, and they all have their origin in the failure of our modern way of life to let the child slowly, without being pushed, work through these first three years while the distinguishing of the self from the non-self gradually emerges.

NAMING THE WORLD

In these first three years, the child will often ask you to name the world for him. A child of two points at objects or asks, "What's that?" By refraining from naming things for the child until he asks, you let the child decide what he wishes to learn.

Most importantly, you can use the opportunity of teaching a word to also teach your child that the world is made of stories, that it is about relationships, not about distinct, separate objects, which fundamentally are illusions anyway. So when you child asks, "What's this?" and points to the bed, rather than merely saying "a bed," rather than creating the impression that we live in a cold world of objects, you tell your child that the bed is the soft place where your wonderful Aunt Millie sleeps when she visits from a long ways away.

Children are not usually satisfied with a single word answer. If you just tell your child, "a bed," you will get repeated "What's that?" questions with no sense of connection. But an answer that infuses the object with meaning might lead to wide eyes, a sense of comprehension and wonder, even sitting on the bed snuggled up telling stories about when you and Aunt Millie were children. Which kind of answer seems to speak more accurately to the soul nature of the child at this age?

MEETING CHALLENGES

One school of thought advocates teaching your child about the objects in the world by describing them to the young child. So a walk on the beach goes like this: "This is the sand, there are the big waves, we don't eat sand and the water is very dangerous and you should never go near it without mommy or daddy." Here is another option: just go for a walk, hold hands when the child wants, let her run, roll around and yes, even put the sand in her mouth and even let her get close to the big waves. Let her experience, without interruption and without editing, all the impressions of the world. Of course, we are not advocating letting your child get swept away by the waves; your job is to ensure her safety, period. But in fact, it has been repeatedly found that when cultures let even very young children explore their own boundaries, for example with knives, they have fewer injuries and accidents than those that don't, and the children grow to have great facility navigating dangers when they are adults.[1]

The expected reaction of a child told never to eat sand or go near waves is, "This guy's not much fun, I'm not sure I trust him, so I'll find out for myself." If, instead, after the child puts sand in his mouth you say, "Yeah, I remember eating sand, yuck!" you will laugh together and develop a real bond of sharing and trust. The child knows you get it, the experience is shared and the appreciation for allowing him to experience the world for himself will be profound. So in addition to assuring the child's safety, you are there to share your story of the world as you experience it.

Another example comes from a wonderful kindergarten program in Denmark. The children mostly play outside and the activities are completely child-directed except for a daily story that the teacher tells the children.

The school has a huge tree on its grounds with many branches to climb on. It is the goal of every child in the program to climb up high in the tree; the only rule (mostly unspoken) is that no one, no child or teacher, helps anyone else climb the tree. Usually the children can get near the top around age five or six.

Children even less than one year old show interest in climbing the tree. Between the ages of one and three, nothing much happens except the children circle the tree, feel its bark and just experience its massive being. You can almost imagine the younger children in small groups marveling as the older ones scurry to the heights, while the younger ones stay below and map out their strategy—in contrast to the modern approach to child development that says, if the child is frustrated with learning to walk then put him in a walker.

At the school in Denmark, the adults do nothing. They let the children circle the tree day after day, week after week, even year after year. No offer of help or advice is ever given. Amazingly, according to teachers at the school, there is no hint of frustration or boredom with this process. What you see is an inner determination.

Then one day, maybe after years, and maybe sooner for some than others—it makes no difference to anyone—the child scales the tree. The entire community literally erupts in joy. Joy, not praise, not "Oh you are so good," or "You are so accomplished." No rewards are given, no prizes, there is just the spontaneous eruption of joy for the child and for those who act as witnesses. No photos or videos are ever taken, yet the children will picture their moment for their entire lives. This is how we want to raise our children, this is the deepest, truest therapy for a whole culture that has attention deficit disorder.

LIFE CHANGES AND THEIR ILLNESSES

Any change in either physical or inner development

THE TEETH AS A MIRROR OF THE SOUL LIFE

Dr. Price showed us that the physical appearance of a person's teeth gives us a picture of the quality of nutrition in that person's diet, even from before conception. Rudolf Steiner put emphasis on the teeth as a mirror of the soul life of the child. (Imagine what that says about the native populations with their wide, straight, white teeth! These are people with a very rich soul life.)

As children grow, the eruption of the teeth signifies a "hardening," an emergence from this watery, undifferentiated state towards the hardened state of adult life in the physical world. By the age of three, the baby teeth are all in, the child knows many words, and refers to himself as "I," a sign that the ego or mental body is beginning to form. The next major milestone in both physical and soul development is the process of losing the first teeth and acquiring the adult teeth. That this happens at all is a miracle; how amazing that we are so complex and fine-tuned to have two sets of teeth, each of which fits the different size and shape of our faces at different stages of our lives.

The "inner" reality is even more fascinating. The human body, especially the bones and teeth, are formed according to the same geometric laws that govern many natural phenomena; but more surprisingly, they correlate in a precise way with the laws that govern music. According to Frederick Husemann, MD, author of *The Harmony of the Human Body: Musical Principles in Human Physiology*, in normal development we have twenty baby teeth arranged in four sets of five (two molars, one canine, two incisors in each of the four quadrants). In the normal adult there are thirty-two teeth, four sets of eight teeth (three molars, three bicuspids, one cuspid and two incisors in each of the four quadrants). As Dr. Husemann points out, the teeth correlate with the two major musical scales in western music, the pentatonic scale, based on five notes and the octave with its eight notes. The pentatonic scale is the predominant scale in folk songs and lullabies throughout the world, songs that are sung for and with young children. Use of the pentatonic scale gives music an ethereal mood and is especially conducive to repetitive songs like children's ditties and Gregorian chants. The music flows, the words don't have to mean anything; such music corresponds well with the soul state of young children. It is the music of the non-differentiated world, the world before naming and counting, the world where there is no difference between the sheet and the body, the me and the mother's breast. Up to the change of teeth, it is as though the child's being, with its pentatonic scale of teeth embedded into the mouth, is constructed to resonate with this type of music. It goes without saying that until the change of teeth, beginning at age seven, this is the music the children should listen to, preferably sung or played on live instruments. Luckily, by their very nature, pentatonic songs are easy to sing or play on simple instruments, such as a recorder or xylophone.

Then comes the change in teeth, the next major developmental step. This is the usual time that children start to experience a different kind of learning, correlating with the stage in human evolution that began the use of numbers and letters. Now is the time to begin reading instruction and introduce the child to classical music.

carries its specific set of challenges and risks. In human development these stages are associated with illnesses that facilitate these changes.

As outlined in the Introduction, the human being has four bodies or levels of activity that link us with the various kingdoms of nature and the four major "elements" of earth, water, air and fire. Each of these bodies must be "born," or go through a kind of liberation in the seven-year cycles of the human being.

The first birth, into the physical body, into the earth realm, occurs during the actual birth process. Frequently, usually in the first year, the child contracts whooping cough (pertussis) or croup, which represents the challenge of overcoming the earth element.

Paradoxically, the earth element resides in the lungs. While it may seem strange to associate the lungs with the earth element, it is through the lungs that we take our first breath and connect most intimately with the world into which we are born. Any birth or transition comes with dangers, but with whooping cough, the child struggles with and eventually emerges the victor for a lifetime over the earth element, the element of the lungs. Not allowing the

---

THE SERIOUS BUSINESS OF PLAY

Only young children know how to play—to occupy themselves with objects while creating an imaginative narration in the mind. While the word "play" is defined as a recreation or amusement, for children, play is a serious business in which adults have no right to interfere. That's right; notwithstanding the advice of countless childrearing experts who advocate "play time" with their children, parents should not share in a child's play activities. Children's play is an activity so foreign to an adult consciousness that no parents can really play with their children.

Consider the young boy playing fort, or the young girl imagining a long sailing trip to distant places. In children's imaginations, they are there, they picture the fort battle, they live their visit to foreign lands. Then adults come along with their rules, their how-to-do-its, their book learning to interrupt the child's imaginative thought patterns. The point of play is not to make something real with rules and books, but to create a world out of inner instincts. Adults generally speaking have too much responsibility, too many disappointments, too much school learning to play. Children should engage in imaginative play, with as many real or made-up props as they can, for as long as they can, until they are as old as possible. Adults do children no service by interfering with this sacred activity.

Note that playing baseball or soccer doesn't count as play. There's nothing wrong with parents throwing a baseball or kicking a soccer ball with their children, but they shouldn't teach young children how to perform specific skills unless the child specifically asks. Then—and this is crucial—briefly and succinctly answer only the question. For example if your child asks how to hold a fastball, show him the grip and nothing more; don't correct him if he is wrong, don't say "good job" if he does it correctly, just keep throwing the ball and let him ask when he wants to know more. More importantly let him spend hours pretending to be Willie Mays, catching the last out in the World Series, off the roof, between the legs— that, for a child, is "playing" baseball. Little league and other organized sports for children is a job—it has nothing to do with play. Organized sports for children should not begin until age seven.

Don't play with your children, just do your stuff—laundry, cooking, gardening, mowing the lawn, bird watching. If you see a beautiful bluebird, it's fine to share this with your child, but don't be disappointed if he wants to look at crickets in the grass rather that watch for birds.

Don't teach them, don't praise them, don't correct them, let them experiment, play, imagine and create the world they want to live in. If they have questions, they'll ask; your job is to answer, no more. Children brought up this way will create a new world, one that works for them and is respectful of all that is around them. That's the purpose of the very serious business of play.

child to go through the "initiation" of whooping cough or croup often sets the child up for a life of struggle with breathing, a fairly accurate description of asthma. (For more on this subject, see Chapters 15.)

Having become master of the earth element, the normally developing child has an illness-free life until the next major encounter, an encounter with the watery realm, which occurs at age seven. Emerging from the undifferentiated, pentatonic, dreamy lullaby world, now is the time to learn and differentiate, to name and number the world. As an aid and a challenge, the child encounters the next archetypal illness, the measles. In measles, there is a huge outpouring of fluids, mucus from virtually every orifice, accompanied by high fever, rash and mouth sores. Measles presents the next great soul challenge for the child.

Three weeks later, the child emerges, like a snake having shed its skin, as lord of the watery realm, rarely to struggle with the mucousy illnesses like ear infections, runny nose or conjunctivitis, ever again. If the child is never allowed to have the measles, he is like a snake that is prevented from transforma-

---

SUPPORTING YOUR CHILD'S DEVELOPMENTAL STAGES

STAGE ONE, 0-7 YEARS:
- During this stage the physical body is taking form; good nutrition is of paramount importance. This is the only stage of life where you can keep most junk food out of your child's diet.
- The child engages in play and should be supported in this activity by a hands-off policy. Don't play with your child!
- Only provide your child with the information he requests—answer his questions without volunteering any more information.
- Gentle discipline using the Time Out method (pages 172-173) may be needed to correct any destructive behavior.

STAGE TWO, 7-14 YEARS:
- With the full anchoring in the physical body, the child can start intellectual activity, learning to read and learning arithmetical concepts in some kind of scholastic setting.
- The etheric body comes into development, often with accompanying illnesses. These illnesses should be honored with non-toxic treatments that support wholeness rather than merely suppress symptoms.
- This is the age when children need heros, adults they look up to, such as a grandparent, teacher or coach—not one of the parents. If you are homeschooling, it is important for your child to have group activities outside the home so that he can become acquainted with adults to admire.

STAGE THREE, 14-21 YEARS:
- During the rocky years of adolescence, the emotional or soul life matures. Parents should not pry into their child's emotional life. Let him share only what he chooses to.
- In medieval times, and even up to the twentieth century, age fourteen was the typical age that male children left home—to become an apprentice, join the military, or simply explore the world. Modern children typically don't leave home until the age of eighteen, but starting at age fourteen, school trips, long sessions at camp and student exchange experiences will support your child's desire for independence.
- Pick your battles! You can't and shouldn't have complete control over every aspect of your teenager's life.

STAGE FOUR, 21-28 YEARS:
- The age when the mental body develops; Steiner stated that no individual should hold a position of authority until he reaches the twenty-eighth year.
- Intense mental activity including advanced studies are appropriate during this period. In fact, some children do better to work for a year or two after high school before starting college studies.

tion—there is a kind of misfitting quality. The child then spends the school years squirming in his own skin, fruitlessly trying to "get out." The problem is, there is no out. At a time when children should be showing an intense interest in the physical world, they may be unfocused. In particularly bad cases, we refer to the condition as ADD or ADHD. Sometimes we see a child with a constantly runny nose, as the process of overcoming the mucousy, watery realm never got completed. The child was unable to meet the challenge, transform and move on.

STORY TIME

There is no more wonderful activity that a parent can do with a child than reading out loud. It's good to set aside time for reading every day, such as before bedtime. Reading material—material that you read to the child and material that the child reads himself—should appeal to her age and stage of development.

For very early childhood, Rudolf Steiner recommended simple, colorful books, expecially those containing ditties and repetitive material. Very young children love repetition, and simple poems and songs. Simple repetitive fairy tales, such as "Robin Hood" or "Goldilocks and the Three Bears," will be heard with delight.

Around age four, more sophisticated fairy tales can be introduced, especially those that provide an image of a benevolent and bountiful world, such as tales that describe the cup that never empties and the wallet of good things that is always full. In the first grade, the illustrated fairy tale should reign supreme. All the experience children of this age need can be found in them, including pictures for letters, colors, songs plays, even counting and arithmetic. Fairy tales such as "Snow White" and "Sleeping Beauty" speak to children of mankind's emotional and spiritual evolution on a very deep level.

As the child grows, the fable becomes more appropriate, in which animals not only speak and enjoy human powers as they do in the fairy tales, but also personify some particular human quality, virtue or vice. Legends of saints, holy men and adventurers lead childen gradually from the archetypal world of fairy tales to the perception of more human qualities in nature and in the individual's relationship with nature, just at the stage when the child is developing that relationship herself. These stories can and should come from all the countries of the world. Children need to be supported in their belief in the magical. Science fiction and computer games are the substitute food for a generation starved of the magical, the unhappy fallout of the humanist education, which feeds children only materialistic concepts.

For age eight, Rudolf Steiner recommended some of the better-known stories from the Old Testament, which provide legend in its highest and grandest form—Noah with the animals, Elijah with the ravens, David with his sling and Joshua with his trumpet. Old Testament stories also provide an allegory of man's journey from paradise to earth, a journey that the children themselves are in the process of making, one they should feel most assuredly is directed by divine guidance.

The ninth year is the perfect time to introduce the Greek myths and stories of life in ancient Greece, as the outlook of ancient Greece, which made man the measure of all things, corresponds to the state of development at the age of nine, when the child embraces his individuality. Norse mythology, which expresses a vigorous individualism, is perfect for age ten. Stories of great historical deeds are also appropriate in this period. At this age children will have outgrown the attraction to fairy tales but will love stories about the Trojan Wars, Robinson Crusoe and Marco Polo. In the twelfth year, as their sense of justice comes to the fore, they will enjoy learning about the Roman Empire, characterized by the rule of law.

At the later ages, the child is probably reading on his own, and access to age-appropriate reading material will encourage and support the habit of life-long reading.

SOURCE: *The Recovery of Man in Childhood* by A. C. Harwood

Most traditional cultures have marked this seven-year change with a ceremony of some sort, to acknowledge the accomplishment. We, unfortunately, often miss it altogether.

The child moves on. Around age nine, we notice a new attitude, a kind of rebelliousness, often epitomized by the child saying "You're not my real parents." Observant adults notice a loss of innocence; a new kind of questioning will often arise at this time. This is the halfway point for the child's physical development. The child has half his adult teeth and is experiencing the last remnants of the non-dualistic consciousness that he will ever experience without "earning" it, without consciously attaining it.

This can be a frightening time for a child; it's painful to leave the garden of childhood, painful to see the objects of the world as discrete, unrelated, cold entities to which he has no connection; the child may even feel that he has no connection to his own family.

Over the next few years, the child may experience a feeling of anticipation; she is heading to the next great transition. The upheaval called puberty happens around fourteen years of age—rather, it *should* happen at that time. Unfortunately, this transition is taking place at earlier and earlier ages in western countries.

Age fourteen marks the emergence of the soul or emotional body. Along with this comes sexual development, the deepening of the voice in boys, and the increased awareness of the emotional realm occurring in girls. Both the physical and soul body change, as the teenager prepares for life as an emotionally mature adult. Of course this transition is rarely smooth, but as an aid comes the dramatic illness of scarlet fever, usually occurring around this time. Often scarlet fever follows strep infection of the throat; it is characterized by a week of fever, and bright red rash, as though the child is literally burning up. This is the birth into the airy or emotional realm.

After the bout of scarlet fever, an emotionally competent young adult emerges, ready to learn about and navigate the mine field of emotional development. Again, this transition is often recognized and cele-

THE SELF-ESTEEM TRAP

One concept of child-rearing, for the generation called the "GenMe'ers," is to constantly praise children, and convince them that they possess unique talents and strengths, that they are "special."

While on the surface such parental behavior might seem to confer advantages on the child in the form of self-confidence and autonomy, unfortunately the opposite often occurs. According to child psychologist Polly Young-Eisendrath, PhD, the child often becomes embedded in what she calls the "self-esteem trap," characterized by excessive self-consciousness, isolation and relentless self-criticism. Instilling the premise that a child is "special" and "different" puts enormous pressure on the child at just the time when he wants most of all to be a part of a group, to be the same, not different from, his friends. The result of well meaning praise may be the child who engages in constant attention seeking; or the teenager who finds ways to dominate a scene by sulking and disengaging.

Of course, it is important to praise children occasionally—when they have conquered the temptation to hit, for example, or behaved particularly well in a restaurant. But excessive praise for normal accomplishments, such as becoming potty trained or learning to use a fork, is a recipe for trouble.

According to Young-Eisendrath, a generation of parenting advice aimed at instilling self-esteem has resulted in children who pressure themselves constantly to be or to have the best, who fear failure and are afraid to take risks, who feel hopeless about the future and dissatisfied with even the most desirable lives.

The greatest gift a parent can give a child is not the feeling of being "special," but the confidence of being normal. Such children very often surprise us in what they achieve as adults.

THE UNCOMMUNICATIVE ADOLESCENT MALE

Puberty marks the entrance into the third phase of a child's life and the beginning of a third major physical transformation. For boys, puberty often ushers in a change of personality. Your once outgoing and communicative youngster may become sullen and taciturn, hardly speaking a word to you for days. Physically, we see a number of changes. Pubic hair begins to develop, followed by the gradual growth of hair all over the body. The musculature of the boy's body starts to develop, growing heavier, thicker and stronger. The voice deepens, the penis enlarges and the production of sperm and semen begins.

Another change that takes place, one that is not visible, is a slight rise in the iron content of the blood. This change is especially striking because it contrasts with the blood changes of adolescent girls, who experience a slight lowering of their blood iron levels at this time. This phenomenon has perplexed the medical profession for many years. No one knows just why this happens, but the fact that it occurs is unmistakable. Researchers have devised many experiments to help them understand how or why these changes come about and in the process have discarded many theories. One explanation was that the decline in blood iron levels in girls was due to loss of blood in the menses. However, studies of girls who never menstruate have shown that this drop still occurs. Other explanations, such as lower activity levels and differences in the diet, also fail to provide a conclusive answer.

Insight can be found in the relationship between the human being and iron, and to the soul changes we undergo during puberty; for it is during this period that the characteristics of the inner life manifest in the physical world. During this phase, boys generally become more inward and withdrawn. Girls, on the other hand, often turn outward. They can become very social, chatty and coquettish. The manifestation of these inner changes—highly "feminine" for girls and "masculine" or "macho" for boys—usually lasts throughout this seven-year phase, after which a more balanced personality emerges.

The challenge of the male lies in balancing the heaviness or inwardness to which he is first subjected at puberty with more buoyant and outward tendencies. According to Steiner, it is during puberty that the emotional body or soul force is born. Consequently, for the first time, the developing man can work with the world of emotions. However, this newborn emotional life finds itself trapped in a world character- ized by the qualities of iron—martial, somber and heavy.

Iron is an interesting substance. It is the only metal found in significant quantities in the human body, and therefore the only metal not called a trace mineral. Instead, it is a substantial metal, substantial not only in quantity but also in its effects. It is the component of red blood cells that carries oxygen throughout the body. Iron is also a component of certain enzyme systems that allow for the transference of oxygen in the cellular respiratory cycle.

Metaphorically speaking, iron is the perfect substance to modulate the process of puberty, and even to physically distinguish man from woman. Increased iron brings more robust life to the youthful frame while its heaviness presages the weightier matters of adult life. Heaviness in the soul is not a pathology, for emotional heaviness leads to depth of ideas and feelings. However, when taken too far, the result can be the uncommunicative, somber, middle-aged man so common in our culture. It is a sign of the biochemical dominance of traits conferred by iron.

An interesting confirmation of the thesis that excess iron causes disease, especially in men, comes in the form of reports that men who donate blood regularly live longer, healthier lives than those who don't. Besides the positive feedback from the altruism involved, regularly losing some blood helps keep the iron stores low and prevents the kinds of oxidative and inflammatory diseases to which men are prone. The ancient practice of bloodletting may indeed have some basis in fact. Men who are too taciturn should regularly donate blood.

brated in traditional cultures through rite of passage rituals, and in our own traditions of Bar Mitzvah, Bat Mitzvah and Confirmation. However, these ceremonies are not enough, as we must always connect the soul development, marked by ceremony, with the physical challenges ushered in by the illnesses.

Many traditional cultures circumvented the illness part and instead put the fourteen-year-old through an intense initiation, often associated with a severe physical challenge. This initiation represents an acknowledgement that the body and the soul must always be treated as one for any real development to occur.

One of the hidden tragedies of modern life, which is happening right under our noses, is the decline in the age of puberty over the past few generations. The decline is particularly acute in African-American girls, with 50 percent of the girls showing sexual development at less than ten years old, and in some cases breast development starts as early as five years old.

THE FOUR HUMORS

Many scholars have tried to categorize the differing personalities of children (and adults), the most famous being Carl Jung, who posited four types, expressing themselves through thinking, feeling, sensation or intuition. Rudolf Steiner accomplished this task by resurrecting the Greek and Medieval concept of the temperaments or four humors. The genius of Steiner is that he correlated the four humors to the four organizing principles, the four "bodies," of the human being.

The choleric personality is one in which the ego body or fire element predominates; choleric individuals have great energy and tenacity, but may lack empathy. The sanguine personality is one in which the emotional or soul body, the air element, prevails over the others; such an individual will have a constant awareness of changing sense impressions or of the undirected flow of ideas. His interests may seem shallow and fickle. Those for whom the life or watery forces predominate are called phlegmatic; this individual takes an interest in what conduces him to personal well-being, he seeks the comfortable complacency that follows a good dinner. Finally, the melancholic temperament characterizes the individual in whom the physical body predominates; such a person feels a certain weight and resistance in reaching the outside world and is driven back upon himself. Every temperament has some virtues and the goal is to avoid the too strong expression of any one temperament, but to amalgamate all the temperaments into the well integrated human being.

When it comes to children, knowing the predominant temperament can be a great help to teachers and parents. It is of no use to force a choleric child, for example, into sanguine activities. Rather, childhood is the time when the child can give full reign to his predominating temperament, to "play it out" so that it does not seek a pathologic expression later in life.

The choleric child will take a deep interest in the world and seeks to be a leader in everything. When he takes up a task, he sees it through to the end. The sanguine personality is the most typical of all children, as the temperament of childhood is one characterized by sanguinity. He is easily distracted and should be forgiven for not completing tasks—it is not in his nature. This is the child who may complain about being bored. More than any of the other personality types, sanguine children need strong adult role models. The melancholic child enjoys his own company; he is receptive and reflective, producing thoughtful school work; he tends to occupy himself and give little trouble, but he can also feel sorry for himself because of some imagined injustice. The phlegmatic child is also content to be left alone and rarely contributes to classroom discussions. He enjoys his food and often appears sleepy. His energy can be aroused, however, by watching other children; he really does care for others and can be stimulated to acts of great unselfishness.

For more on this fascinating subjet, see *The Recovery of Man in Childhood*, by A. C. Harwood.

There are many reasons for this, soy formula and soy foods with their heavy estrogen load being foremost. But the unacknowledged reason is our inability to honor natural cycles and rhythms, the unfounded belief that sooner is better. Literally from birth we push anything that can be pushed; in Head Start and similar programs we teach the children to read, use numbers and work with their heads, even play with computers, well before their inner development has any ability to integrate these things. We have separated out in our science, in our medicine, and even in our religion the body from the soul with the result that neither realm is healthy.

Whenever we find the timing varying from the archetypal human pattern—puberty starting around ten to twelve years old—assuredly illness will follow. The particular illnesses vary—sometimes they manifest as menstrual problems, other times as soul disorders, such as anorexia, eating problems, drugs and alcoholism. All are consequences of the increasing disconnection between the timing of development compared to the archetypal patterns that we need to honor for optimum health.

Finally, we come to the time when our octave teeth, the wisdom teeth or third molars, emerge. This occurs around the age of twenty-one, or on completion of the third cycle. With the wisdom teeth, we complete the scale—the child now has four sets of eight teeth—and can enter the period of adulthood.

This new stage correlates with our modern age and modern stage of consciousness. We become fully differentiated and ready to embark on our life's work. Part of our future path involves work to achieve the re-integration that we vaguely remember from our first year of life. Unfortunately, very few western individuals have room for their wisdom teeth these days—they are often extracted. One must wonder how the lack of wisdom teeth affects our soul and mental life.

SEX EDUCATION

It is best for the child that the rudiments of sex education begin early, so that the basic facts may be presented in the most appropriate way by the parents, and not learned from television, the Internet or from friends. In any event, around the age of three, children will begin to ask questions about where babies come from, and they deserve answers, not evasion.

There are a number of books designed just for this task. Two that receive high marks from parents are *Where Did I Come From?* by Peter Mayle and *It's Not the Stork* by Robie Harris (although the stork is a beautiful image of the the soul brought to earth from supersensible worlds). These present just enough information to answer a child's questions without getting into areas that might cause embarrassment or dismay.

School is the place to present more detailed information about sex and reproduction, starting around the sixth or seventh grade. (Unfortunately, many girls get their first period sooner than that, so this is something that mothers will need to explain to them at an earlier age.) The material should be introduced in small, same-sex groups, not in large assemblies of boys and girls. The menstrual cycle can be described as one of the cycles of nature. Both boys and girls will find interest in the various rites of passage into adolescence from around the world.[2] Sex education should always be presented in the context of how to have healthy children.

The danger of sex education lies in the risk it poses of destroying the sacredness of sex. In our society this has already happened. No matter how much we try to protect our children, they all have had access to much information that damages our efforts to present sex as part of a loving relationship. Still, the concept of sex as a sacred act between loving individuals can be presented to children as they grow older; and a careful explanation of the biology of sexual function need not exclude an appreciation for a more exalted concept. Parents can do a lot for their teenage children by expressing disapproval not about sex itself, but of idle gossip about the sexual forays of their friends.

The age of twenty-one marks the end of the third cycle. Normally at this time we graduate from college and move out of our parents' house. We begin work and are allowed to vote and drink alcohol. Again, many cultures celebrated the end of childhood with a ceremony or initiation, of which the college graduation is an example.

Not surprisingly an archetypal fourth illness often occurs around this time. This illness is called mono (mononucleosis), characterized by an intense sore throat, swollen glands and spleen, and profound lethargy. The young adult may have encountered mono through sexual contact (it used to be called the kissing disease). Mono is usually thought of as an adult experience but it literally takes us a step back into the early days of childhood as we become temporarily bed-ridden, like a small child, forced to eat soft foods due to the pain and swelling in the throat.

The illness of "mono" is aptly named as it marks the birth of the fourth body, the ego or mental body, the individuality of the human being. It provides the initiation process needed to complete the final step of childhood. With proper care and rest the child emerges from this experience full of vitality, ready to meet his destiny as an adult in the "real" world. If the experience is not handled well, nor seen as a transition step, it often devolves into months or even years of low energy, chronic sore throats and low vitality.

THE ROLE OF ILLNESS

This brief description shows us that we need to shift our view of illness; illness is not something to be avoided or suppressed, but honored as an integral part of our developmental process. Of course, we need to take steps to prevent the illness from having serious consequences, which usually involves the right diet and specific medicines. When we allow the illness to manifest while we nourish our bodies at the same time, the illness runs its course as required, leaving us stronger than before.

When honored as important initiation processes, these illnesses help us with the full integration of our four bodies: the earth body born at our physical birth and ushered in with whooping cough; our watery nature at age seven and ushered in with the change of teeth and measles; our emotional or air body with scarlet fever at puberty; and finally our human spirit or individuality coincident with mono at age twenty or twenty-one, when we come into full adulthood and our wisdom teeth come in.

Development seen in this light presents itself as a progressive integration rather than a series of disconnected steps. When the integration is cared for and honored in the proper way with good nutrition, the right medicines and care for the soul, the stage is set for the child, now a young adult, to stride towards his or her destiny, confident to meet the challenge of whatever lies ahead with the patience, dignity and the quiet determination of the fully integrated adult.

FOR FURTHER INFORMATION

The Ascent of Humanity by Charles Eisenstein

The Recovery of Man in Childhood: A Study of the Educational Work of Rudolf Steiner by A. C. Harwood.

The Harmony of the Human Body: Musical Principles in Human Physiology by Frederick Husemann, MD

The Self-Esteem Trap by Polly Young-Eisendrath, PhD

Chapter 11
Child Spacing & Birth Control

Dr. Weston Price described the careful nutritional preparation practiced by traditional peoples throughout the world; and this preparation was lavished not only on the first child but on all subsequent children as well.

Among the peoples throughout the South Seas and Africa, it was considered shameful to have a child more than once every three years. The practice of child spacing allowed mothers adequate time to replenish their nutritional stores after the stress of pregnancy, thus ensuring that every child born into the community was robust and healthy.

For example, among the Ibos of Nigeria, "it is not only a matter of disgrace but an actual abomination, for an Ibo woman to bear children at shorter intervals than about three years. . . The belief prevails strongly that it is necessary for this interval to elapse and thus be in a thoroughly fit condition to bear another child. Should a second child be born within the prescribed period the theory is held that it must inevitably be weak and sickly, and its chances jeopardized."

In South America, the Indians of Peru, Ecuador and Colombia understood the necessity of proper spacing between children. "The numbers (of pregnant women) are remarkable in view of the fact that hus-

bands abstain from any intercourse with their wives, not only during pregnancy but also throughout the period of lactation—far more prolonged with them than with Europeans. The result is that two and a half years between each child is the minimum difference of age, and in the majority of cases it is even greater."

Among the Melanesians and Polynesians, Price noted that after the birth of a child, the husband was not supposed to cohabit with his wife until the child could walk. If a child was weak or sickly, the people would say, speaking of the parents, "Ah, well, they have only themselves to blame."[1]

The Trobriand Islanders honored a taboo against sexual intercourse between the sixth month of pregnancy until the child's second birthday in order to put adequate spacing between children.[2]

In pre-colonial Africa, children were born at least three years apart. It was considered taboo to engage in sexual activities during breastfeeding and pregnancy, and breastfeeding lasted at least two years. African women believed that sexual activity during lactation would lead to the contamination of their breast milk, causing the baby to become ill and possibly die.[3] As many tribes were polygamous, the burden of abstinence fell mostly on the women; husbands had relations with wives who were not pregnant or breastfeeding.

While many cultures relied on abstinence to ensure optimum spacing between children, other groups practiced various methods of birth control, using herbs and pessaries that remained secrets of the womenfolk.

Even in the Northern Hemisphere, folk wisdom mandated adequate spacing between births. For example, a parenting school in Russia that is teaching parents to raise children as was done traditionally in Russia stipulates that children be born three and one-half to five years apart. The founder of the school claims she was taught this practice by her grandmother, who lived almost one hundred years and came from a remote Siberian village.[4]

WHAT THE SCIENCE TELLS US

Just as science has confirmed the dietary practices of nonindustrialized peoples, studies have also shown the wisdom in spacing your children at least three years apart.

Limited research suggests that a pregnancy within twelve months of giving birth is associated with an increased risk of problems with the placenta—either placental abruption (the placenta partially or completely peeling away from the inner wall of the uterus before delivery) or placenta previa (the placenta attaching to the lower part of the uterine wall). A pregnancy within eighteen months of giving birth is associated with an increased risk of low birth weight, small size for gestational age and pre-term birth .[5]

Research on optimal birth spacing from fifteen developing countries in Africa, Latin America and Asia looked at the association between birth intervals and perinatal, maternal, and adolescent health outcomes, using a database of over two million pregnancies in eighteen countries.

These findings indicate that spacing births between three and five years has the greatest positive health impact on perinatal, neonatal, infant, child, maternal, and adolescent maternal health in both developing and developed countries. Interestingly, the risks for both mother and child increase after an interval of five years.[6]

According to a study by the Centers for Disease Control and Prevention the recommended interval between pregnancies is eighteen to twenty-three months.[7] Those who became pregnant within six months of giving birth had a 30 to 40 percent greater chance of delivering a premature baby or a child small in size. The risks also increased significantly for mothers who waited ten years. These women were twice as likely to have undersized babies and had a 50 percent greater chance of delivering prematurely.

Confirmation of the importance of child spacing for adequate vitamin A comes from a European study, which found that one-third of women with short birth intervals or multiple births had borderline deficiencies in retinol. "If the vitamin A supply of the mother is inadequate," they warned, "her supply to the fetus will also be inadequate, as will later be her milk. These inadequacies cannot be compensated by postnatal supplementation."[8] Maternal vitamin A status is key to avoiding birth defects.

Finally, a 2011 study suggests that children born after shorter intervals between pregnancies are at increased risk of developing autism; the highest risk was associated with pregnancies spaced less than one year apart.[9]

Birth spacing can have an effect on the quality of mother's milk as well. For example, levels of fat in a mother's milk will decrease with each baby unless she takes special care to consume high levels of nutrient-dense fats between pregnancies, during pregnancy and during each lactation.[10]

BIRTH ORDER AND IQ

A number of studies have indicated that oldest children tend to have higher IQ scores, including a recent study from Norway involving nearly two hundred fifty thousand draftees ages eighteen and nineteen years old. First-born children had higher scores than younger siblings.[11]

The usual explanation for higher intelligence in the first born is greater attention from the parents; another is that older siblings "tutor" their younger brothers and sisters, thereby reinforcing their own learning.[12]

But the most likely explanation is better nutritional

stores in mothers giving birth for the first time, and depleted nutritional stores in subsequent births. Women who put our nutritional principles into practice and who ensure enough space between children to recover from the pervious pregnancy report that all their children develop and speak at the same rate, and all do well in school.

PSYCHOLOGICAL EFFECTS

The spacing between the births of children can affect a child's emotional as well as physical health. In a national survey of more than seventeen hundred teen-age boys, for example, researchers found that children had a more negative view of themselves and their parents when their closest siblings were around two years apart. However, if the space between siblings is under one year or over four years, the negativity disappeared.

When children are born within about a year of each other—not something we recommend for nutritional reasons—the older child does not seem to experience a "dethronement" from the position of the parents' sole focus. However, if the first-born has reached the age of two by the time the younger child is born, those feelings of resentment are more likely to emerge.

Such feelings of "dethronement" are less likely to occur if the first child is nearing the age of four before the second child comes along.[13]

Viewed from Steiner's perspective, it makes sense that children need optimum attention and care until the point where the Ego or Mental Body emerges, around the age of three years. After that point, a new sibling diverts the parents' attention, allowing the older child more freedom to develop on his own.

In addition, there is much less occasion for jealousy and resentment when all the children in one family can enjoy the same nutritional head start. Instead of the first child showing more intelligence or talent than the younger siblings, as is the most usual situation, all the siblings are likely to do well in school and sports.

We also have the mother's emotional state to consider. She will have more time to devote to each child if the previous child has reached the stage of relative independence. And certainly, her emotional health and equilibrium will depend to a large extent on having the opportunity to recover nutritional stores.

PREGNANCY AFTER MISCARRIAGE

Miscarriage is a difficult, often heartbreaking, occurrence for most women, especially women who

---

THE PILL AND NUTRITIONAL DEFICIENCIES

Taking oral contraceptives depletes users of key nutrients including folic acid, vitamins B_2, B_6, B_{12} and vitamin C, as well as zinc.[14] These nutrients are critical for the development of the baby, including the optimization of baby's intelligence. Thyroid hormones are also depleted by the Pill;[15] thyroid hormones are crucial to optimal development of intelligence in the fetus. Drug companies include a statement in their handouts about the Pill warning women to avoid conceiving within six months of discontinuing it.

Another problem with the Pill: it depletes gut flora,[16] leaving both mother and child more at risk for digestive problems. Many women report the development of severe Candida overgrowth from taking the Pill. Digestive disorders due to disrupted gut flora have a strong tie to learning disabilities, behavior problems and autism.[17]

To ensure a healthy baby (and a healthy mother), women who have taken the Pill need to favor foods rich in vitamins A and E, B vitamins, essential fatty acids, magnesium and zinc.[18] Foods containing iodine and vitamin D are also recommended, as well as lacto-fermented probiotic foods. Our advice to eat liberally of superfoods like cod liver oil, butter from grass-fed cows, raw milk, liver, eggs from pastured chickens and wild seafood for at least six months before conception is especially important for women who have been on the Pill.

have been trying to get pregnant for a long time. The temptation to try to get pregnant again is great. However, miscarriage represents a strong signal that a woman's body is not yet ready for pregnancy.

We recommend waiting one year after a miscarriage before attempting another pregnancy. That year should be focused on the most nutrient-dense diet possible. Such preparation will support fertility and ensure the optimal environment for the fetus, not to mention may prevent the heartbreak of another miscarriage.

NATURAL BIRTH CONTROL

Prolonged abstinence for the spacing of children is not something that modern couples can accept. But the punctuated abstinence of the fertility awareness method of birth control is the ideal method for spacing children.

Fertility awareness involves knowing which days you can and can't get pregnant, and avoiding sexual intercourse on the days you are likely to conceive—or, if you want to get pregnant, making sure you have intercourse on the days you are likely to conceive. Much more accurate than the rhythm method, fertility awarness involves four important measures: calendar, morning temperature, mucus quality and cervix position. These are charted every day to determine the best days for avoiding and having intercourse.[19] The method is about 95 percent effective, as effective as most of the other contraceptive choices.

But it is not for everyone. It requires excellent com-

BREASTFEEDING FOR BIRTH CONTROL

Breastfeeding groups advocate breastfeeding not only for infant and maternal health, but also for natural child spacing.[20] With exclusive breastfeeding, most mothers do not menstruate—called lactational amenorrhea—for at least the first six months after the birth.

Breastfeeding did seem to facilitate child spacing for some traditional groups. For example, Canadian researcher Otto Schaefer claimed that prolonged lactation of about three years among the Eskimos kept the family size small; when bottles and formula became available to the Eskimos via the trading posts, family size increased. Wrote Dr. Schaefer: "As something of a diversion while I was in Baffin Island in the mid-1950s, I made calculations that indicated that the intervals between siblings shrank in direct relation to the mileage of the family from the trading posts. The shorter the distance, the more frequently they had children. The effect of rapid development of communications and the consequent movement of former camp Eskimos into large settlements is reflected in the more than 50 percent jump in the Eskimo birthrate in the Northwest Territories alone. . . "[20]

However, in the Southern hemisphere, traditional methods of birth control and child spacing relied on abstinence rather than breastfeeding, even though women typically nursed their infants for two years.

Modern women should not rely on breastfeeding to prevent pregnancy before they are ready to have another child. Lactational amenorrhea is likely to persist after six month only when the mother spends all her time with her baby and breastfeeds almost exclusively, not something we recommend. Further, you will ovulate before you menstruate, so may get pregnant even though your period has not appeared.

Even if breastfeeding is going well, you have plenty of milk, and your period has not appeared, it's wise to begin Fertility Awareness charting shortly after the birth.

If you do get pregnant while still nursing, it's best to phase out the breastfeeding as soon as possible, so that your body can concentrate its efforts on nourishing the next baby. You can nourish your existing child with homemade formula and nutrient-dense baby food.

munication between partners, and full acceptance and cooperation of the father. And some women are simply not organized or disciplined enough to carry it through effectively. Many couples object because it takes the spontaneity out of sex.

Of the many alternatives, those that involve hormones are to be avoided, as much for the health of subsequent children as for the health of the mother. Birth control pills, hormonal implants and intrauterine devices (IUDs) that emit estrogenic hormones should not be considered options.

Barrier methods include condoms (male and female), diaphragm, cervical cap and the contraceptive sponge. Spermicides, a form of chemical contraceptive that works by killing sperm, are often combined with barrier methods of contraception for greater effectiveness. However, use of spermicides exposes women to any chemicals these may contain. A better choice is antifertility herbs used with a plain condom. According to Susun Weed, in *Herbs for the Childbearing Year*, these include stoneseed root, jack-in-the-pulpit root, thistles, wild carrot seed, rutin and smartweed leaves.

A final choice is the copper-emitting IUD. Unfortunately, the plain IUDs, emitting neither hormones nor copper, are no longer available. The IUDs in use today either emit hormones or have copper wire wrapped around the stem and the arms, which emits copper ions that act as a spermicide.

The danger of these IUDs is copper overload in women who are zinc deficient. If you opt for a copper-emitting IUD, be sure your diet contains plenty of red meat and shellfish to supply plentiful amounts of zinc.

Of course whatever method of contraception you choose to ensure adequate space between your children, your diet during this intervening period should follow our recommendations. A diet containing cod liver oil and rich in nutrient-dense foods like liver, organ meats, animal fats, butter and egg yolks, whole raw milk or cheese—all from grass-fed animals—and lacto-fermented foods to encourage the proliferation of beneficial gut flora will ensure the blessings of not just one, but a family of healthy children.

FOR MORE INFORMATION

Garden of Fertility by Katie Singer.

Honoring Your Cycles by Katie Singer.

Herbs for the Childbearing Year by Susun Weed.

Chapter 12
The Illnesses of Childhood

The remedies and therapies for childhood illnesses presented in this book go very much against the mainstream view, which fundamentally treats symptoms with drugs. Acceptance and application of the therapies that we present depends on whether parents understand certain core issues. It is our experience that the better parents understand the philosophy on which these treatments are based, the better will be the outcome for their children.

In whatever task we take up, we all perform better when we are confident and well-grounded in the core philosophy of the work and have a firm belief in what we are doing. It's hard to be a confident baseball pitcher if you are not well grounded in your mechanics and intentions of throwing a baseball. It's hard to teach a course if you are not well grounded in the subject matter. It's hard to make sound choices in a relationship if you are never sure of the feelings or intentions of the person with whom you are interacting.

In the choice of medical therapies, we are dealing with deep philosophical issues, issues that reach to the core of our culture's belief systems. This challenge should not put us off, for the trouble we face as a culture—whether we are referring to our economy, the ecology, our way of raising children or our state of health—stems from unexamined core beliefs. We need to bring these subconscious assump-

tions out into the open so we can choose how we want to see the world and what decisions we make in it.

There are basically two ways of viewing the world. In our culture we believe in science, science as a core belief system. We believe that we should make decisions based on objective science, that is, the conscious, unbiased study of an objective reality "out there." We believe that we can study this world out there without affecting the results of the study, compile our findings in the form of numbers or statistics, and then generate some conclusions about how the world out there works and how we should act in that world.

The cultures that Weston Price studied had a very different viewpoint. For them, the answers about how to treat illness, how to eat for good health, about which herbs worked best for which conditions, came not from "out there" but from "up there," from a supersensible world accessed by a different consciousness than the waking consciousness we use to operate in the physical world.

For example, the Australian Aborigines believed that the physical world was merely a reflection of "dreamtime." In their worldview, the answers to life's riddles were solved by asking questions in this dreamtime mode and then listening for answers. Imagine a debate about why a child has fallen ill

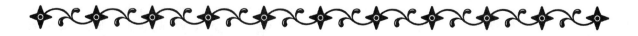

between advocates of these two divergent ways of thinking, then imagine the different treatments we might apply depending on which philosophy we embrace.

What modern, "scientific" man needs to understand is that the proofs we rely on are only proofs because we use the same underlying philosophy to test our hypothesis as we use to generate the hypothesis in the first place. And today our science, in its attempt to remove anything subjective from its work—in other words, by trying to remove everything that makes us human—finds itself at odds with modern quantum thought. Quantum mechanics has shown that experiments are influenced by the experimenter, so that no answer we get in science is entirely objective.

Modern science attempts to eliminate all "meaning" from our experience—but that is exactly what's on a parent's mind when he or she visits the doctor with a sick child. Parents yearn for someone to put the illness in a context that makes sense to them, that helps them see the illness as a result of definitive causes. Instead the doctor usually tells them that the illness their child is suffering is simply something that "happens" to the child, that it is not due to poor diet or lifestyle choices; certainly few health professionals will tell parents that their child's illness is a process that might be beneficial. Instead parents get the fatalistic answer that illness is caused by germs or genes, and the best way to deal with it is to take a drug that gets rid of the symptoms.

The choice of drugs for particular symptoms is made by assessing certain "scientific" studies that isolate a symptom and then determine which drug or drug combination is statistically best able to get rid of the symptoms. Such an approach provides no meaning, no big picture, no body wisdom at work, no direction towards wholeness. That's because we eliminate the possibility for meaning in the scientific point of view; we don't look for relationships and wholeness, and in fact we assume that relationships and wholeness are the stuff of fairy tales. The trouble is that the fatalistic "scientific" point of view is actually not very scientific; at least not if we equate science with the search for truth.

CONFLICTING PARADIGMS

One example will serve as the paradigm for the entire philosophy of pediatric medicine. The job of a doctor is—or should be—to distinguish between the therapy and the disease and never mistake the one for the other. By way of illustration, imagine that you get a splinter in your finger and can't remove it. After a while pus will form around the splinter. The decision on what to do next depends on whether you believe the pus is the disease or the therapy.

In medical school, we learn that pus is "caused" by certain bacteria, which have certain properties and which can be killed by certain antibiotics. Medical students learn that infections are bad and need to be suppressed.

However, it is obvious from our example that the pus is actually a response our body makes to rid itself of an invader, in this case the splinter. Gradually the pus will push the splinter out. The pus is the therapy, not the disease.

The respective courses of action required, depending on whether you believe the pus is the disease or the therapy, will lead to different outcomes. If you subscribe to the pus-is-bad theory and use antibiotics, then the outcome will be repeated attempts by your body to clear the splinter, repeated episodes of pus, until the pus either gets the splinter out or your body gets tired of the thwarted attempts and encapsulates the splinter in a cyst or tumor. If, however we see the pus as a therapeutic attempt by the "wisdom" of the body to remove the splinter, then we do not suppress it but guide it towards getting the splinter out, restoring the health of the finger and restoring the patient to a state of optimal well-being, at least with regard to the splinter.

These philosophical choices have huge consequences, consequences that may affect your child for her entire lifetime. This pus-splinter dynamic plays itself out many times every day in every doctor's office in the "civilized" world.

Consider the smoker, a person who is essentially putting little splinters in his lungs every day. Periodically, usually about twice a year, he gets "bronchitis," a reaction of mucus in the bronchial tubes, along with cough, fever and body aches. The fever and body aches are side effects from chemicals produced by the immune system during an inflammatory response.

During bronchitis, bacteria and viruses can be present in the lungs or bronchial tubes. The question is, are these microorganisms causing the bronchitis? Or, are the bacteria and viruses a side effect of the bronchitis? We know from studying compost piles and the forest floor that bacteria are scavengers; they digest unwanted debris and from this we can deduce that it is not the bacteria that are making the unfortunate smoker sick, rather, the bacteria are helpful, clearing unwanted debris.

The symptoms of fever and achiness are side effects of the immune response. And what is this immune response? Nothing more than his body's attempt to flush out the little splinters from his lungs. The smoker's "illness" is the therapy.

The decision the smoker needs to make is whether to use antibiotics to kill the infection or allow the illness to rid his body of toxic debris. If he takes the latter course, he may be able to live a long life in spite of his smoking habit, especially if his diet provides plentiful amounts of protective nutrients. If he suppresses his twice yearly bronchitis with antibiotics, and does this for thirty years, those splinters are likely to become encapsulated into a tumor, and he will end up with lung cancer. Each time the bronchitis is successfully "cured" with antibiotics, the body's attempt to restore wholeness is thwarted.

In fact, the high fever that our smoker experiences twice yearly is a very effective therapy against cancer. We know that spontaneous remissions of cancer often follow serious infections accompanied by high fever; indeed, induced infections have been known to cure cancer. Coley's toxins involve a treatment that brings on high fever, as do hyperthermia treatments with bacteria used in German cancer clinics; these fever-inducing methods have been effective in many cases of cancer. Other treatments involve giving substances our immune systems produce during the course of infections, such as interleukin-2 and tumor necrosis factor.

In recent years, doctors have been asking whether the suppression of fever in children results in a predisposition to cancer later in life, and even whether fever during childhood is the body's strategy for creating immunity for life to this dreadful disease.

Pediatric medicine, which largely treats "infections"—ear infections, bronchitis, tonsillitis, measles and so forth—must confront this philosophical debate. Is the body possessed of innate wisdom that strives towards wholeness, or do children get sick because they are attacked by random microorganisms which should be killed as swiftly and thoroughly as possible? It turns out that the answer to this question can be gleaned from the very way that humans are put together.

THE THREEFOLD PLANT

The conventional description of matter since the time of Newton, at least until quantum physics came along to confuse us all, says that all matter, all stuff, is composed of atoms arranged into molecules. The atoms themselves have a tiny but dense nucleus composed of neutrons and protons, which are encircled by even tinier, fast-moving electrons. Different atoms are made of different numbers of these three basic particles; the configuration is very much like our solar system with a nucleus like the sun and electrons arranged in discrete orbits or shells circling around the nucleus.

In fact, most of an atom's volume is just space, that is, nothing. This means that matter is predominantly space, or nothing. Many esoteric spiritual traditions teach that substance is merely an illusion, which makes sense when we realize that atoms contain mostly empty space. But try as you may, you cannot stick your hand through a table, through the nothing that makes up the atoms of a table. That's because, although the substance may be an illusion, that substance creates a force or energy field that has the appearance of solidity. The energy fields of all the atoms in a table create an overall force field or signature that we experience as a solid table.

The practice of medicine deals with human beings, so it is important to consider the energy field of the human being—although very few doctors actually do this. We need to consider how the energy field of a human being manifests and ponder what relevance this energy field has to the treatment of sick children.

It should be noted that the materialistic, scientific view of life is new to human evolution. Among primitive peoples, and until the 1600s in Europe, the predominant—in fact the only—philosophy of medicine was rooted in an energy-based or qualitative outlook on life. Native American practices, African shamanism, Chinese medicine and Medieval texts all shared a belief in an energy or spirit as a pervading reality in the universe as well as in the human body.

Until the modern age, all these cultures shared a qualitative outlook on life. They believed that a conscious spirit pervaded the universe, that it moved and condensed to form the substances of the world, including plant, animal and human forms. Their "research" was directed at understanding how this energy moved and what its different qualities were. Everything in the world manifested certain qualities of the pervading spirit—the tree was wise, the eagle cunning, the river lilting, and so on. Traditional peoples were concerned about their relationship with the substances of the earth and about how families or tribes could interact with these substances in a healthy, respectful, cooperative way. Traditional man would consider it absurd to merely objectively observe a tree, and to deny that the tree has intention and qualities.

This view changed slowly and progressively until its culmination in the Renaissance period in Europe, when for the first time in history humans began to see the stuff of the world as "just" a collection of molecules, essentially devoid of attributes. Modern man refers to the old outlook as "animism," deriding it as hopelessly out of touch, damning it as "unscientific" and best relegated to the dustbin of history.

Philosophically speaking, we are still in the grips of this matter-based philosophy. Trees are just big collections of lignan to be clear cut as needed. Rivers have no inherent life of their own so can be dammed up or manipulated at will.

STUDIES ON FEVER SUPPRESSION

Until the invention of aspirin and other fever-suppressing drugs, doctors believed that fever helped the body, and they actually used "fever therapy" to treat such ailments as syphilis, tuberculosis and even mania.[1] New findings are now calling fever suppression into question. These studies show that fever stimulates antibody production specific to the infection, stimulates the production of interferon, stimulates the production of more white blood cells, and even directly kills invading organisms through heat. Consider the following scientific studies:

- A study published in the journal *Surgical Infection* looked at patients admitted to a trauma intensive care unit. The subjects were randomized into "aggressive" and "permissive" groups. The aggressive group received a fever-reducing drug and a cooling blanket; the permissive group received no treatment unless body temperature exceeded 40 degrees C. There were 131 infections in the aggressive group (out of 961 patients) and 85 infections in the permissive group (out of 751). More important, there were seven deaths in the aggressive group and only one death in the permissive group.[2]

- A study published in the *Journal of Allergy and Immunology* followed over eight hundred children from suburban Detroit, Michigan. Clinic records from their first year were extracted for episodes of fever, antibiotic use and respiratory infections. The researchers found that children with fevers before age one year were less likely to demonstrate allergic sensitivity at ages six to seven years.[3]

- A study published in *Nature Immunology* showed that elevating the internal temperature in mice to mimic fever, increases the number of immune cells that are recruited to the lymph nodes, where these cells are "educated and armed" to seek out and destroy offending pathogens.[4]

- Several scientific papers have documented the regression of tumors in patients who contracted a serious infection and had a high fever.[5] How much better to develop an immunity to cancer by having the occasional fever during childhood.

In the sphere of human relationships, this materialism interprets the sadness of a friend as a condition of low seratonin. We think this even though our "soul" doesn't buy this explanation for one minute. We ache for our sad friend, even though science tells us there is no such thing as sympathetic feelings—or maybe it's just a bit too much dopamine in our brains.

Fortunately, not every Western philosopher and scientist agreed with the prevailing view of a mechanistic world composed of matter alone and lacking quality or spirit. The pre-eminent scientist and thinker of the early 1800s, Johan Wolfgang von Goethe, did not embrace the mechanistic views that contemporaneous science adopted during his time, and he denied rationality's superiority as the sole interpreter of reality. Rudolf Steiner began his career as a Goethe scholar and named the building he created to house the Anthroposophical society the Goetheanum in deference to Goethe. Goethe wrote the play *Faust*, considered one of the most insightful and dramatic depictions of modern man's inner life; and he created a theory of optics and color that is still in use in the world of art. Goethe is credited with many other achievements in philosophy and thought.

At the end of his life, Goethe was asked to name his most important achievement. He replied, "I discovered the *Urpflanze*," the archetypal plant. In his book *Urpflanze*, he brings the old theory of animism into a modern scientific frame of reference. His theories can serve as the basis of a renewed spiritual-scientific medical practice, where these two seemingly divergent ways of seeing the world do not conflict but work together.

So what is the nature of *Urpflanze*? According to Goethe, through a series of transformations, all plants emerge from seed to leaf; then out of the leaf are formed the root "sphere" and the flower "sphere." Goethe used the word "sphere" because while plants have literal roots and flowers, these are not as crucial as the dynamic underlying their formation. In other words, in any plant, first comes the leaf or green "sphere," which is the real essence of "plant." It is this shape and color that immediately tells us we are looking at a plant as opposed to an animal. Then the green, leafy realm transforms itself "downwards" into roots (typically white roots) and the "upwards" into flowers (typically colored) and then into fruits (typically sweet) with seeds.

When we see a three-part living object with these characteristics we are "moved" to recognize it as plant. The *Urpflanze*, the archetypal, ideal or perfect plant, has green leaves and stems, white roots, and colored flowers within green sepals, with these three realms in perfect balance. These three realms correspond with the earth (the roots), the air (flowers with their scents) and the sun (the leaves drawing nourishment from sunlight).

This perfect plant does not exist in nature, but Goethe was able to see it in his "mind's eye," to

WHEN HOME REMEDIES ARE NOT APPROPRIATE

TRAUMA: If your child has a serious injury, head for the emergency room. Modern medicine really does have a lot to offer when it comes to treating trauma, and when we ignore these gifts, bad things can happen. When your child falls out of a tree and has a concussion or a bone is sticking out through his skin, you don't want to treat him at home.

EXTREMELY HIGH FEVER: Most fevers play a beneficial role in your child's health but an extremely high fever (over 104 degrees) can be a dangerous situation for a young child and you may need to get emergency care. (For treatment of fever, see page 227.)

TROUBLE BREATHING: This is another situation that calls for quick action. If a child is unresponsive, limp in your arms or has glazed eyes, you need to get help. Dial 911 or hurry him to the emergency room.

CHILD HAS SWALLOWED POISON: Your child has gotten into the dishwashing powder, anti-freeze or other poison? Get him to the emergency room at once.

see how it was created from the transformation of the leaf "realm," and to realize that this is the true nature of the plant. The perfect plant exists not in nature but as a blueprint or energetic field behind the plant, and every individual plant is a variation of this blueprint. The insights that come from this concept lead to a true understanding of the plant-based medicines used to treat or support various medical conditions throughout the ages. Even our current "science-based" medicine derives 70 percent of its drugs from plants.

Consider a carrot, and compare it to our archetypal plant. Archetypal plants are divided into equal parts or spheres with the color normally manifesting in the flower domain. If we observe the carrot from a Goethean point of view, that carrot will tell us that it has decided to go its own way, to do things differently; it doesn't want to be the perfect plant, it wants to exhibit carrot-ness. Its energy is focused on putting color, sweetness, even a bit of smell in the root realm. What is so interesting about this type of analysis is that it allows you to predict and understand the world in a new way, even without direct experience. Knowing that the carrot focuses its energy into the root realm, you might guess that the carrot has wispy leaves and colorless, insignificant flowers—which it does.

The carrot is telling us, "My energy is in my roots, I have no time for that mundane leaf thing or for speaking to your so-called emotions with a beautiful flower. I am about the earth and nutrition." And, it is no surprise that carrots are loaded with nutrients for animals and humans, specifically nutrients that nourish the sensory region of the human being. (We'll discuss the corresponding threefold human below.)

Now, let's consider the rose. Clearly the rose is all about the flower, the airy, emotional realm of the plant. It has a flower of perfect harmony, loaded with color; the flower dominates the life history of the plant. Just to make things even more dramatic, the quintessential rose is deep red, the color of mammalian blood. Even if we are a bit dense, we can't help but notice the rose's connection with the human heart and the human emotions of romantic love. It shouldn't come as any surprise therefore that the rose has no relation to such mundane endeavors as food, it is hunting bigger game—love. And, for

those who have eyes to see, the rose will even teach you a bit about this game of romantic love.

Unquestionably the second main feature of the rose is its sharp thorns, so in case you think that romantic love is all about sweetness and joy, let us just say the rose has a different story to tell. Almost everyone who has been in love has felt love's thorns.

Each plant has a different story to tell for those who will listen and observe. As we discuss how to treat different illnesses in children we will try to understand the different plant medicines from this perspective; and we can use this perspective for mineral-based and even animal-based medicines as well. Everything we see in this world has a story to tell and in many cases its story is related to the human story, just as is the case for the carrot and the rose. Should such anthropomorphizing, should this return to primitive animism, be discarded as "unscientific?"

To my continual amazement, what really happens when we use this energetic, archetypal model as our compass, is that modern science actually begins to make more sense, to become streamlined and even predictable. It becomes no surprise that carrots contain large amounts of carotenoids, which have a therapeutic relationship to the human sense organs.

Moreover, when we take the subjective Goethean point of view, rather than the objective scientific point of view, when we enter into a relationship of listening with awe to the carrot, we are far less inclined to accept toxic conditions for growing carrots. Rather, we become willing to provide a loving, organic or biodynamic environment for them to thrive and express their full nature. Providing non-toxic growing conditions serves as a gesture of thanks to the carrot for "choosing" to participate in our nutrition and health. That is the relationship to the world that ultimately provides health for us all, not the distance and separation so characteristic of our modern age.

THE THREEFOLD HUMAN

Just as the plant has three spheres, so does the human being. It was the famous European physician and alchemist Paracelsus who first delineated the three spheres in the human being, who referred to the "threefold man." Unlike the plant, which has its sensory system located in the roots, the human sensory organs lie primarily in the head; and while the plant's reproductive system points upwards, the human reproductive system lies in the lower part of the body and points downwards.

In essence, the three spheres of the human being are flipped over from those of the plant. But in both man and plants, the sphere that mediates between the sensory sphere and the reproductive sphere, circulating nutrients and fluids, lies in the center—in the leaves and stems of the plant, in the heart and lungs of the human being. The plant is rooted in the earth and strives towards the heavens, while the human being is rooted in the heavens and strives towards the earth.

Over the years many philosophers have taken up the threefold concept; Rudolf Steiner gives the three-fold concept center stage in his teachings about the human being.

The three spheres delineate the head, the heart and the abdomen, but they refer not so much to anatomical features as to qualities. Just as the color realm of the plant belongs archetypally in the flower, likewise we can ascribe qualities to the different spheres of the human being. For example, the head region is the center of the nervous system. It is the area of crystallization, of clarity—think of the clear cerebral spinal fluid or fluid in the eye. They are characterized by stillness and coolness. The head should not move much when we talk—in fact, we begin to feel nauseated if we move our head too much—and it feels much better to put a cool cloth on one's forehead than a hot water bottle. In contrast, the metabolic region is characterized by movement due to its association with the limbs, transformation (as of food into nutrients), activity, warmth and chaos.

The middle realm serves as the mediator between these two extremes, as well as the bearer of the quality of rhythm. We are most healthy when our heart beat is rhythmical, our breathing is regular and our entire lives are characterized by a comforting rhythmical flow. By the same token, the child should experience an enjoyable rhythm between unregulated free play and a fixed schedule of meals, sleeping and story telling.

Paracelsus described the threefold realms through the Medieval metaphor of the three basic elements—salt, sulfur and mercury. Salt, a quintessential crystal represents the head realm. Sulfur, a picture of movement and activity, represents the metabolic realm; and mercury or quicksilver, the messenger god who mediates between the human and the divine realm, represents the region of the heart and lungs. These pictorial images allow us to conjure up vivid images of the forces at work behind these three realms.

Also, just as there is an archetypal or perfect plant, likewise there is an archetypal or perfect human being, which can be the guiding compass in our medical practice. This archetypal human being does not exist of course, but serves as a kind of blueprint or force field. Disease can be seen as a moving away from the harmonious balance of the perfect man; therapy is the attempt by the doctor or the body to restore balance.

SHEPHERDING THE PROCESS

Before we move on to the application of these concepts to childhood illnesses, we need to explore one more idea, one that is crucial to the right practice of medicine, and in particular pediatric medicine. That is, the human being starts out as "all head." The shape of the head sphere is circular or egg-like and its activity is stillness and reflection. Gradually through life we grow upright, with limbs that can move and act in the physical world. In fact, one can immediately distinguish the young child from the old man; the child is more head, the old man more limb.

As we "grow up" we actually grow down into our limbs; over time we go from a state where the limbs move randomly, as in the newborn child, until we are a young adult, when we can do amazing figure skating or classical guitar playing with perfect control over our limbs down to the tips of our fingers. This is the crux of the transformation project we call "growing up;" it is a progressive mastery of our metabolism and limbs until we become a full participant with our thinking (head), feeling (heart) and doing (limb) regions in the outer world.

The task of pediatric medicine is to shepherd this process so that the child arrives at adulthood without impediments. Of course, each child arriving at adulthood will have his own individual balance between the realms, but it should be one that is a reflection of his particular destiny and not a result of illness which he may have to spend the rest of his life trying to overcome.

Let us keep these concepts in mind as we describe individual illnesses in the following chapters, recognizing that imbalances between the three realms underlie the key diseases that our children experience. Once we understand the overall picture and the particular forces behind each illness, the appropriate therapy will become obvious.

These therapies will aim not to eliminate symptoms but to restore balance or wholeness as we honor each young person's attempt to claim and master his or her own body.

Chapter 13

Treating Infectious Disease
Colds, Fevers & Congestion

We start life in the uterus as a fertilized egg, as a sphere living in a watery realm. If all goes well, we will end life about ninety years later, in a desiccated, shrunken body in which the limbs predominate and the sphere of the head is relatively small. Along the way we have many dangers to overcome, many transformations to undergo, many metamorphoses to accomplish.

The main role of pediatric medicine is to guide these transformations; to provide true healing while always keeping these transformations in mind. Illness has many causes, and its manifestation can be extremely complex. But one way of looking at all childhood diseases, and in fact diseases at all stages of life, is to acknowledge that they represent a condition where something is either out of place or occurring at an inappropriate time.

Consider the child who is not kept warm enough, who has consistently eaten food lacking sufficient life forces, whose food has been subjected to the techniques of modern food processing, or who even grows up without the unconditional love that is every child's birth right. Or, consider the child growing up in our modern, technological age with all its business, stress and challenges. Compare this modern child to a child of our more primitive ancestors, to the children studied by Weston Price. Their environment was non-technological, they were loved and nurtured by entire villages, and they consumed the purest, most healthy food imaginable.

Many have noted that our modern environment is one that can easily overstimulate the nervous system of a young child. It is also obvious that in the very early years, when the child is building his metabolism, establishing his gut ecology, strengthening his ability to digest his food and transform it into his own substance, certain predictable types of imbalances are likely to arise.

In our concept of the threefold man, it is the head that should be still, cool and clear while the abdomen, seat of digestion and metabolism, should be warm, cloudy and active. Many illnesses in children involve imbalances of these spheres. An overstimulated nervous system can create a premature hardening or crystallization of the head sphere. In essence, the child becomes too old, too soon, unable to enjoy childhood to the fullest. In later life we see this excessive crystallization—the medical term is sclerosis—in many of the typical adult diseases. We see gallstones (concretions in the gall bladder), arteriosclerosis (hardening of the arteries), osteoarthritis (hardening of the joints), chronic obstructive pulmonary disease (hardening of the lung tissue) and even cancer with tumors that can feel as hard as stones. It is normal to get drier and more hardened as we age, but too much too soon results in illness.

Sclerosis or rigidity, of both body and soul, is the enemy of young children. Their task is to remain open, flexible, full of choices and possibilities. At the same time they are trying to master their digestion, to focus sufficient warmth forces into the metabolic sphere for the complete breaking down of their food.

So, imagine the earliest hint of this sclerotic force in a young child, and imagine it in the head where the force archetypally originates. The body in its wisdom finds this intolerable and works to dissolve the congestion, to restore balance, warmth and flexibility to an area that has become too hard and cold. The healing forces of the child's body will always use warmth and dissolving mechanisms to re-establish balance. This is what we call the common cold. The virus is incidental, for like all micro-organisms, viruses are scavengers that digest the breakdown products of the inflammatory process.

The four cardinal symptoms of this "cold" are strategies the body uses to dissolve sclerosis and their side effects: warmth or fever, fluids or mucus, muscle pain and redness of the tissue. The forces of the blood contribute to the redness and fever while the forces of metabolism contribute to the formation of pus, a classic dissolving gesture. Muscle pain and stiffness are side effects from by-products of the inflammatory response.

Modern scientific thought is in total agreement with the belief that the symptoms of a cold are not the result of an infection but rather stem from the immune system response. Conventional medicine recognizes the fact that cytokines and white blood cells are brought to affected areas, and it is our body's response to these compounds that cause the symptoms of a cold. We know this because when we inject bacteria or viruses into a healthy person and then prevent them from mounting an immune response, they will not exhibit any symptoms of sickness. The symptoms are clearly and unequivocally the response.

It is true that we respond to some stimuli and these stimuli can include an "invasion" of micro-organisms from outside. But children who are in balance normally do not get sick when exposed to germs.

TREATING FEVER

Once the sickness begins, our job as parents and healers is to guide the process to its health-restoring conclusion. Obviously we can do this only when we clearly understand the underlying dynamics. We must keep in mind the fact that the sickness is the body's therapy, therefore we must work with it, not merely suppress symptoms.

So what can we do to work with the illness and not thwart its healing process? First, since an over-stressed or over-active nervous system is the basic dynamic leading to illness, we can put the child in a calm, peaceful, under-stimulating, restful environment. The child should be kept warm in layers of natural fiber clothes and blankets; the room should be free of all electric appliances, entertainment, music and anything else that would "appeal" to the senses. The shades should be drawn so the child is not stimulated by bright light. The child should be kept still—her metabolism is already working hard, she doesn't need any other forms of movement. Above all, the child should hear the calm voice of her parents or caretaker.

During illness, the metabolism is already working hard and doesn't need to be burdened with digesting food. A sick child should eat only soup made from rich bone broth, either plain or cooked with a few vegetables, and with a bit of coconut oil or coconut milk mixed in the broth. If the child is really sick, you may be able to give the broth only one or two teaspoons at a time. Avoid raw juices as these are actually hard to digest and not an appropriate food for children, sick or well. The natural instincts of the child make this easy as a sick child will usually reject most food, and certainly any cold foods like vegetable juices.

Foods rich in vitamin A are important because fever and inflammatory process rapidly use up vitamin A. Depletion of vitamin A in children with high fevers can result in blindness or seizures, so giving drops of high-vitamin cod liver oil to maintain vitamin A status is vital. Use the syringe that comes with the bottle to give four or five drops morning and evening.

As the child recovers, you can add other nourishing, easy-to-digest foods, such as smoothies made with whole yogurt, egg yolks and honey; creamed soups or a thin gruel of soaked oatmeal. You can add a little finely chopped liver to soups or prepare a simple liver paté, rich in vitamin A. Custards made from egg yolks and cream are also good. When the child's appetite returns, well-cooked brown rice with plenty of butter is an excellent choice.

The next step is to ensure the child clears his bowels at the onset of an illness. After all, constipation is a form of sclerosis of the metabolism. Often this clearing will happen naturally as many childhood illnesses are accompanied by diarrhea. If the child is constipated, stewed prunes will often work; if not,

a glycerin or Dulcolax suppository can be quite effective.

Once these steps have been taken, and a hot water bottle is put into the child's bed, the next step is rest in the presence of a confident, peaceful mother.

Tylenol (acetaminophen) is often the first thing given to children with fevers. Besides lowering fever when it shouldn't be lowered, drugs like Tylenol are toxic to the liver, causing hundreds of cases of acute liver failure each year. The compound is also found in over-the-counter cold remedies and pain relievers. For children, there is an added danger: the

TREATING VERY HIGH FEVER

If a child's fever is very high—over 103 degrees—then you need to take steps to bring it down. A cool water enema is one good way to do this. Nobody likes to give them but they are a very effective remedy for high fever. You can get an enema bag from any pharmacy for about ten dollars and they're easy to administer. Place a thick beach towel and a washable pillow in the tub. Lay your child on his side without taking clothes off. Slide their pajamas down a little. Coat the enema nozzle with a little coconut oil. Place 1/2 to 1 quart luke warm filtered water in the bag and insert the enema nozzle. Your child will start to feel pressure and will want to go to the toilet—the water usually doesn't run out. Then gently put him on the toilet and let him go. This will usually bring the fever down by a degree or two.

High fevers—those that range between 104 and 105 degrees—are not dangerous in themselves, but they make the metabolism run very fast and increase the risk of dehydration. Blood sugar often drops, which can lead to convulsions. Your child can sip 50 percent diluted fresh fruit juice to keep tissues hydrated and blood sugar levels in the normal range. If your child will not take anything, you can administer about 4 ounces diluted fruit juice rectally using a bulb syringe. The body will absorb it rectally. It won't run out. This may save your child a trip to the emergency room.

Should you feed or starve a fever? Food will naturally drop a fever within about twenty minutes and this drop will last for an hour or two. If your child will eat a few bites, by all means give him food, but don't force food if he doesn't want it. And you don't have to give your child a lot of food. Just a few bites of scrambled egg or a few sips of broth can bring that fever down a bit. It will not make the fever go away but may bring it within the 102-103 degree range.

Remember that high fever rapidly uses up vitamin A. Be sure to give about 1/2 teaspoon high-vitamin cod liver oil every day that your child has a high fever. You can use an eyedropper for this, giving drops under the tongue.

Sulphur is important for the proper modulation of fever. Broth with egg yolks and some garlic beaten in will supply the child with sulphur.

Whatever you do, don't give Tylenol or other NSAIDS (non-steroidal anti-inflammatory drugs). Use of these drugs to suppress high fever has been linked to autism (see pages 227-228).

If your child's very high fever is resistant to any of these methods, it's best to get him to the emergency room.

possibility of developing autism spectrum disorder (ASD), as acetaminophen depletes sulfur.

NATURAL MEDICINES

There are also natural medicines that can be given, medicines that work with the process of a fever or a cold, not against it. These medicines come in three basic types. First are anthroposophical "potentized" or homeopathic medicines indicated for the various types of childhood illnesses; second are herbal medicines; third are food-based medicines made by Standard Process.

Potentized medicines are the gift of Samuel Hahnemann, founder of homeopathy. Homeopathic medicines are produced by a process of progressive shaking and diluting, whereby the gesture or blueprint of a substance is extracted from condensed or "frozen" matter. The technique extracts the "gesture" or the particular forces of any substance into an accepting medium, usually water, alcohol or some form of sugar. We then simply match the force of the substance with the imbalance of the sick child.

Herbal medicines represent another way of extracting "forces" from plants, usually by macerating them and then soaking them in alcohol. The difference is that in homeopathic potentization we are specifically activating the force part of substance, whereas in herbal medicine we choose to make the active, physical, therapeutic ingredients of the plant available. Potentized medicines are gentler and therefore best for very young children; herbs are more powerful and can have drug-like effects, albeit more complex and usually gentler than those of conventional drugs. We must be sure that we are using herbal medicines in a way that cooperates with the illness rather then merely suppresses symptoms.

Standard Process medicines include mixtures of plant extracts, minerals like calcium and magnesium, animal organs such as thymus gland, and other food substances, like kelp or sesame oil. These are more appropriate for older children, that is, two to three years old, who are more able to metabolize food. These medicines work to strengthen the tissues that are participating in the healing process.

HOMEOPATHIC APIS BELLADONNA

This is the potentized mixture of an extract from the honey bee and the plant *belladonna*, also known as deadly nightshade. If colds and fevers are caused by "hardening" or sclerosis due to excessive head or nerve activity, the condition requires dissolution by warmth and fluids. *Apis*, the honeybee has a strong relationship to the crystalline realm with its gesture, that is, construction of a hive of perfectly shaped six-sided crystals or combs. It is as though the bees live in a perfect crystalline womb. In this womb, as if to relate it to the human being, the bees work together to create an internal constant temperature inside the core of the hive of exactly 98.6 degrees, the exact temperature of the healthy human body. *Apis* is one of the classic homeopathy remedies for infec-

---

SUMMARY FOR COLDS, FEVER AND CONGESTION

INFANTS: Give only potentized medicines. Best choices are Meteoric Iron *Prunus* from Uriel Pharmacy, 2-3 pellets every two hours until the child is better; also *Apis belladonna,* also from Uriel, at the same dose although it is best to alternate these two medicines throughout the day. Also give Echinacea Glycetract from Mediherb, 1 teaspoon, 3-4 times per day. The only other medicine is 1/2 teaspoon per day of high vitamin cod liver oil (see Sources) for its vitamin A and D content, both of which help with various acute illnesses. Cod liver oil may be given to infants with an eye dropper or syringe.

CHILDREN AGES 1-2, in addition to the remedies for infants, you may also give elderberry-thyme syrup from True Botanica (see Sources), following the directions on the bottle.

CHILDREN OVER AGE 2: In addition to the medicines described above, give Congaplex by Standard Process (see Sources), 2 capsules every 2 hours, until the child is clearly better. If your child can swallow tablets, instead of Echinacea Glycetract, give Echinacea Premium tablets from Mediherb, 1 tablet, 4 times per day.

tions and fever; it seems to be saying, "I will help sick people find their way back to healthy warmth and perfect crystallization," exactly the "purpose" of the illness in the first place.

As for the *belladonna* component, this plant lives in dark, swampy areas, and out of this swamp creates a deadly poison that changes our consciousness (as shown by the wide pupils, altered pulse rate, and other physiological changes that follow the ingestion of the chemical atropine in the *belladonna*). It also stimulates our mucus to run. These gestures interact with the other two components of any inflammation, that is the fluid involvement (mucus and pus) and the pain (change in consciousness). In this one remedy we gently show the child the way to resolve the acute inflammation and work with the four manifestations of illness to restore balance.

HOMEOPATHIC METEORIC IRON PRUNUS

One of the most glaring absurdities of our modern medical approach is the fact that we seem to have little or no awareness of the human being as a biological entity deeply embedded in the rhythms and patterns of nature. We are literally created out of the soil that nourishes the food we ingest, yet when was the last time your doctor inquired about the nature of the soil your food grew in? Doctors don't ask these questions even though they know that many illnesses stem from mineral imbalances, for example, anemia from iron deficiency or poor immune system function due to zinc deficiency. The minerals must come from somewhere; ultimately they must come from the soil.

Similarly, extensive research has shown us how healthy biorhythms relate to hormone production, to cortisol, melatonin, endorphins and other hormones, all of which contribute to our health and sense of well-being. Again, it is a rare modern physician who inquires about the rhythm of a patient's day, or helps the patient create a healthy pattern of eating, working, relaxing, exercising and sleeping.

Meteoreisen or meteoric iron, the potentized extract of a meteor that has fallen to the earth, helps to connect us with the cosmic rhythms in which we are immersed. Illnesses that are a reaction to sclerosis may be said to be a reaction to too much winter, a time when coldness and contraction are most ap-

parent in the world of nature. The opposite impulse is, of course, summer, when the world bursts forth with color, smell, abundance and warmth. We might say that summer is the cure for winter. The problem, however, is that if we only had the condition of summer in our bodies, we would dissolve in a fit of metabolic frenzy. Too much summer results in out-of-control pus and inflammation that can actually dissolve our tissues. This is the ultimate danger for any sick child, an excessive inflammatory response creating an actual threat to his well-being.

In the world of nature, there is a turning point where the exuberance of summer starts to turn inward and, as any sensitive person can feel, autumn begins. The event that marks this transformation is the Persdie meteor showers, which happen mid-August, when the cosmos rains down little bits of iron onto the earth. Some of these bits get through intact, can be found and made into a medicine that helps to stem the tide of summer. The medicine does not stop inflammation, rather it guides it back into the healthy stream of the human being.

The *Prunus* component of this medicine comes from the blackthorn plant, which produces an iron-rich fruit. This plant-based iron works along with the meteoric iron to help bring the child back to healthy balance. The combination of meteoric iron and *prunus* is meant to help the child finish the illness. Too often we see children get over the initial acute symptoms and then go on to have fatigue, or a persistent runny nose that can go on for weeks. Often this will even lead to the cycle of repeated ear infections or other exacerbations. The combination of meteoric iron with *prunus* will help your child complete the illness, so you can truly say "now my child is better."

ECHINACEA

Echinacea is perhaps the premier herb used in acute medical care. The alkylomides in echinacea stimulate white blood cell proliferation and movement,[1] which is the primary defense of our cell-mediated immune response. The plant puts most of its energy into its root system, which is also the part of the plant richest in these immune-stimulating alkylamides. We particularly recommend the alkylamide-rich echinacea found in the Mediherb products—you know they are rich in alkylamides because these compounds make your tongue tingly and slightly numb when you ingest them.

Give echinacea as close as possible to the onset of the illness, in relatively higher doses initially then tapering down as the child improves. Contrary to some reports, the herb can also be taken long term with good effects, as the immune stimulation seems to remain active over time.

For young children who can't swallow tablets, use echinacea glycetract from Mediherb; the acute dose is one teaspoon in water or a small amount of juice three or four times per day. For children who can swallow tablets use echinacea premium tablets from Mediherb, one tablet four times per day. Echinacea is also in *Andrographis Complex*, so if you are able to get your child to swallow the *Andrographis* tablets, then you can omit the echinacea.

ELDERBERRY-THYME SYRUP

Sometimes herbs are best described through the gesture of the plant from which they originate; other times it seems best to describe the components of the herb or its traditional use. Elderberry, thyme and oregano extracts, the principal components of this medicine, are all traditional plants valued for their anti-microbial effects and their mucolytic properties. In other words, these herbs help keep pathogenic viruses and bacteria under control and keep mucus flowing so the body can get rid of it.

Even though we submit that microorganisms are not the root cause of colds and other inflammations in children, we still need to guard against excessive growth of these microbes. Overgrowth of bacteria and viruses is rarely a concern in a child with a simple cold, but we can still apply this medicine as a kind of insurance policy. Used early in the course of any acute illness, this remedy aids the child as his body works to restore balance and wholeness.

CONGAPLEX

For older children, the Standard Process medicine Congaplex is appropriate. It contains calcium lactate, which stimulates white blood cell activity, and thymus gland extract to strengthen our immune response.

With these natural medicines, your child can recover from colds, fevers and congestion without any undesirable side effect, but rather as a stronger child than he was before.

Chapter 14
Ear, Nose & Throat
Ear Infections, Tonsillitis, Strep Throat, Bronchitis, Pneumonia, Sinusitis & Whooping Cough

As with colds and flu, it is important to understand the dynamics of common childhood infections in the ears, nose and throat. When we have a cold or flu, we ache all over; we suffer from mucus, cough and fever, but with no localized effects. In contrast, in illnesses of the ears, nose and throat, while we still might feel sick all over, the main focus shifts to a specific location.

Conventional medicine generally holds that colds and flu have a viral etiology, while illnesses of the ears, nose and throat are caused by bacteria. However, this distinction is not absolute; bronchitis, for example, can be viral in origin. The curious thing about the viral-bacterial distinction is that with the possible exception of strep throat, there is very little data that a physician can use to know whether a particular inflammation is "caused" by a virus or a bacteria.

In reality, the sequence of events in most acute illness (that is, illness that tends to resolve on its own) is first, an overall sense of sickness, often accompanied by fever and body aches, and then mucus, with specific symptoms showing up in one or more areas of the body. The localized infection will either resolve or become more serious; in the latter case there may be severe localized pain with redness and perhaps pus in the middle ear space or fluid in the lungs.

Current medical convention calls the first stage a viral infection and the later localized stage a bacterial infection, but obviously both stages are part of the same dynamic.

As with colds and flu, it is helpful to view these illnesses as ones in which strong metabolic forces come out of their boundary (which is the abdomen) and "invade" the areas of the head and chest with an intensity that results in illness—when the fluids of the head, which should be clear, become cloudy with mucus. The underlying reason for this is an excessive and premature sclerosis in the head realm, often combined with an anatomic predisposition to infections in that area. Nutrient deficiencies are also a factor, which put the child in a weakened state.

In all the illnesses described in this chapter, the basic treatment is the same as for colds and flu. This means the child should rest as much as possible, dress in warm clothing or bedding made of natural fiber, and consume a diet consisting mainly of broth-based soups containing vegetables and some coconut milk or oil, with small amounts of protein. Stewed fruit, with or without cream, can be added as the condition improves. The regimen should include one-half teaspoon of high vitamin cod liver oil per day. It is important to ensure daily evacuation of the bowels.

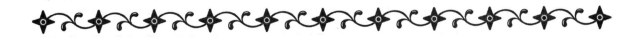

BRONCHITIS and PNEUMONIA

The diagnosis of bronchitis or pneumonia is made when a sick child has either a harsh raspy cough (bronchitis) or a deep, wet, cough with mucus (pneumonia). As there is no clear distinction in many cases between these two situations and because they have the same treatment, we will discuss them together. Ultimately the distinction between them can only be made by listening to the child's chest or by taking a chest x-ray, which is actually rarely necessary.

Specific treatments for bronchitis and pneumonia should augment and guide the metabolism in resolving the inflammation. The key components include accentuating warmth in the chest, detoxifying through the liver and gall bladder, and using herbs to stimulate white blood cell activity and release mucus.

With this basic plan, we have seen hundreds of cases of bronchitis and pneumonia resolve without the need for antibiotics. In fact, the child is actually strengthened in the process, the tendency to future chronic infections and asthma is lessened; children are actually brought to a healthier, stronger state by successfully overcoming this illness. (For dosages

---

PNEUMONIA VERSUS ASTHMA

A vivid story from Dr. Cowan's days in medical school on a pediatric rotation demonstrates the underlying dynamics—usually hidden—behind bronchitis and pneumonia. In this case, however, the cause practically stared the doctors in the face. The patient was an eight-year-old overweight child, not very healthy, living with two parents who smoked and did not follow good health practices. The child suffered from severe asthma. He was on daily oral steroids and bronchodilators, yet still his asthma was not controlled. He was wheezing on exam at every doctor's visit and had limited activity and constant shortness of breath.

Then one day he was admitted to the hospital with a one-hundred-four degree fever and pain in his right chest area; a chest x-ray showed a virtual white-out of the right lower lobe of his lung, signifying a bad case of pneumonia. Amazingly, he was not short of breath on examination and had no wheezing!

Pediatric textbooks actually recognize the fact that bacterial pneumonia often "dissolves" asthma—sometimes only temporarily, sometimes permanently. We know that asthma is associated with the production of spirals and crystals in the lung tissue and we know that the lungs and chest area of a chronic asthmatic child gradually become more spherical in shape as the disease progresses. In other words, the chest area becomes more like the head, or the head realm encroaches on the chest, even forcing the chest to be still, like the head. Pneumonia in these cases is like a revenge of the metabolism, a dramatic, even a dangerous attempt to flush this "head" out of the chest.

This story does not have a happy ending. The child was given strong IV antibiotics, which "cured" him of the pneumonia, and then they put him right back on all his inhalers and steroids. He suffered from severe asthma for as long as the hospital kept track of him.

This story dramatizes both what is right and what is tragic with modern medicine. The right part is that we can reliably treat even the worst cases of pneumonia, even in a compromised host. An illness that could have killed this child, and that has undoubtedly killed many children in the past, has been rendered manageable. The tragedy is that we have almost no understanding about the underlying dynamics of this situation and therefore no way to resolve the pneumonia without giving back the asthma. Pride in medical accomplishments has blinded us to the bigger picture.

We are not suggesting that we will never need antibiotics to manage a case of pneumonia, but unless we look deeper, we are condemned to go from one disease to the next, and in the process our children get sicker and sicker.

of recommended medicines for illnesses of ears, nose and throat, see the Summary on page 236. For sources of the various medicines, see Sources.)

Accentuating warmth in the chest is accomplished with compresses, a traditional method now unfortunately disdained by modern Western medicine. In this case, we can use mustard compresses, an age-old treatment for pneumonia. The purpose of the mustard is clear—mustard is perhaps one of the "hottest," that is most metabolically stimulating, plants known. It is a perfect remedy to increase the heat in the chest, dissolve the underlying sclerosis and flush out toxins. See Appendix I for a full description of the mustard compress.

Clearing toxins from the liver and gall bladder is an important component of any treatment for acute illness. The liver eliminates metabolic wastes and exogenous poisons through processes called conjugation and glucuronidation, among others. Then the gall bladder excretes these wastes out the bile duct into the intestines to be evacuated. Any time there is increased metabolic activity, as in infection and inflammation, there is a need to increase the excretion of wastes.

The liver-gall bladder system can be compared to a system for handling household garbage. First we bag the garbage (the role of the liver as it attaches toxins to various compounds), then we take it to the compost pile (the gall bladder). We can stimulate this process by giving liver herbs to the sick child (to help bag the garbage) and bitter herbs (to help carry it to the compost).

The herb *Andrographis* will serve for both the bagging and the eliminating. Known as the king of the bitters, *Andrographis* is similar in effect as an antibiotic, even though it has little antimicrobial effect. Rather, by stimulating the liver-gall bladder detoxification pathways, it addresses the underlying dynamics of the infection.

White blood cells, the critical component of our cell-mediated immunity, digest and clear invaders through the elimination channels of mucus and rashes.

The Mediherb preparation *Andrographis Complex*, which mixes the herb *Andrographis* with echinacea, a white blood cell-stimulating herb, is the basic treatment for all the infections in this chapter. It comes in pills, which should be given every two hours at the start of any serious infection.

You can also give Congaplex (described in Chapter 13) until improvement is seen.

Another remedy is sesame oil, which contains sesamin, an anti-oxidant shown to stimulate the activity of white blood cells. Sesame oil capsules can be obtained from the company Standard Process.

Clearing the chest is accomplished by the mucolytic (meaning "to make the mucus flow") and expectorant herbs contained in the Mediherb preparation Bronchafect. This can be given as a liquid or in tablet form. As the situation resolves, the dose can be lowered and given less often.

THE FLUIDS OF THE THREE REALMS

Each of the three realms in the body has its specific fluid. Lymph is the cloudy fluid of the metabolic system; it collects wastes and poisons and carries them out of the body. Blood is the fluid of the rhythmical system; it takes oxygen and nutrients to all the cells in the body, and also carries carbon dioxide and wastes away. The fluid of the head is the cerebro-spinal fluid.

Blood is either red or blue depending on where it is in the rhythmical cycle of circulation. The cerebro-spinal fluid should be clear; likewise the mucus of the head region is clear when we are healthy. When the mucus in the head region becomes cloudy, it is a sign that the qualities of the metabolic system have taken over the head, usually in an attempt to prevent sclerotic tendencies in that realm, and impart more of the moving, cloudy characteristics of the metabolic system.

EAR INFECTIONS

Otitis media, or middle ear infection, usually begins with a cold and progresses to congestion in the nasal passages, including the Eustachian tubes. As a result, fluid collects in the middle ear space behind the ear drum, which then eventually serves as a culture medium for various bacteria to grow. Symptoms of pain in the ear come next. In some cases this is followed by rupture of the ear drum and fluid drainage out of the ear canal. This rupture is not serious; it just represents more exteriorization or "housecleaning" and is actually quite safe. In rare, serious cases, the infection does not exteriorize but spreads into the mastoid bone and even into the meninges of the brain, causing the dreaded complication of meningitis.

The controversy of whether ear infections require antibiotic use has raged since the early 1960s. Antiobiotics have side effects and the condition usually resolves without them. In a meta-analysis of more than two thousand children with otitis media, ear pain resolved spontaneously without antibiotics in two-thirds by twenty-four hours and in 80 percent by day seven.[1]

Generally speaking, pediatricians in Europe have adopted a "timing" approach to otitis media, meaning they let the illness run its course for ten days and only then give antibiotics to those who still have symptoms of ear pain and fever. This approach dramatically lowers the re-infection rate; it also lowers the incidence of chronic glue ear, a condition in which the middle ear is filled with thick fluid, often leading to a recommendation of ear tubes insertion. Most importantly, the ten days' wait does not increase the risk of complications.

This approach, used in Dr. Cowan's practice for over twenty-five years in conjunction with ten days of natural medicines for resolving ear infections, has eliminated complications (meningitis or mastoiditis), and rarely results in a child developing glue ear or requiring tube insertions.

The other factor to note in ear infections is that just as in all other infections in the head, there is a significant component that relates to the facial bone configuration. Children with wide facial bone development have plenty of room for drainage of their ears, air flow around their tonsils and drainage of

---

OTITIS MEDIA VERSUS OTITIS EXTERNA

Otitis media refers to an infection of the middle ear. This almost always follows or is associated with a cold or fever. The child is usually congested and there is nothing unusual about the appearance of the ear. Other signs of sickness, such as cough or sinus congestion, are common.

Otitis externa refers to an infection of the outer ear or ear canal. Rarely is such an infection associated with a cold or fever. Often called "swimmer's ear," it usually follows swimming in polluted waters, exposure to excessive humidity or some kind of abrasion or cut in the skin of the ear.

Both conditions can be painful, but with otitis externa, movement of the outer ear can cause severe pain. While there may be pain with otitis media, movement of the outer ear does not cause pain. In addition, with otitis externa, the ear canal can become red and inflamed, and is often narrowed; discharge from the ear is also common.

Home treatment of otitis externa involves ear drops: vinegar diluted with equal parts water works best, 1-2 drops in the ear, 4 times per day.

If the canal is closed, treatment by an ear, nose and throat doctor will be necessary. The physician will insert a wick into the ear and will prescribe a drug for the infection and inflammation, usually Cortisporin Otic Suspension, which is formulated for the treatment of superficial bacterial infections of the external ear canal.

their sinus passages. Therefore, as Price found, the triad of tonsillitis, ear infections and sinusitis rarely, if ever, occurs in these children. And while the facial structure of the child cannot be changed, the diet that creates good facial structure in the formative period can still offer substantial protection in children with less-than-optimal facial structure. In the child prone to ear infections, it is particularly important to avoid concentrated sweeteners, fruit juices, processed foods, and above all, pasteurized milk. Even if you can't get raw milk, it's best to completely remove pasteurized milk from the diet of children susceptible to ear infections. However, usually the diet can include butter, cream and cheese (preferably raw cheese).

The principles of treating otitis media are the same as for bronchitis and pneumonia, with the same basic medicines, except in this case we need a different compress treatment, and instead of Bronchafect we use a different therapy, one that specifically drains the ear space.

For local treatment of the ears, we need to remember that acute diseases are self-limiting; therefore we can expect they will resolve on their own. Our job as doctors and parents is to help ensure that they are resolved completely and to help mitigate the pain and discomfort. Above all, we need to take steps to ensure that the disease does not get "stuck."

With ear infections, all of these goals can be furthered by the simple use of onion packs over the ears at the first sign of ear pain or congestion. As well as having antimicrobial effects, onions make mucus run—as anyone who has ever cut into an on-ion has observed. This is what we want in the ear. While it's obvious that you don't need to touch your eye with an onion to make mucus run, with an onion compress we can accentuate the effect by holding the onion directly on the affected ear. This will keep the mucus from getting "stuck" in the middle ear space. The onion will actually pull some of this excess fluid out from behind the drum and, by lowering the pressure, often dramatically helps with the pain. (For details on the onion compress, see Appendix I.)

As with bronchitis and pneumonia, ear infections require medicines for supporting liver and lymph systems. These include *Andrographis Complex* from Mediherb, Congaplex from Standard Process and Sesame Oil Capsules from Standard Process.

For clearing the ears, instead of Bronchafect, which specifically loosens mucus in the chest, we use *Apis Levisticum* from Uriel pharmacy and *Euphrasia Complex* tablets from Mediherb. *Apis,* the honeybee extract, is described on page 228.

Added to the *Apis* extract is *Levisticum*, a homeopathic remedy for otitis media extracted from the lovage plant. The lovage plant looks like a giant celery plant; it has many gestures or qualities, but the main one for our purposes is the glue-like sticky latex in its roots. Following our concept of the three-fold organization of plants, we can conclude that the story of the lovage plant is the story of how to live with a protein-rich, gluey fluid in the head. Pus in the head: that is the story or gesture of Levisticum. In otitis media we have this same pus in the head, which we don't want to become the dreaded glue

---

ILLNESS AS A STEPPING STONE

Dr. Cowan still remembers the vivid experience of his young son having an infection in both ears, sleeping all night with onions strapped onto his ears, and waking up in the morning without pain or congestion. Without saying anything to anyone, he went into the kitchen, cut an onion into slices and bandaged up both ears of his "doll."

Then, he sat down to draw a pine tree, which he had done dozens of times before; but that morning, for the first time in his life, he drew red apples on the tree. It was as though overcoming the ear infection brought a kind of fulfillment or next step in his life (represented by the apples), which he then expressed, as children often do, in his drawings. This story portrays the essence of what acute illness can accomplish and what the medical system should honor.

SUMMARY FOR DISEASES OF EAR, NOSE & THROAT

BRONCHITIS and PNEUMONIA
- Mustard compresses to clear the chest (see Appendix I).
- *Andrographis Complex*, from Uriel Pharmacy, 1/4 of a pill dissolved in hot water for small children, up to 2 tablets every 2 hours for adolescents. When there is clear improvement the frequency and amount can be gradually reduced.
- Congaplex by Standard Process, 2-3 capsules, 4 times per day until improvement is seen.
- Sesame oil capsules from Standard Process, 2 capsules, 3 times per day.
- Bronchafect by Mediherb, liquid 1/2 teaspoon every 2 hours for small children, or in tablet form, up to 2 tablets every 2 hours for adolescents. As the situation resolves the dose can be lowered and given less often.

EAR INFECTIONS
- Onion compress to clear the ears (see Appendix I).
- *Andrographis Complex*, 1/4 of a pill dissolved in hot water for small children, up to 2 tablets every 2 hours for adolescents. When there is clear improvement the frequency and amount can be gradually reduced.
- Congaplex by Standard Process, 2-3 capsules 4 times per day until improvement is seen.
- Sesame oil capsules from Standard Process, 2 capsules 3 times per day.
- *Apis Levisticum* from Uriel Pharmacy, 3-5 pillules every hour until the situation starts to resolve.
- *Euphrasia Complex* from Mediherb, 1 tablet dissolved in hot water or swallowed, 4 times per day until the situation is resolved.
- For children who won't take tablets (*Andrographis comp.* or *Euphrasia comp.*), use Ear Formula Drops from Uriel Pharmacy, 2-10 drops orally (not in the ears!) every two hours until symptoms clear, then 4 times per day for 2 weeks.

TONSILLITIS
- Gargle with hot salt water to soothe the throat.
- *Andrographis Complex* from Uriel Pharmacy, 1/4 of a pill dissolved in hot water for small children, up to 2 tablets every 2 hours for adolescents. When there is clear improvement the frequency and amount can be gradually reduced.
- Congaplex by Standard Process, 2-3 capsules 4 times per day until improvement is seen.
- Sesame oil capsules from Standard Process, 2 capsules 3 times per day.
- *Apis Belladonna* with mercurio, especially if there is strep present, from Uriel Pharmacy, 5 pills under the tongue every 2 hours until better, then 4 times per day until all symptoms are gone.

SINUSITIS
- Steam inhalations to clear the sinuses, with either a drop of eucalyptus oil in the water or, if that is too caustic for the child, an infusion of chamomile tea in the water (see Appendix I).
- *Andrographis Complex*, from Uriel Pharmacy, 1/4 of a pill dissolved in hot water for small children, up to 2 tablets every 2 hours for adolescents. When there is clear improvement the frequency and amount can be gradually reduced.
- Congaplex by Standard Process, 2-3 capsules 4 times per day until improvement is seen.
- Sesame oil capsules from Standard Process, 2 capsules 3 times per day.
- *Euphrasia Complex* from Mediherb, 1 tablet dissolved in hot water or swallowed, 4 times per day until the situation is resolved.

OPTIONAL FOR ALL CONDITIONS
- Pleo-Not homeopathic penicillin preparation from Sanum, 5-10 drops directly under the tongue, first thing in the morning, continued for 2 weeks or until all symptoms are resolved.

ear. Lovage given homeopathically can clear the pus in a healthy way.

In addition to *Apis Levisticum, Euphrasia Complex* is excellent for treating congestion and inflammation in the head. Therefore, it is a fundamental remedy for ear infections, sinusitis and tonsillitis. The components of *Euphrasia Complex* include echinacea, euphrasia (otherwise known as eyebright) and goldenseal, a very potent bitter herb with antimicrobial properties. These herbs in combination serve to drain mucus and other toxins, keep the microbial growth in check and restore healthy mucosal tissue.

Another option for treating ear infections, especially in young children who can't or won't take tablets (*Andrographis Complex* or *Euphrasia Complex*) is Ear Formula Drops from Uriel Pharmacy (see Sources).

TONSILLITIS

The issues and dynamics with tonsillitis are basically the same as with otitis media. For direct soothing of the throat, the patient can gargle with hot salt water. Use water as hot as the child will tolerate, about one tablespoon unrefined salt per cup of water, several times per day.

The medication treatment is also the same with the exception that instead of *Apis Levistecum* for the ears, we can use *Apis Belladonna* with mercurio from Uriel Pharmacy, especially if there is strep present.

Mercury is an old homeopathic remedy for illnesses of the throat and tonsils. Interestingly, the Greek god Mercury was the patron of physicians, a tradition that has continued to this day—the symbol of physicians is the staff of Mercury or Hermes.

In its non-toxic homeopathic form, mercury keeps mucus congestion from getting "stuck" in one place, in this case in the lymphatic tissue of the tonsils. Furthermore, in alchemical medicine it is said that mercury rules the lymph, the fluid of the metabolic system, which collects wastes and poisons and carries them out of the body.

It is no surprise then that ancient wisdom correlates

healing with a healthy lymphatic flow. When the lymph is free of "garbage," wellness ensues.

The danger of tonsillitis, particularly when associated with strep, is that without treatment with antibiotics, rheumatic fever will develop. The facts show, however, that rheumatic fever was in dramatic decline for unexplained reasons before the introduction of penicillin. Over the last few decades few cases of rheumatic fever have occurred, even in those populations that typically eschew the use of antibiotics. In our experience with hundreds of cases of tonsillitis and strep throat treated for up to ten days without antibiotics, we have yet to encounter any complications like rheumatic fever.

SINUSITIS

In sinusitis, we are again often dealing with the unfortunate consequences of poorly formed facial bones and a lack of room for proper airflow in and around the sinus passages, nor for proper drainage from the sinuses.

For direct application, instead of compresses, use steam inhalations with either a drop of eucalyptus oil in the water or, if that is too caustic for the child, an infusion of chamomile tea in the water. Steam inhalations will often help to loosen the congestion, encourage drainage and resolve the pain. This can be done as often as needed. (For a full description, see Appendix I.)

Follow the basic treatment as for tonsillitis and ear infections, including the use of *Euphrasia Complex* to resolve the mucus congestion.

HOMEOPATHIC PENICILLIN

Another homeopathic preparation for treating bacterial infections like otitis media, bronchitis, pneumonia, sinusitis and tonsillitis is the homeopathic form of penicillin called Pleo-Not. This medicine has been shown to improve the ability to counteract simple bacterial infections. The preparation is available from a company called Sanum (see Sources).

WHOOPING COUGH

Whooping cough, otherwise known as pertussis, is the one "old-time" children's disease that is still very much around. Dr. Cowan has treated hundreds of cases during his career as a physician, including his own three children. In fact, his youngest child got whooping cough when he was around eight weeks old, giving him the distinction of being the youngest person Dr. Cowan had ever seen with this illness.

The lesson here is that of these many hundreds of cases, all are alive and well, with no lasting repercussions from having gone through what is, in truth, a pretty dramatic illness. Children do die from whooping cough, and the mortality rate of eight-week-old children is said to be around 10 percent. Of the hundreds of children with whooping cough seen in Dr. Cowan's practice, none were given antibiotics, only the natural medicines described herein.

Unfortunately, during the last ten years, parents have come under much greater pressure to give antibiotics, and most parents now give their children an antibiotic (usually erythromycin) as soon as the case is confirmed.

It's hard to blame them. Whooping cough is a truly dramatic event. It usually comes in mini-epidemics, usually in early fall or late spring. Investigations of the various outbreaks over the years have shown that both fully vaccinated children and partially or unvaccinated children get the disease.

In classic whooping cough, for the first two weeks the child suffers only a mild to moderate runny nose, usually with clear mucus. There is usually little or no fever and the child is only moderately ill. This is the infectious phase as the bacteria said to cause whooping cough are present but don't actually cause the difficult part of the illness; rather in about two weeks, as they are dying off, they leave behind a toxin that binds to the lining of the lungs and stimulates paroxysms of coughing.

This usually starts at about two weeks from the onset of the first symptoms, and it is dramatic, especially in young children. The coughing fits usually occur at night and culminate in a long outbreath and then a deep whooping inbreath (hence the name). This can go on all night, night after night for anywhere from two to ten weeks. The child is usually in a fair amount of distress, often exhausted from coughing all night, unable to sleep and seemingly unable to catch his breath. Sometimes the coughing paroxysms are so intense they even can cause them to vomit or burst blood vessels in their eyes.

After the paroxysm stage is over, the resolution phase again lasts about two weeks, the runny nose often comes back, the coughing episodes gradually subside and the child slowly recovers. Sometimes there is a post-pertussis phase, often lasting even a year, where every cold will push the child back into the coughing paroxysms. These are always less dramatic and shorter lasting than the original event. Adults can get whooping cough as well, but its

SUMMARY FOR WHOOPING COUGH

- *Drosera comp.* from Uriel Pharmacy, given at 3-10 drops—a minimum of 3 drops for children three and under, 4 drops for a child of age four and so on up to 10 drops for a child of ten or older.

- *Cuprum aceticum comp.*, from Uriel Pharmacy, given at 3-10 drops—a minimum of 3 drops for children three and under, 4 drops for a child of age four and so on up to 10 drops for a child of ten or older, alternating with Drosera comp.

- Amla-Plus vitamin C, 3-4 tablets per day

- *Andrographis comp.* from Uriel Pharmacy, 1 tablet 4 times per day until all the symptoms are gone.

- Plantain Spruce cough syrup from Uriel Pharmacy, 1 full tablespoon 4 times per day.

- Plantain Beeswax Cough Relief Ointment from Uriel Pharmacy on the child's chest and back, 4 times per day as long as the coughing persists.

manifestation in adults is not nearly as dramatic as with young children.

The first question is why would we even consider exposing our children to such a frightening illness—why not give antibiotics at the first hint of whooping cough?

The best answer is that the older wisdom points to the fact that overcoming pertussis is the best way to prevent a child from developing asthma in later childhood. (Also, a natural case of whooping cough gives natural immunity for twenty to thirty years; the pertussis vaccine gives immunity for three years at most.) It is as though there exists, as Rudolf Steiner suggested, an air body, which needs to be wrestled with and integrated for the child to be fully incarnated and healthy.

The meeting with the air, as ancient Greek theory suggests, is the archetypical encounter with the physical realm, which is why it is often the first illness the child encounters, as first we must learn to breathe.

If we thwart this encounter, we risk a life of asthma. Back in the early part of the century almost everyone got whooping cough and there was almost no asthma—ask your grandparents! Now almost no one gets whooping cough and asthma is rampant. This is not a coincidence. If we can safely guide our children through the dangers of whooping cough, we get the best of both worlds, and that is the goal of this therapy.

The first step of the strategy is to remain calm and resolute in your choices. This illness tests the mettle of any parent; the child needs to know you are strong and confident and able to guide him through the challenge of whooping cough. The environment in the house should therefore be calm, with lots of fresh (but not cold) air in the house and the child's

WHOOPING COUGH VACCINE FAILURE

Whooping cough is a scary illness, the thought of which often sends parents running to the doctor to vaccinate their children.

However, new research reveals that whooping cough rates are *higher* among vaccinated children compared with unvaccinated children. This is based on a study led by Dr. David Witt, an infectious disease specialist at the Kaiser Permanente Medical Center in San Rafael, California.[2]

In early 2010, a spike in cases appeared at Kaiser Permanente in San Rafael, and it was soon determined to be an outbreak of whooping cough—the largest seen in California in more than fifty years. Witt had expected to see the illnesses center around unvaccinated kids, on the assumption that they are more vulnerable to the disease. "We started dissecting the data. What was very surprising was the majority of cases were in fully vaccinated children. That's what started catching our attention." The same article also admits that these vaccines have never been tested for long-term effectiveness.

The fact is that whooping cough rates have been rising since 1991, the same year that the new purified acellular vaccine (DTaP) was introduced. There were over twenty-seven thousand reported cases of whooping cough in 2012, up from just under eight thousand in 2000,[3] with very low numbers in 1980.[4] The new vaccine replaced one that caused adverse reactions in up to half the children receiving it. DTaP does not seem to cause as many acute reactions, but the statistics support the accusation that the current whooping cough vaccine is actually causing, not preventing, pertussis, by keeping the disease in circulation.

There are no studies on the severity of whooping cough in vaccinated compared to unvaccinated children, but one mother reports that when an outbreak of whooping cough occurred at her children's school, two of her children had mild cases. Three children in the school died; they had all been vaccinated.[5]

room. A strong air filter that cleans the air to operating quality may can be very helpful (see Sources).

The child should be kept warm at all times, and well hydrated with soup and coconut juice; his activity should be very subdued and quiet.

There are two homeopathic medicines that work well for whooping cough, both from Uriel Pharmacy. The first is *Drosera Complex* given at three to ten drops—a minimum of three drops for children three and under, four drops for a child of age four and so on up to ten drops for a child of ten or older. These alternate every two hours the child is awake with *Cuprum Aceticum Complex*, given at the same dosage (see Sources).

Drosera is a mixture of the common homeopathic remedies used for whooping cough, and copper is an anti-spasmodic that lessens the coughing spasms.

Amla-Plus vitamin C can be given in a dose of 3-4 tablets per day, as well as *Andrographis Complex* from Mediherb, 1 tablet 4 times per day until all the symptoms are gone.

Plantain Spruce cough syrup from Uriel Pharmacy (see Sources) one full tablespoon four times per day, will soothe the throat.

Finally, rub Plantain Beeswax Cough Relief Ointment from Uriel Pharmacy (see Sources) on the child's chest and back, four times per day as long as the coughing persists.

These home remedies were all Dr. Cowan gave to the hundreds of whooping cough patients he has seen over the years. They worked in the past and they still work today. Whooping cough does, however, need the help and guidance of a physician who has seen it before, so it is important to learn in your early visits whether your pediatrician has this experience.

Chapter 15
Allergies, Asthma & Eczema

We now turn our attention from the acute or self-limiting diseases of childhood to the more chronic illnesses so common in modern children. The incidence of asthma, allergies such as hay fever, food intolerances and allergic skin conditions like eczema has increased tremendously during the last fifty to eighty years. Just a few decades ago, these conditions were rare. In contrast, a recent report indicates that asthma affects 25-30 percent of children living in certain disadvantaged Chicago neighborhoods.[1] Conventional treatment for asthma calls for steroid inhalers, which children carry with them at all times. Side effects of these inhalers include growth retardation and lowered bone density.

When one factors in the number of children taking medications for allergies and eczema, or for attention deficit disorder and behavior problems, we can see that it has become more common than not for a child to be taking a daily pharmaceutical medication—all of them with serious side effects.

This dramatic shift in the disease patterns of a large population over such a short time frame—just two generations—obviously has nothing to do with genetic changes. Our genetic material would take hundreds if not thousands of years to change this much. Clearly, the answers to these diseases can be found in the many dietary and lifestyle changes that have occurred during the last fifty years.

When we try to tease out which factors are different in the lives of children, and which of these factors may be accounting for the increase in these chronic illnesses, we find many possibilities to consider. One has to do with a fundamental change in the way children grow up. Until the late 1960s and early 1970s, much of children's lives happened outside in the company of peers and away from the watchful eyes of any adult. Most of the games we played and most of the socializing was self-organized or organized with other children in the neighborhood. We were sent out to live our lives in the parks and streets and occasional wild places. During the summer, children were out all day and got really dirty, and came in only to eat and then go to bed.

In contrast, one or two generations later, children rarely play any game that isn't adult supervised, rarely run in a pack with their friends; they have schedules to follow most of the time. Or, they are home in an air-conditioned environment watching television or playing computer games. What has changed is the culture of childhood, which in spite of the best efforts of any particular family, is difficult to overcome.

THE HYGIENE HYPOTHESIS

The relevance of this change in rates of childhood illness has to do with what is called the hygiene hypothesis. That is, modern life is a lot more "clean"

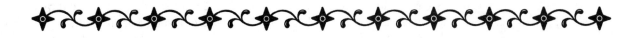

than at any time in the history of our species. We are exposed to fewer germs and less dirt; children have fewer close contacts with their peers; children have less contact with animals and farm environments; Mom cleans everything with antimicrobial wipes. Today our lives are lived indoors in an ostensibly clean and germ-free environment.

As a consequence of this, we actually become weaker and more powerless against the microorganisms we do encounter, and our immune systems don't get the essential "exercise" they need, which is what happens when they frequently encountered dirt and germs. Our immune systems therefore become both weak (susceptible to foodborne illness) and overreactive (with asthma, allergies and eczema).

Asthma, allergies and skin rashes are essentially illnesses of intolerance to the world, and they force us to ask what is going on these days between children and their environment. What really is making them sick?

The modern view point sees the world "out there" as something "other" or foreign, whereas indigenous peoples lived within the natural world, considering themselves one with nature. In contrast, we see the world out there as distinct and separate, something to be observed, feared and overcome. The challenge for modern man is to strike the right balance between being overcome with infections and overreacting, with allergies, asthma and eczema as a result.

Modern medicine is rife with war images—we "fight" or "beat" diseases like cancer and arthritis. The fundamental relationship between man and his diseases is one of antagonism, with clear winners and losers. If the world wins we get an infection; if we win, managing to avoid germs and dirt, we get an overreactive immune response and the illnesses we are discussing. It's as though we project certain principles onto the world and ourselves, then we live to see this projection play out in our lives.

Indigenous people had a different point of view and hence a different projection; they lived their lives in the lap of a nature, which although awesome in its power, was fundamentally part of the family. In that projection, there would be no reason to overreact to keep nature out, hence their immune systems were calm, and immune diseases were virtually unknown.

Of course diet plays a role in immune diseases. The very nutrients that were so plentiful in primitive diets—vitamins A, D_3 and K_2—are critical for supporting the immune system. And primitive peoples did not consume foods that depleted the body's immune resources, such as sugar, white flour and industrial fats and oils. Milk-drinking cultures consumed raw milk, and raw milk is designed to build the immune system; pasteurized milk and milk products require the body to mount an immune response every time they are consumed, leading to exhaustion of the immune system.

BACTERIA: MAN'S BEST FRIENDS

During the last few decades, scientists and doctors have been forced to dramatically revise their views on bacteria. Modern research has discovered that only a very small number of microorganisms are pathogenic, that is, able to make us sick. The vast majority of bacteria are beneficial, in fact, we cannot live without them. Beneficial bacteria live on and inside our physical bodies. We now know that there are more bacterial cells residing in our gastrointestinal tract, our gut, than there are cells in our body.

It is thought that the fetus resides in a sterile environment inside the womb; whether or not this is true, we do know that his skin and gut get colonized with the mother's microorganisms as he goes through the birth canal. If the mother has beneficial gut bacteria, beneficial organisms will also colonize her birth canal and vagina; baby will start life with the great gift of healthy gut bacteria. If the mother has a preponderance of bad micro-organisms in her gut—such as candida and yeasts from excess sugar consumption or antiobiotic use—her baby may start off life prone to digestive problems, yeast infections and thrush, with allergic diseases not far behind.

The myriad species of bacteria, fungi and viruses that baby picks up during the birth process colonize the spaces, linings and the crevices in the child's intestinal tract. They also set up a "bank" in the appendix, where a few of each species hide out to recolonize should the gut bacteria be wiped out by a bad case of diarrhea or a course of antibiotics.

This is an ingenious dance that occurs in our guts, an intimate ecological cooperation down to the cellular level. Neither we nor the micro-organisms can exist on our own.

As baby grows, he undergoes—or should undergo—a daily replenishing of the gut flora, first from mother's colostrum and milk, then with raw and cultured food products, like raw cow or goat milk, kefir, yogurt and lacto-fermented foods. Along the way, he eats a goodly amount of local dirt, sucks on stones, swallows river water, puts his face up to animals and shares some germs with his friends. In our ideal scenario, these are all local foods and bacteria that serve to implant the local ecology directly into the child's intestinal tract. It is not surprising that indigenous peoples feel such a kinship with their place, as their place is literally within them.

The place where most of our intestinal bacteria lodge is in the small intestine, which is organized in a very interesting way (see below).

We have millions of little hair-like villi lining our entire gastrointestinal tract, and all of these hair-like structures are covered with a biofilm of micro-organisms.

The healthy gut contains from five to seven pounds of beneficial organisms organized into a biofilm. The functions of this biofilm are manifold. It helps with digestion of food, secretes vitamins that we absorb into our bloodstream, makes anti-bacterial, anti-fungal and anti-viral substances that mitigate

the growth of pathogens, and maintains the intestinal lining in good health. When the bacteria of the biofilm die, they provide the bulk of the stool. The biofilm plays a role in general detoxification, produces feel-good chemicals, and performs many, many other vital functions. This list of functions shows that without healthy gut flora, life is simply not possible.

Imagine this healthy gut system as a luxuriant meadow in which the villi are analogous to the soil and the gut flora to the grass. When the soil is healthy and thick with lots of humus, it supports a thick grassy layer on top, and we know that the meadow is strong and healthy. However, if somehow the grassy layer is disturbed, either by overgrazing, herbicides, or conversion of the meadow into a grain field, the soil becomes exposed. The next inevitable step is soil erosion. Big cracks will develop in the soil, then contaminants start to seep into the ground water. Eventually the entire organism—the farm, the locality, the earth—become affected.

The same scenario can play out in the human gut. The biofilm may become disrupted by poor diet, antibiotics, vaccinations or fluoridated and chlorinated water. The good flora may not thrive due to a lack of good flora from birth; also, the "soil," that is the intestinal wall with its millions of villi, may not have been well constructed to begin with. Without plentiful fats, cholesterol and fat-soluble vitamins in the pre- and postnatal diet, the cell-to-cell junctures of the gut are likely to be weak. This is tantamount to holes or cracks in the soil, which allow allergenic proteins into the blood stream.

In cases of disrupted gut flora and poor condition of the gut wall, the villi become damaged and flattened, and can no longer do their job.

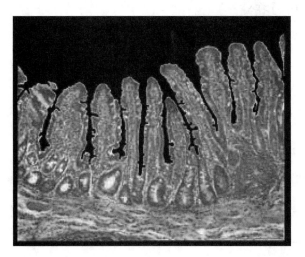

Healthy villi produce enzymes called disaccharidases, which break down the complex carbohydrates found in grains, potatoes, sweet potatoes and milk products. With damaged villi unable to produce these enzymes, digestion of these types of foods becomes very difficult. The body becomes plagued with immune system dysfunction, allergies, skin rashes and asthma. Behavior and learning problems often accompany this type of dysbiosis (see Chapter 16).

GUT AND PSYCHOLOGY SYNDROME

The treatment for this intestinal dysfunction is called the GAPS diet. GAPS stands for Gut and Psychology Syndrome. The diet was developed by physician Natasha Campbell-McBride and originally came out of work suggesting an association of autism with an inflammatory condition of the gut wall. As a result of a variety of causes, including vaccine-induced inflammation, small holes are formed in the gut wall, which allow various toxins to leak into the blood stream from inside the gut. These toxins are at least partly responsible for the neurological symptoms seen in autistic children.

On learning of this research, Dr. Campbell-McBride embarked on a program to heal the intestinal tract of her autistic son and then of other patients who came to her with autism and similar problems. The relevance to our current chapter is that the GAPS theory provides a cogent explanation for the underlying dynamics of allergies, asthma and eczema.

When the gut flora is disrupted, the villi become blunted, the gut wall becomes porous, and toxins are absorbed into the bloodstream. The body then produces antigens that the child reacts against. What this means is that the question normally asked in conventional medical circles, that is, how to stop the inflammation on the skin (eczema), in the lungs (asthma) or in the bloodstream (allergies) is the wrong question. This, of course, explains why there is no answer to the causes of these conditions, and no directions on how to heal them.

Because conventional doctors don't ask the right questions, conventional medicine never heals any chronic disease. In fact, most doctors don't believe it is possible to cure chronic disease, and they may even deride those for whom it is the goal. The usual antihistamines, desensitization shots, cortisone creams and inhalers never cure the child of any disease. They may stop the symptoms, but as any doctor or parent knows, when you stop the drugs—usually because of their many side effects—the symptoms will come back, often worse than before.

The real tragedy of this situation is not that conventional medicine can't actually cure any of these diseases but that doctors have lost the ability to consider it possible. To cure a disease means to change the conditions in the patient so the symptoms do not arise, even after the therapy is over. Curing a disease is fundamentally an educational process, a growth process, a leading of the patient to a new and better way of life.

So, the process unfolds like this. First we harm or don't plant healthy grass (gut flora), then the soil (villi) erodes, then cracks (leaky gut) form in the intestinal wall, then we absorb proteins (antigens) that don't belong in our blood stream. The body then targets these proteins with immune system antibodies and then eliminates these antigen-antibody complexes with an inflammatory response either through the lungs (asthma), the skin (eczema) or with mucus (allergies)—the same illness, the same dynamics, just a different site of action.

CAUSES OF GUT DYSBIOSIS IN CHILDREN

- Failure to have proper implantation of micro-organisms at birth, either because of imbalances in the mother's vaginal flora or C-section.

- Antibiotic use, either by the mother in the perinatal period or by the child.

- Chlorinated water.

- Vaccinations, which have a dramatic adverse effect on the health of the gut flora.

- Improper diet, in particular the failure to use local cultured foods in the child's diet; use of pasteurized dairy products; and inclusion of processed foods in the diet.

- Overcontrol of the child's environment, including limited exposure to dirt, animals and other people.

- And finally, the philosophical failure to understand the true relationship between the human being and everything else "out there," thereby projecting fear and antagonism onto the natural world, which instead deserves our awe and humility.

As the villi deteriorate, they make lower amounts of disaccharidases, which means the child will be unable to fully digest such common and enjoyable foods as milk (even raw milk), grains (even properly prepared grains), legumes, potatoes and sweet potatoes. These undigested foods become food for the ubiquitous pathogens that also live in our gut, such as *Candida albicans*, resulting in the proliferation of this species and the progressive exclusion of healthy microflora. Now we are monocropping, and instead of a healthy biodiverse gut ecosystem that includes a small amount of candida, we have fields of candida.

Sometimes we can see direct evidence of this overgrowth as in thrush, anal redness or superficial skin infections. Other manifestations of candida overgrowth may be more subtle. In any case, the candida crowds out diverse flora, synthesizes poisons which get absorbed and interfere with immune function, and prevents the healthy flora from making a myriad of compounds that otherwise keep us healthy.

The inevitable result is chronic illness, poor digestion and nutrient deficiency. The child gets weaker, the viscious cycle continues—more candida, blunted villi, fewer disaccharidases, more candida, worse gut flora, more blunting, and on and on. The child may become a very picky eater, insisting on only those simple carbohydrate foods, which his candida yeasts crave, but that make his condition worse. Abnormal behavior patterns are common. Chronic illness like this never gets better on its own, and the GAPS theory explains why. Healing these conditions involves breaking this vicious cycle.

THE GAPS DIET

To recap, the overarching goal of therapy for asthma, allergies and eczema is to stop the introduction of antigens into the bloodstream. Then the body will not need to create inflammation at various sites to eliminate the immune complexes. In other words, we need to heal the leaking gut and restore the ecology to our intestinal tract. Specifically, this means healing the villi and restoring the gut flora. Or, to use our analogy, we need to restore the soil and replant grass seeds.

The first step is to eliminate all processed foods for good, and temporarily remove all foods containing disaccharides and complex carbohydrates; that means all grains, potatoes, sweet potatoes, parsnips, seaweeds (with a couple exceptions) and unfermented (even raw) milk. In severe cases, characterized by a strong immune response, even fermented dairy products need to be excluded from the diet for about one month as we work through the introductory stages of the diet and slowly restore the gut lining and flora. Ghee rather than butter should be used during the early stages of the diet.

The second step is to adopt a nourishing traditional diet with a specific emphasis on bone broths made from long simmering of cartilaginous bones. There is no better tonic for intestinal and digestive disorders, and hence for allergic conditions. The specific amino acids and gelatinous matrix of the broth nourish, soothe and protect the delicate intestinal lining. It is the number one food needed for restoring a healthy gut ecosystem.

Cholesterol-rich foods such as ghee (and later butter), egg yolks, liver paté and fatty meats will help heal the gut wall—the cells of the gut are especially rich in cholesterol. Arachidonic acid, found only in animal fats, helps produce tight cell-to-cell junctures. Cod liver oil, to supply vitamins A and D, is an important component of the GAPS diet.

The next component consists of probiotic and lacto-fermented foods such as sauerkraut, beet kvass, marinated fish and then cultured dairy such as yogurt and kefir made with raw milk. (The fermentation process breaks down the lactose in milk, hence the sour taste.)

Important in this process is to do some of the lacto-fermenting in your own home (see Recipes); this hands-on preparation is an important part of connecting with place, one of the secrets of indigenous peoples and a lost art in our modern world.

In addition, most children will need an appropriate probiotic given in gradually increasing doses. Our aim is to carefully and systematically bring back the healthy bacteria that should colonize a healthy gut. (See Appendix II.)

Depending on the severity of the condition, the child will need to follow the GAPS diet for a couple of weeks (in some cases of mild dermatitis) to two years (with a severe case of asthma). In some cases, we see an initial improvement of the major symptoms in a few days, in other cases it may take a few months.

It should be noted that this diet is difficult—but temporary. The goal is to heal the gut and return to a diet that includes grains, potatoes and raw dairy products. It is most helpful if the whole family can do the diet at the same time, with one caveat: because the GAPS diet provokes die off and detoxification, it should not be followed by pregnant and nursing mothers.

When we replace the pathogens in the gut (predominantly candida) with healthy bacteria, we will naturally provoke a dying off of the fungal organisms. This can result in diarrhea, fatigue, achiness, headaches and many other unpleasant symptoms. When this occurs, as it inevitably does, we slow down the increase of the probiotic supplement or lacto-fermented foods, keep the diet very simple and go slowly. In some cases, we need to use specific antifungal medicines to help in this process, such as oral Nystatin, which requires the guidance of an experienced physician.

Fundamentally the GAPS diet addresses on an individual level the root cause of these allergic-immune disorders. It helps us reconnect and restore our sense of place and our inner ecology. Many patients will discover a true healing with this protocol, meaning that they overcome their eczema, asthma or allergies, and are then able to move on to the basic traditional diet without any other food restrictions. Nevertheless, the patient will always need to focus on nutrient-dense foods, include lacto-fermented foods on a daily basis, and go easy on problematic foods like grains. (For details on the GAPS diet, see Appendix II.)

The following are specific treatments for eczema, asthma and allergies. Doses are listed in the text box on page 247. (To obtain the various remedies, see Sources.)

ECZEMA

For eczema and related skin rashes, along with the GAPS diet, cod liver oil and a probiotic supplement, it can be helpful to take an oil mixture that contains multiple seed oils, such as evening primrose oil, coconut oil and flax seed oil. The blend we recommend is YES Essential Fatty Acid Blend.

As an aid in the detoxification process we can give sea vegetables in capsule form, which serve to bind heavy metals and other toxins and promote their excretion through the bowels. A good choice is Seagreens for oral consumption.

In addition, seaweed baths are helpful to directly soothe and nourish the skin. The Aalgo baths in particular exfoliate the skin, allowing it to breathe and regenerate more quickly.

When the eczema seems to be temporally related to one or more vaccines, positive results may be obtained with *Thuja Thymus Complex* from Uriel pharmacy (see Sources) at a dose of three pellets sublingually first thing in the morning. Thuja is the specific homeopathic antidote for vaccines and the thymus extract helps to stimulate the thymus gland (which makes T cells, a major player in our immune response) to normalize the immune response.

A final remedy is Dermatrophin, the Standard Process protomorphogen of the skin. A protomorphogen is extracted from the same tissue type as that involved in the underlying illness (in this case, the skin); it binds the antibodies produced and allows them to be excreted through the feces instead of causing inflammation in the skin.

An excellent topical treatment is Dermrash cream from Dr. Kang Formulas. The principal ingredient is *Sophora*, a shrubby plant used as an herb in Chinese medicine to counteract allergies by stabilizing the mast cells (the cells that produce histamine). We have seen severe cases of eczema clear up with the sole remedy of applying this cream.

One final note about eczema: we must be careful to watch for infections of the skin. If this occurs, the medicine of choice is *Andrographis Complex*.

ASTHMA

When considering specific remedies for asthma, in addition to the GAPS diet, it is instructive to consider the difference between asthma and pneumonia (see page 232). Simulating the condition of pneumonia can greatly improve the situation for an asthmatic child. During an acute asthma attack, we can do this by putting mustard compresses on the chest, as the mustard carries the sulfur or metabolic "message" strongly into the child's lungs. This should be done until redness of the skin occurs, which depends on the potency of the mustard. Do the compresses daily until there is clear improvement (see Appendix I).

We can also use the Mediherb preparation Bronchafect, which acts as an expectorant and contains phlegm-loosening herbs.

Many acute asthma episodes follow an upper respiratory infection; the recommendations for upper respiratory infection (see page 232), including the food guidelines, apply in these cases as well.

Acute asthma is a potentially life threatening condition and should always be treated in conjunction with a physician well versed in the treatment of the asthmatic patient.

For the nonacute stage, we follow the entire GAPS protocol including the cod liver oil, with a probiotic. YES Essential Fatty Acid Blend at a dose of two capsules twice per day. If the diet brings clear improvement, no other medicines are necessary.

As soon as possible on the GAPS diet, introduce whole raw milk, which several studies have shown to provide powerful protection against asthma.[2] Some cases of asthma have cleared up with the simple addition of raw whole milk to the diet. Pasteurized milk and pasteurized milk products should be completely avoided.

If more help is needed, give Pneumotrophin, the Standard Process protomorphogen of the lung; and Phytocort, a mixture of licorice, ganoderma and sophora from Allergy Research. This preparation has proven efficacy in the treatment of pediatric asthma;[3] it combines the anti-allergy effects of ganoderma (the reishi mushroom) and sophora with the cortisone-stimulating effect of licorice.

By helping the child's body to produce more cortisone, licorice decreases the need for pharmaceutical cortisone as in prednisone or steroid inhalers. Phytocort is given at a dose of one to three capsules four times per day, often for six months.

TREATMENT SUMMARY FOR ALLERGIES, ASTHMA & ECZEMA

In addition to the GAPS diet for all these conditions, specific medications are as follows:

ECZEMA
- YES Essential Fatty Acid Blend, 2 capsules, 2 times per day.
- Seagreens sea vegetables, 1-2 capsules, 2 times per day.
- Aalgo sea vegetable baths to exfoliate the skin.
- *Thuja Thymus Complex* from Uriel pharmacy, 3 pellets sublingually first thing in the morning.
- Dermatrophin by Standard Process, 1 tablet, 3 times per day, ideally between meals.
- Dermrash topical cream from Dr. Kang Formulas.
- *Andrographis Complex*, from Uriel Pharmacy, 1-2 tablets per day for skin infections until the problem is resolved.

ASTHMA
- Mustard compresses on the chest.
- Bronchafect by Mediherb, 1 teaspoon every 2 hours until there is clear improvement.
- YES Essential Fatty Acid Blend, 2 capsules, 2 times per day.
- Pneumotrophin by Standard Process, 1 tablet, 3 times per day.
- Phytocort from Allergy Research, 1-3 capsules, 4 times per day, for about 6 months.
- Chiropractic treatments.

ALLERGIES
- Culturelle from Allergy Research, 1 capsule each morning.
- Echinacea by Mediherb, 1 teaspoon daily of the liquid preparation, or 2 tablets, for 3-6 months.

Some cases of asthma have improved dramatically with chiropractic treatments.

Conventional treatments for asthma, such as the rescue inhalers and preventative inhalers, should be assessed on a case-by-case basis, always keeping our sights set on the ultimate healing of the situation balanced by the short term need to quickly resolve dangerous symptoms.

ALLERGIES

The basic GAPS diet is the foundation of treatment for such conditions as hay fever and allergic rhinitis. Often the diet readily brings clear improvement and no other treatments are necessary. It is critical for the diet to contain plentiful fats, so that blood sugar does not drop between meals.

In some cases it is helpful to change the probiotic. The probiotic Culturelle from Allergy Research is a proven immune tonic and is given instead of the GAPS probiotic, at a dose of one capsule each morning.

The other beneficial medicine for allergies is echinacea by Mediherb, given long term. Echinacea is an immune modulator; it brings both an overactive or under-active immune response into a normal balance. The medicine is usually given long-term, at least three to six months, before significant relief is seen.

FOR FURTHER INFORMATION

Gut and Psychology Syndrome: Natural Treatment for Autism, Dyspraxia, A.D.D., Dyslexia, A.D.H.D., Depression, Schizophrenia by Natasha Campbell-McBride

Chapter 16
Neurological Disorders
Autism, Epilepsy, Dyslexia, ADD & ADHD

Autism is the disease of our era. Recent surveys indicate that the incidence of austistic spectrum disorder has reached one in every one hundred children and as many as one in seven boys. So-called experts—perhaps we should say spin doctors—question whether these figures represent a real increase or whether we are just more sophisticated in our diagnosis. They also reassure us that many children with autistic spectrum disorders can be helped with conventional therapies, urging parents to "seek out professional help as soon as possible."

In the clever doublespeak of our modern era, the implication is that in former times, doctors were just not savvy enough to diagnose autism. After all, we are at the pinnacle of human evolution today, so we can't admit to an actual increase in a disease that is tantamount to the soul's turning its back on the world. This is the same bromide the public gets about hay fever, allergies, childhood cancer, diabetes and virtually all of the other current diseases playing havoc with our children.

NOT HARD TO DIAGNOSE

The fact is, it is not hard to diagnose an autistic child. Physicians in previous generations, before all the x-rays, CT scans and blood tests, were, if anything, much more astute diagnosticians than modern doctors; they had no choice but to observe and examine

their patients, habits that are almost extinct in our HMO-based practices. To think that these parents and doctors could not spot a child with autism—or hay fever or asthma—strains all credulity. No, the doctors are not really smarter today, something really is going on, and it is obvious that our current way of life is not working for our children. Many seem to reject all contact with our culture, often in the stark way of an autistic child.

Jaimen McMillan, movement specialist and founder of the movement therapy system called Spacial Dynamics® (see Sources), got his initial inspiration as a result of working with autistic children in a therapeutic home in Germany. As he worked and lived with children in this home, he realized that most autistic children have similar movement patterns. While hard to describe in words—and yet obvious when you see it—their heads, which should be still, move too much and their limbs and hands seem to have a jerky, repetitive or poorly flowing quality. Their movements lack the purposefulness that we expect from movement; instead, they exhibit lots of random swaying motions. In many cases, the mouth moves too much and one hears repetitive speech, but with no obvious intent to communicate with another person through this speech. McMillan's hypothesis was that autism is a movement disorder, and he developed many exercises to retrain the movements of these autistic children, greatly facilitating their recovery.

AUTISM: THE CONVENTIONAL VIEW[1]

Autism is characterized by impaired social interaction and communication, and by restricted and repetitive behavior. The conventional view of autism treats the disease as a disorder of neural development and looks for its cause in the brain, as a condition that affects information processing by altering how nerve cells and their synapses connect and organize.

There are three recognized disorders in the autism spectrum (ASDs), the other two being Asperger syndrome, which manifests as impaired social interaction without the delays in cognitive development and language, and pervasive developmental disorder, not otherwise specified (commonly abbreviated as PDD-NOS), which is diagnosed when the full set of criteria for autism or Asperger syndrome are not met.

Generally, parents usually notice signs of autism in the first two years of their child's life. The signs usually develop gradually, but some autistic children first develop more normally and then suddenly regress. Many parents report regression after a vaccination, but these observations are dismissed by conventional physicians.

Autistic individuals display many forms of repetitive or restricted behavior, which the Repetitive Behavior Scale-Revised (RBS-R) categorizes as follows.

- Intentional compulsive behavior, appearing to follow rules, such as arranging objects in stacks or lines.
- Sameness or resistance to change; for example, insisting that the furniture not be moved or refusing to be interrupted.
- Ritualistic behavior involving an unvarying pattern of daily activities, such as an unchanging menu or a dressing ritual.
- Restricted behavior that is limited in focus, interest, or activity, such as preoccupation with a single television program, toy, or game.
- Self-injury with movements that injure or can injure the person, such as eye poking, skin picking, hand biting, and head banging.

About half of parents of children with ASD notice their child's unusual behaviors by age eighteen months, and about four-fifths notice by age twenty-four months. Failure to meet any of the following milestones is considered an indication of autism, with further testing suggested:

- No babbling by twelve months.
- No gesturing (pointing, waving, etc.) by twelve months.
- No single words by sixteen months.
- No two-word (spontaneous, not just echolalic) phrases by twenty-four months.
- Any loss of any language or social skills, at any age.

Conventional treatment of autism involves various psychosocial interventions. . . and drugs. More than half of U.S. children diagnosed with ASD are prescribed psychoactive drugs or anticonvulsants, with the most common drug classes being antidepressants, stimulants and antipsychotics, but no known medication relieves autism's core symptoms of social and communication impairments.

Diagnosis of autism has greatly increased during the last twenty years. The conventional view is that this increase is an artifact of more inclusive diagnostic criteria. But any veteran teacher can tell you that this condition was unheard-of, or at least extremely rare, until the 1990s.

In our three-fold model of the human being, the proper realm of movement is the metabolic or limb area, in contrast to the nerve-sense realm of the head which in healthy people mostly remains still. To understand what is happening with the autistic child, try spending just one day—or even one hour—with the limbs as still as possible and the head in constant motion. Even after just a few minutes, you will have a clear sympathy for the trials of autistic children.

In autistic children the three-fold dynamics are flipped upside down; the metabolism ends up in the head, creating the constant movement that is only proper for the legs, arms and hands. Because the head is not good at movement, the movements are unhealthy—repetitive, jerky and without purpose. This is the pattern we encounter in most autistic children. And while the head moves constantly in an unnatural way, the metabolism, specifically digestion, is severely inhibited.

The idea of a connection between the digestive tract and the brain and nervous system is by no means new. In 1998, Michael Gershon, the head of gastroenterology at Cornell Medical School wrote a book called *The Second Brain*, pointing out the similar physiology of the brain and the intestines right down to the receptors embedded in the tissues of each organ. Rudolf Steiner once commented that the brain is simply coiled up intestines crowded into the dome of the skull.

Therefore, if we want to understand the dynamics behind autism we must search for answers in the metabolic realm, or more specifically into how the proper activity of the gut realm seeps into the brain and nervous system region, in essence poisoning our children's brains.

This brings us to the GAPS diet, described in Chapter 15 and in Appendix II, which was originally developed as a treatment for autism. The diet works to seal the gut and stop the leakage of the metabolism into a realm where it doesn't belong: the head. The details of the GAPS theory and treatment even lead into an understanding of which chemicals are the ones that leak and clearly identify a disorder in the gut ecology as the metabolic "culprit" in autism.

We can even understand the controversial relationship between autism and vaccines as one in which the mercury, aluminum, formaldehyde, and other toxic excipients contained in the vaccines, in conjunction with the inflammatory response provoked by the vaccine administration, when coupled with weak "borders" (that is, the gut wall and the blood-brain barrier) gain access to the nervous tissue and create serious damage. All of this naturally follows when we look at autism as a movement disorder originating in an unhealthy and porous metabolism.

A DIET FOR A DISEASE

As with asthma, allergies and many other chronic diseases, modern medicine insists that there is no cure for autism. Germane to our discussion of autism and other supposedly incurable diseases is the fact that there is only one disease considered curable by conventional pediatricians. There is only one disease where a parent can take a child to a conventional pediatrician, describe the child's symptoms, get the appropriate tests and diagnosis and then hear the doctor say, "I know a diet that can cure your child of this disease." By "cure" we mean that you can do this diet for about two years then make a transition to a "normal" diet and not have the disease come back.

The disease we are talking about is epilepsy, and the diet is a high-fat diet called the ketogenic diet. You will never hear of a curative diet suggested for ear infections, asthma, eczema, not even for diabetes (the recommended diet for diabetics is not meant to be curative). Like a sore thumb, the ketogenic diet for epilepsy sticks out as an anomaly in medicine; it is the one area where conventional medicine recognizes, albeit reluctantly, that a dietary intervention can cure a disease.

The ketogenic diet has been part of conventional medical therapy for over fifty years and is still used at the Stanford and Johns Hopkins medical centers. The diet is based on the recognition that the brain uses two types of "fuel." The usual fuel is glucose, derived primarily from the breakdown of dietary carbohydrates and secondarily from the metabolism of proteins; only when there is no glucose available will the body shift to its back-up fuel, which is ketones. Ketones are the break-down products of fat metabolism, and when the body is deprived of carbohydrate sources it will begin to use ketones as fuel. (This is a different process from the one called ketosis, which is a dreaded complication of uncontrolled diabetes.)

This switch from glucose to ketones as fuel can be documented because when the brain is using ketones as fuel, ketones will be found in the blood and urine. The amazing finding, which is as yet unexplained in conventional medicine, is that very soon after this shift in fuels is made, and the child's brain is running on ketones, the brain wave pattern shifts. In 40-80 percent of cases, the EEG patterns reflect the cessation of seizure activity in the child on the ketogenic diet. This brain pattern persists as long as the child remains on the ketogenic diet, which—

TOXINS IN THE GUTS OF AUTISTIC CHILDREN[2]

ALCOHOL: The production of alcohol by candida and other yeasts results in what is called "auto-brewery syndrome," first described by a Japanese doctor in the 1970s. Today, this phenomenon is well known. Gut dysbiosis can result in a chronic state of semi-drunkenness, which is particularly devastating to young children.

ACETALDEHYDE: The liver converts alcohol into acetaldehyde, an extremely toxic substance. Anyone who has experienced a hangover knows what acetaldehyde does. It causes hundreds of devastating effects on the body. Acetaldehyde attaches itself to various proteins in the body, changing their structure. The immune system then starts attacking these foreign proteins with antibodies. Thus acetaldehyde in the body creates auto-immunity. And because acetaldehyde attaches itself to a lot of proteins that are the working sites for various nutrients in the body, these nutrients cannot fulfill their functions. The most common deficiency that can result is vitamin B_6 deficiency. Tests show that B_6 is present in the bloodstream, but the receptors for it do not work. Vitamin B_6 deficiency is linked to the problems we see in autistic children—learning disabilities, hyperactivity and dyslexia—and in schizophrenics as well.

DERMORPHIN and DELTORPHIN: A New York biochemist named Alan Freedman found these two frightening substances in the urine and blood of autistic children. These are identical to the toxins found on the skin of Amazonian frogs. The local tribes dip the end of their darts on the skin of these frogs in order to paralyze their enemies—these are extremely potent neurotoxins that cause paralysis. The interesting thing is that it is not the frog that produces the toxin but a fungus that grows on the skin of the frog. The suspicion is that the autistic child grows that fungus in his digestive system and the fungus produces the toxin. This may account for some characteristic muscle tone abnormalities and movement without purpose seen in many autistic children.

GLUTEOMORPHINS and CASOMORPHINS: Gluteomorphins and casomorphins are partially digested proteins. Gluteomorphins come from gluten found in grains and casomorphins come from the casein found in dairy foods. Gluten and casein are large molecules that are hard for even normal people to digest. In children with damaged, porous and leaky gut walls, these proteins do not get digested properly but are partially broken down into peptide chains whose structure is very similar to the structure of heroin, morphine and other opiates. These substances are absorbed in that form and have a similar effect on the brain as heroin and morphine would have.

Autistic children are often put on a gluten-free/casein-free (GFCF) diet. It is a tragedy that this diet has been pronounced as "the" diet for autism and schizophrenia because removing grains and dairy foods only removes two toxic substances from the body—gluteomorphins and casomorphins. While about 30 percent of children do show improvement with the GFCF diet, it doesn't deal with all the other toxins, it doesn't heal the gut and it doesn't change the gut flora. The majority do not show any improvement at all, and those who show some improvement then reach a plateau and the parents end up in a nightmare situation where if the child gets hold of even a crumb of bread or steals a cracker, there is a huge regression. This happens because the gut is still damaged, the gut flora is still abnormal, the gut wall is still leaky and porous. All the toxins are still flowing into the brain and nervous system.

embarassing as this fact may be to the medical profession—is a diet extremely high in fats like cream, egg yolks and butter. Miraculously, after about one and one-half years, the change becomes permanent. At this point, even if the child goes off the ketogenic diet and resumes a more "normal" diet, he will not suffer from seizures. Thus we have a true dietary cure for epilepsy, something that conventional medicine does not recognize in any other illness.

In working with children, one can't help but notice that young people on the ketogenic diet seem healthier overall; they seem calmer, more focused and have a clarity that is unmistakable, all reflected in the EEG brain patterns. Some have commented that the brain wave pattern of a child on the ketogenic diet resembles that of an experienced meditant in a state of deep meditation or relaxation.

But the story of the ketogenic diet gets even more interesting. Recent research over the past decade has shown that Alzheimer's disease or dementia is associated with a state of insulin resistance in the brain cells. In other words, the brain puts up a resistance to the uptake of glucose in order to protect it from excessive glucose exposure. The problem for the brain cells is that since the glucose is the main brain fuel, the end result is a kind of brain starvation, resulting in the well-documented atrophy of the brain cells, with loss of connection associated with memory loss.

As the phenomenon of insulin resistance in the brain became clear, scientists began searching for a back-up fuel for the brain cells, in particular a fuel that could traverse the blood-brain barrier. That search inevitably led back to the ketogenic diet coupled with the use of medium-chain triglycerides, the main type of fat in coconut oil, which is readily used by brain cells for fuel. There are now many reports of the successful use of the ketogenic diet along with large doses of coconut oil (or commercially prepared solutions of medium-chain triglycerides) in the treatment of Alzheimer's dementia.[3]

DIET & TECHNOLOGY IN THE MODERN AGE: THE PERFECT STORM FOR AUTISM

A number of factors can take the blame for our modern epidemic of autism, all coming together as the perfect storm for this dreadful condition.

- Lowfat, low-cholesterol diets during pregnancy and lactation prevent the baby's brain and gut from forming properly.

- Antibiotics in the mother's diet before conception and during pregnancy prevent the colonization of baby's gut with beneficial flora; antibiotics given to the child from infancy wipe out beneficial gut flora.

- Overuse of ultrasound during pregnancy.

- Heavy metal exposure from pollution, amalgam fillings and other sources.

- Soy infant formula, which prevents the proper development of the digestive and nervous systems. High manganese levels in soy formula can poison the brain; the symptoms of manganese toxicity are very similar to those of austim.

- Standard American Diet (SAD) for growing children, especially the substitution of vegetable fats and oils for animal fats; such a diet will be lacking in the nutrients needed for proper neurological development. The SAD also lacks lacto-fermented foods needed for the proper colonization of the gut.

- Strong electromagnetic fields from cell towers, smart meters and high-tension power lines.

- Vaccinations, often the straw that breaks the camel's back.

- Use of Tylenol to treat fever following vaccination, depletes sulphur needed for detoxification.

Like a spring flower that just insists on popping up whenever it can, the ketogenic diet is popping up as a treatment for more than just neurological diseases. Recently discussion of the diet is showing up in the pages of oncology journals. For years, the main diagnostic tool for the oncologists in diagnosing met- astatic cancer, that is, cancer that has spread beyond the original tumor, is to do a PET scan. In a PET scan, radioactive glucose is injected intravenously in the cancer patient; this glucose is preferentially taken up by the cancer cells. Doctors can locate the site of the new, metastatic cancer growth by the ra-

VITAMIN A, VITAMIN D & ARACHIDONIC ACID FOR MENTAL HEALTH[4]

Clinically defined psychiatric disorders afflict just under half of Americans for at least one period of time during their lives. Depression and anxiety often occur together and also often occur in conjunction with physical ailments such as inflammatory bowel disease and asthma. The lifetime prevalence of depression, anxiety, impulse control problems and substance abuse disorders is twice as high for people born after 1945, when Americans began the switch from animal fats to vegetable oils, than for those born earlier, and the proportion of Americans suffering from three or more disorders—nearly a fifth—has more than tripled for the post-World War II generations.

Personal success depends on confronting challenges with focused, goal-oriented behavior rather than hiding from such challenges in self-defeat, while at the same time restraining the impulse to spend and consume all the fruits of one's labor in the present in order to build something greater for the future. Science is now showing us that key nutrients available from animal fats and organ meats are criticial for the biochemical pathways that protect us against depression and other mental disorders, and support focused, goal-oriented behavior. These key nutrients are arachidonic acid, vitamin A and vitamin D, which cooperate to promote mental health by regulating the adrenal hormone cortisol and the neurotransmitter dopamine through the potent central nervous system regulators known as endocannabinoids.

Arachidonic acid is an elongated omega-6 fatty acid found primarily in eggs and liver and in smaller amounts in all other animal fats including butterfat. Healthy adults can also synthesize small amounts from omega-6 linoleic acid, found in both plant oils and animal fats. Vitamin A, however, is necessary for this conversion and also helps carry out dopamine signaling more directly. Vitamin A is present in large amounts in liver and cod liver oil and in small amounts in egg yolks and butterfat.

Vitamin D directly interacts with vitamin A in many contexts and is critical to maintaining blood and tissue levels of calcium. Calcium is a central regulator of arachidonic acid metabolism in virtually every type of cell, making vitamin D essential for proper handling of this nutrient. Vitamin D is present in large amounts in fatty fish and cod liver oil and in small amounts in the fats of land animals. We also obtain vitamin D when we are exposed to sunlight that is directly overhead, which at most latitudes is available only during the summer months.

Arachidonic acid is the direct precursor to the endocannabinoids. Endocannabinoids regulate the adrenal response to stress, mediated primarily by the hormone cortisol, which is responsible for the fight-or-flight response; they also regulate the production of dopamine in the brain, which is responsible for the motivation to sustain goal-oriented effort over time. By curbing the excess production of cortisol and supporting adequate production of dopamine, endocannabinoids help prevent excess tension, anxiety, burnout and feelings of self-defeat, and help support the confrontation of challenges with the attitudes necessary for success.

The role of these critical fat-soluble nutrients eclipses all other factors in the raising of children blessed with the ability to maintain sustained goal-oriented behavior and a happy outlook on life. Cod liver oil, organ meats, animal fats, egg yolks and butter in the diet of your growing child are key to robust mental health and success in life.

dioactive signature of the sugar that accumulates there. Some researchers began to wonder whether you could starve cancer cells by withholding all forms of sugar, since cancer cells in essence live off the ingested glucose, thereby stimulating their own growth and starving their "host." The obvious therapeutic step would be to withhold fuel from cancer cells by cutting off glucose (that is, sugar) and since you have to feed the host something, and since cancer cells can't metabolize ketones, why not the ketogenic diet? Not surprisingly, there are reports that this strategy does in fact work; the tumor starves and the host—the patient—thrives.[5]

The surprising success of the ketogenic diet, for conditions as diverse as epilepsy and cancer, leads to more questions. What if the main fuel for the brain is actually ketones, and glucose is the backup? What if the natural diet for human beings is a high-fat diet, the high-carbohydrate diet serving as a poor substitute?

When you examine the dietary habits of indigenous peoples studied by the painter George Caitlin, the explorer Vilhjalmur Stefansson, Weston Price and others, it becomes clear that the healthiest humans lived on diets akin to the ketogenic diet, in which the predominant source of energy came from fats. These diets did contain some carbohydrate foods, and may not have been as high in fat as the therapeutic ketogenic diet used for epilepsy; but what emerges from these considerations is the fact that a diet based on carbohydrates is the anomaly.

In disease situations, we may need to consume more fat than the amount found in traditional diets, which in essence forces the patient to "learn" how to use fats as fuel. Once established, the lesson of the ketogenic diet in epilepsy shows that a fundamental change has occurred, which will not regress even when returning to the more conventional mixed-fuel approach. The important message here is that metabolizing fats seems to be a "skill" we lose at our own peril; temporarily forcing the issue seems to have great benefit in a number or diseases that are common in our modern lives.

MEETING OUR DESTINY

In discussing the nervous system, Rudolf Steiner insisted that our division of the nervous system into sensory and motor branches was misguided. He claimed that all nerves are sensory and that the nerves that "control" movement are actually just sensing the movements that originate in the metabolic-limb system. The metabolic-limb system correlates with the soul properties of the will, or of activity. Out of ourselves we move, our nerves sense the movement and integrate this into our purpose and intention. The movements originate in the metabolism, in the gut, which is the place to look and to heal the various movement disorders discussed in this chapter.

Jaimen MacMillan, founder of Spacial Dynamics®, describes the origins of movement as actions coming through us, which use our bodies as their "vehicle." In essence we are moved by the world to action. So where are we being moved? We are moved to seek our destiny, our unique path in life, which calls to us from out there in the world. For those who have ever fallen in love, you will understand the distinction between moving and being moved—for love calls to us as a powerful force that does not originate within, but comes from the outside.

For the truly well adjusted person, the sense of destiny, of being moved in a certain direction, feels powerful and actually irresistible, as if there is simply no other choice. And while not everyone is called by destiny to accomplish some great work, everyone is called to live out his or her unique story, always in relationship to others and the world. In autism, and to a lesser extent in other neurological disorders of childhood, this sense is tragically lost. The individual without a destination is like a ship simply listing on the seas. The destiny is still there, the story is there to be lived, but the sensing of the story is cloudy rather than clear. By applying the therapies and the thinking outlined in this chapter, we can bring clarity to the vehicle of our children's bodies, in particular strengthening their metabolic-will forces. Such clarity would constitute a true healing for these otherwise tragic and all too common illnesses of our times.

To summarize, autism and related neurological disorders arise when the metabolism has "lost its place," and invaded the head. This may result in full-blown autism, or in variations like attention deficit disorder (ADD) and attention deficit hyperactivity disorder (ADHD). Specific symptoms may reflect the effects of particular neurotoxins produced in the gut on particular parts of the brain.

We still have much to learn about these conditions but the overall treatment required is now clear. We need to first detoxify from toxic metals, yeasts and exogenous morphines, restore gut ecology integrity and switch the fuel source of the brain from glucose to ketones or medium-chain triglycerides.

Fortunately, these goals are not mutually exclusive; rather, they are aspects of the same therapy. A low-carbohydrate diet, high in fat, including butter or ghee, coconut oil and cod liver oil, not only provides needed fuel for the brain, it also kills the fungal infections in the gut, provides building material for the intestinal wall, nourishes the immune system and provides the elements needed for detoxification. In short, a modified GAPS diet low in carbohydrates and rich in fats outlined in Appendix II provides a rational therapy to address the underlying causes of neurological diseases in children.

Since every child will have slightly different manifestations of these illnesses, access to a health practitioner well versed in these therapies is essential. To find such practitioners, check the GAPS website at www.GAPS.me or contact the nearest local chapter of the Weston A. Price Foundation (www.westonaprice.org).

Most importantly, this outline will give parents faced with these devastating illnesses information about genuinely helpful therapies, which in many cases have completely turned around situations that otherwise carried a dismal prognosis.

Let us now turn to specific therapies for neurological conditions, always used in conjunction with a high-fat GAPS diet. For doses of recommended medications, see the sidebar below (for sources of medicines and therapies, see Sources).

AUTISM

In autism, we often have to deal with the ramifications of heavy metal exposure as a precipitating cause. This leads us to choose a gentle chelation therapy, that is, therapy that captures toxins and moves them out of the body, at the same time remembering that healing the gut and restoring optimal nutrition is the best chelation therapy of all.

TREATMENT SUMMARY FOR AUTISM, EPILEPSY, DYSLEXIA, ADD & ADHD

In addition to a high-fat diet GAPS diet, the therapy for these conditions is summarized as follows:

AUTISM
- For heavy metal detoxification, Seagreens or Longvida curcumin, 1 capsule, 2 times per day. This treatment can be applied for the long term.
- For fungal overgrowth, oral Nystatin, Diflucan or both, always under the care of a qualified physician.
- A milder treatment for fungal overgrowth is Lauricidin, given according to the directions on the jar.
- After several months on the above therapies, a broad spectrum anti-parasitic drug, Vermox, 100 mg twice per day for 3 days and then repeated in 2 weeks.
- Spatial Dynamics movement therapy.

EPILEPSY
- *Acidum sulfuricum e vitiolo D3* by Weleda, 10 drops, 3 times per day.

DYSLEXIA, ADD and ADHD
- Extra Lesson™, used widely in Waldorf schools.
- Spatial Dynamics movement therapy.
- Let nature and the child's natural instincts serve as the main educators.

A good strategy for chelation involves the use of sea vegetables and curcumin (also called turmeric), both shown in many studies to be effective and gentle chelators. Seagreens and Longvida curcumin, both by Nutrivene (see Sources) can be used long term at the dose of one capsule each, twice per day.

Many autistic children will need antifungal treatment with either oral Nystatin, Diflucan or both; these treatments should always be given under the care of a qualified physician.

A milder antifungal therapy is the coconut oil extract monolauren sold under the name Lauricidin, which acts as an antifungal agent, as well as providing medium-chain fatty acids used by the cells as fuel. This is given according to the directions on the jar.

Many will benefit from treatment with a broad spectrum pharmaceutical anti-parasitic drug like Vermox, or Pin-X, 100 mg twice per day for three days and then repeated in two weeks. Anti-parasite treatment should never be given as a first step, and should always be undertaken with the supervision of a physician. And remember that salt is necessary for the production of hydrochloric acid, our first defense against parasites. We all need plenty of salt in our diets, and that includes the autistic child.

Finally, we should address directly the movement component of this disorder. For this, the best way is to work directly with a Spatial Dynamics practitioner, who can also give guidance as to the best home "exercises" and movements to use. The general theme is that the less mechanical the movements the better. This means that the less the life of an autistic child is based on machines of any sort—including computers, the ultimate image of pure "head"—and the more the movements come as result of direct contact with nature, the better. Long walks, playing in a stream or meadow, playing with animals, bugs, plants, helping out on a farm—these are the activities that can heal the movements of the autistic child. More barefoot, fewer shoes; more trees, even to just lean against them, less brick and concrete: nature with its flowing movements and calm rhythms is the therapy for the unnatural movements of the autistic child.

NEUROLOGICAL DISORDERS IN THE ELECTROMAGNETIC AGE

Many scientists have correlated the increase in autism and attention deficit disorders with the increasing use of electromagnetic devices such as cell phones, WiFi, smart meters and microwave ovens. According to Dr. Andrew Goldsworthy of the Imperial College London Department of Biological Sciences, signals too weak to cause heating can nevertheless cause damage by removing calcium ions from cell membranes in the brain. The resulting disruption of brain biochemistry leads to neuro-excitation of the brain cells, making emotional contact and concentration difficult. Goldsworthy also postulates that the background of electromagnetic signals makes it difficult for the brain to prune spurious connections, a process that normally happens as the child grows. As a result, the child may be left with a defective hard-wired mindset for social interactions.[6]

It is difficult to escape the background of electromagnetic signals that constantly bathes all of us, but some steps will mitigate the load. Don't use a microwave oven, do your best to avoid the installation of a smart meter to read your electricity and gas usage, use landlines not cell phones in your home, and avoid living too near to a cell tower or high-tension power lines. In addition, turn off WiFi in your home at night; avoid using fluorescent bulbs, dimmer switches or electric blankets; and keep all electronics including electric alarm clocks away from your child's bedroom at night.

Good nutrition can help protect against the effects of electromagnetic radiation, especially choline from egg yolks and liver and cholesterol from animal foods, especially animal fats. Arachidonic acid found in animal fats and organ meats will support the formation of tight cell-to-cell junctures in the brain. The wireless revolution is not going to go away, and certainly many children grow up with normal brain function and behavior in spite of the electromagnetic background. Avoiding excesses of exposure and good nutrition are obviously key to protecting your child.

EPILEPSY

Epilepsy, otherwise known as seizure disorder, comes in many types and variations (to describe them all is beyond the scope of this book). Unlike the other illnesses described in this chapter, epilepsy is an archetypal human disease, one that has been part of the human condition for millennia. It is also the one neurological disease that doesn't seem to be increasing at the same alarming rate as the others we are discussing.

Epilepsy was of such a concern in Europe during the Middle Ages that the famous physician Paracelsus spent a good part of his life developing a cure. Paracelsus was an alchemist, a word that conjures up shadowy connotations, but which in those days placed him at the pinnacle of the scientific community. Alchemists were the nuclear physicists of their era, as concerned then as today with the nature of matter and of life.

Through a fairly complex alchemistic process, Paracelsus was able to convert sulfuric acid into a medicine that he claimed cured epilepsy. While it is not clear how it works, Rudolf Steiner gave some insight when he noted that a seizure results from the higher "bodies" getting stuck in an organ, not being able to emerge, thereby creating a kind of inner tension, which then bursts forth as an explosion of "energy," manifesting as a seizure. He then went on to say that the rational therapy would be to dissolve the overly "coarse" coating of the organs to allow the soul and spirit of the patient to freely flow in and out of their organisms. He is speaking of boundaries, just as we do with the GAPS diet, but boundaries which in this case need to be made less dense and more porous.

Steiner suggested using the sulfuric acid compound discovered by Paracelsus to gently dissolve these coarse boundaries and restore the patient to good health. Thanks to the long and patient work of physician Dr. Bertram von Zabern, we now have access to the same preparation developed by Paracelsus many centuries ago. It is sold through Weleda under the name *Acidum sulfuricum e vitiol D3* and is given at a dose of 10 drops three times per day. In many patients, along with the low-carbohydrate, GAPS protocol outlined above, a very significant lessening or even elimination of the seizures can occur.

DYSLEXIA, ADD and ADHD

In addition to the above information about the cause of neurological disease in general and also the movement disorder component of neurological disease, dyslexia and the conditions of ADD and ADHD urge us to come to grips with the important distinction between education and school. Education—the natural human urge to progressively learn more about everything to do with ourselves and the world around us—is fundamental to human existence and has been our quest since the dawn of time.

School, or at least the western version of mandatory public education, is a new invention which in the U.S. began in the mid 1800s. At that time, children on Cape Cod, Massachusetts were taken at gun point to undergo the grand social experiment we call schooling. While couched in terms of laudable goals (as with many misguided social programs), namely universal public education, the early theorists were unmistakably clear in their intentions—which was to prepare children for life as obedient participants in an industrial, factory-based, machine-oriented economy.

Universal education has been very successful in attaining this goal—but it failed miserably at creating an educated populace. In fact, before there was any school to speak of, in colonial U.S., the literacy rate was near 100 percent, and the best seller was Thomas Paine's book *Common Sense*. Today it's unlikely that 10 percent of Americans could really grasp the revolutionary concepts that Paine eloquently laid out in this book. The will, the ability, the interest in understanding complex ideas is lacking—such thinking is just too hard for most of today's young people.

That is more or less what the child with learning disorders is telling us: "It's just too hard to focus on this; let me be entertained instead." The phenomenon of the learning disabled child is a dramatic warning that we need a new view of education, one that either doesn't involve school, or if it does, in a much different way than school is currently constituted. I would encourage all parents with dyslexic children to let nature and the child's natural instincts serve as the main educators.

ADD and ADHD are conditions that exhibit aspects of a movement disorder, particularly in their "purposeless," unfocused movements. In others the illness manifests as an inability to focus or concentrate on any given subject or task, while in still others there are prominent allergic or gastro-intestinal symptoms.

All of these issues cry out for healing of the GI tract using the GAPS low-carbohydrate diet outlined above.

In addition, dyslexic, ADD and ADHD children need help with remedial movement training, as they have often skipped the usual developmental stages of childhood, such as crawling. They can be aided by doing a therapy that takes them back through these stages, such as that found in the work of Extra Lesson, used widely in Waldorf schools for these children. They can also work with a Spacial Dynamics practitioner (see Sources).

Finally, learning disabled children cry out for "nature" therapy. The rhythms of nature are the true therapy for the unfocused, disjointed inner world of the dyslexic and attention-deficit child. Returning to participate in nature's natural slow and patient rhythm often has dramatic effects on the healing of these children. While this is often a difficult therapy to organize, as the awareness of this dynamic increases, more and more programs and camps are becoming available. Parents should choose schools, summer camps and other programs that emphasize nature therapy and working with animals as much as possible.

FOR FURTHER INFORMATION

Gut and Psychology Syndrome: Natural Treatment for Autism, Dyspraxia, A.D.D., Dyslexia, A.D.H.D., Depression, Schizophrenia by Natasha Campbell-McBride

A Different Kind of Teacher by John Taylor Gatto

Deschooling Society by Ivan Illich

The Art of a Healing Education, A Compilation of Articles containing five articles on the Extra Lesson, the Pedagogical Law, Working with a School Doctor and addressing the Higher Nature of the Child, available from www.healingeducation.org

Chapter 17
Remedies for the Illnesses of Childhood

The following summary of various illnesses that tend to afflict children is meant to serve as an adjunct for the basic therapy: a healthy diet. That means a diet based on the principles outlined in the cookbook *Nourishing Traditions* and taught by the Weston A. Price Foundation; or, in cases of severe digestive disorders and neurological problems, the more restrictive GAPS diet for a period of time necessary for the gut to heal and the symptoms to resolve.

Bone broths, cod liver oil, eggs and butter from pastured animals, raw milk if tolerated, lacto-fermented foods and frequent organ meats in the form of paté, liverwurst or cooked lamb, calves or poultry liver—these form the basis of the diet that supports good health on every level. All industrial oils and sweeteners should be avoided. Fruits and vegetables should be organic whenever possible.

Many of the infectious diseases listed in this chapter will be accompanied by a fever—remember that fever is a child's best friend and should be allowed to run its course, unless it gets very high. (For details, see Chapter 13 on Infectious Disease.)

For sources of recommended medications, see Sources.

ACID REFLUX

Just a few decades ago, no one considered acid reflux a problem in children Now every infant who spits up is given acid blocking medicines for his supposed reflux. The reality is this condition is rare in healthy children. However, acid reflux does occur in unhealthy children nowadays, often in children born to mothers who have eaten a lot of modern wheat products and pasteurized dairy foods.

Doctors prescribe a variety of medications such as antacids (Mylanta and Maalox), given with each feeding; acid blockers such as Zantac, Pepcid, Tagamet and Prilosec; and motility medicines, which work by increasing muscle tone and therefore tightening the lower esophageal sphincter muscle; or they increase the movement and muscle tone of the stomach and upper intestines. This class of drugs includes Urecholine (bethanechol), Reglan (metclopramide) and Propulsid (cisapride). Side effects of these various medications include poor digestion (due to decreased stomach acid), cramping, diarrhea, restlessness, twitching, fainting and even cardiac arrhythmias. Obviously, these drugs are not a good solution to the problem of acid reflux.

Fortunately, modern research gives us a clue to the cause of acid reflux and suggests a dietary treatment without harmful side effects. A paper published in *Alternative Therapies* from the Duke University Department of Gastroenterology showed that the gastro-esophageal sphincter pressure, that is the pressure that keeps the stomach contents from refluxing into the esophagus, is controlled by insulin.They found that putting patients on a low-carbohydrate diet was a reliable treatment for most individuals with reflux.[1] It follows from this that sugar is the main culprit in the diet of a child who suffers from reflux. The solution is to eliminate the excess carbs in the child's diet (and in mom's diet if she is breastfeeding) and use bone broth and lacto-fermented vegetables in the context of a healthy diet, rich in animal fats.

To support the digestive process, for children over age two, one-half teaspoon of Swedish bitters mixed with a little water can be given morning and evening. This will take care of the vast majority of reflux problems. Using these dietary methods, Dr. Cowan has never needed to put a pediatric patient on antacids in all his years of practice.

For infants who are colicky or seem to be in discomfort on eating, the solution is to add a little extra cream or cultured cream to the homemade formula, and reduce the amount of lactose slightly. Using the liver formula, or adding a little grated liver, rich in vitamin B_{12}, to the milk formula may also give relief. Although conventional medical thought denies a connection between B_{12} deficiency and acid reflux,

it makes sense that the muscles of the esophagus and stomach need adequate B_{12} to work properly.

If you are breastfeeding, be sure to feed at least twenty minutes on each side, to ensure that baby gets the fat-rich hind milk. Mom should increase her consumption of animal fats and organ meats, and avoid excess carbohydrates, especially sugar.

Sometimes all that baby requires is to be properly burped. Hold him upright with his chin on your shoulder and gently stroke his back up and down. This will quickly bring up trapped air and give baby relief. Keep him upright for awhile; avoid putting him down in a horizontal position immediately after feeding.

Chiropractic and osteopathic treatments can also help—sometimes one gentle adjustment is all it takes to resolve acid reflux and colic.

ANAL ITCHING

Eating too much sugar can cause itchy bottoms from candida.

However, the usual cause of anal itching is pinworms. Adult pinworms live in the intestine and colon. At night, the female adult worms deposit their eggs outside the rectum or anal area. The presence of pinworms can be confirmed either by visually checking the anus or stool, or by doing the scotch tape pinworm test.

WHEN HOME REMEDIES ARE NOT APPROPRIATE

TRAUMA: If your child has a serious injury, head for the emergency room. Modern medicine really does have a lot to offer when it comes to treating trauma, and when we ignore these gifts, bad things can happen. When your child falls out of a tree and has a concussion or a bone is sticking out through his skin, you don't want to treat such emergencies at home.

EXTREMELY HIGH FEVER: Most fevers play a beneficial role in your child's health but an extremely high fever (over 104 degrees) can be a dangerous situation for a young child and you may need to get emergency care. (For treatment of high fever, see page 227.)

TROUBLE BREATHING: This is another situation that calls for quick action. If a child is unresponsive, limp in your arms or has glazed eyes, you need to get help. Dial 911 or hurry him to the emergency room.

CHILD HAS SWALLOWED POISON: Your child has gotten into the dishwashing powder, antifreeze or other poison? Call the poison hotline (800-222-1222) or get him to the emergency room at once.

For a visual test, shine a flashlight on the anal area. The worms are tiny, white and threadlike. If none are seen, check for two or three additional nights. You can also visually examine the stool, where pinworms will look like small white threads.

The best way to diagnose this infection is to do a tape test, preferably in the morning before bathing, because pinworms lay their eggs at night. Firmly press the sticky side of a one-inch strip of cellophane tape over the anal area for a few seconds. The eggs stick to the tape. The tape is then transferred to a glass slide, sticky side down. Your practitioner needs to examine the slide to confirm the presence of eggs.

The tape test may need to be done on three separate days to improve the chances of detecting the eggs.

If pinworms are found, give one tablet of Vermox, or over-the-counter Pin-X antiworm medication. It is very important to repeat the treatment in two weeks.

If pinworms are not found, the best solution is meticulous anal hygiene including rinsing the anal region with water, then drying well, after each bowel movement until the problem resolves. Application of coconut oil may help.

ANEMIA

If your child has a pale complexion, seems listless or unnaturally tired, or is fearful and clinging, it's best to do a blood test for anemia. Left untreated, anemia can lead to mental retardation; mild cases result in lack of energy in children, who should be bouncing and robust.

The conventional treatment for anemia is iron supplements, which often make matters worse and frequently cause constipation. Much better to treat anemia with diet.

For simple iron deficient anemia, the solution is to give liver once a day (usually as a liver purée or paté) plus red meat at the other two meals. In addition, give well cooked dark greens or beets served with plenty of butter, some dark fruits like prunes or figs, along with nettles tea. Molasses in gently heated raw milk may also be helpful.

Avoid sugar and all refined carbohydrates; whole grains should be made by the sourdough method or properly soaked in an acidic medium to neutralize iron-blocking phytic acid (see Recipes).

Cofactors for iron absorption include vitamin A and vitamin C. Be sure your child is getting his half teaspoon of high-vitamin cod liver oil per day; for vitamin C, take one tablet of Amla-Plus vitamin C daily.

If diet alone does not resolve the problem, try Floradix liquid, one-half teaspoon in a litle water, twice daily. Another good choice is Fe-Max from Mediherb, at a dose of one teaspoon, twice daily.

BOILS

Boils can be a vexing problem; they are usually caused by a strep or staph infection of the skin. Boils with significant pus should be drained by a physician, after which *Andrographis Complex*, from Mediherb should be given, one to two tablets fourtimes per day.

Hot compresses can be used to facilitate the ripening of the boils and compresses with raw honey over the area will help resolve the infection.

BUG BITES AND STINGS

The main thing to know about bee and wasp stings is the difference between a local reaction and an allergic reaction. By definition, an allergic reaction is a reaction that happens at a site not connected to the original sting.

This means that if you get stung on the wrist and your whole arm swells but nothing else, this is a local and therefore harmless (albeit unpleasant) reaction. If you get stung on the foot and your mouth swells, no matter how much or little swelling in the foot there is, this is an allergic reaction.

This simple fact, which is so misunderstood by laymen and even doctors in emergency rooms, provides the basis for the therapy. Local reactions are always harmless and need no treatment except perhaps ice packs and homeopathic *Apis*. Benadryl, antibiotics and similar medicines should not be given, they do no good in this situation; however three to four tablets of Amla-Plus vitamin C taken twice a day or even more frequently may greatly help reduce swelling and the general feeling of irritation.

On the other hand, an allergic reaction needs to be treated with urgency and care. Benadryl should be given and if there is any sign of breathing issues the child should immediately do an EpiPen injection or go to the nearest emergency room.

For mosquite bites and small bites of unknown origin that are itchy or swollen, apply chickweed gel topically and take several tablets of Amla-Plus vitamin C.

For protection against insects, use the nontoxic insect repellent products from Badger Balm, or a natural product called Buzz Away. Avoid all commercial insect repellents containing DEET or other harmful insecticides. Studies have shown that DEET leads to brain cell death and behavioral changes in rats after frequent and prolonged use. This exposure causes neurons to die in regions of the brain that control muscle movement, learning, memory and concentration.[2]

BURNS

Burns are categorized by the degree of thickness of the burn. A first or second degree burn leaves the epidermal layer intact, whereas with a third degree burn, otherwise known as a full-thickness burn, the entire epidermal layer is gone. The important point is that the epidermal layer does not regenerate.

Burns that blister are almost always second degree-burns; and, if a burn hurts, it is not a full-thickness burn because third degree burns destroy the nerve endings as well as the epidermus. Full-thickness burns always need immediate attention, and many require skin grafts to properly heal.

Unless extensive, non-full-thickness burns can be treated at home. The best treatment is to immediately give Traumeel drops every fifteen minutes while the child is awake; the next day you can decrease the frequency to every hour while awake.

Then, without disturbing the blisters, run the burned area under cold water until it stops burning. After that, apply aloe gel or fresh aloe juice from an aloe

plant onto the entire area and cover loosely with light gauze. (It's good to keep an aloe plant in your house for this very reason. Simply cut open a fleshy leaf, squeeze out the juice and gently apply it to the burn.) Change the gauze and reapply the aloe twice daily, keeping the blisters as intact as possible until they are completely healed. If signs of infection such as pus develop, then have your child examined by your pediatrician.

Nutritional support is important for burns. The diet should include plenty of eggs for protein, bone broths and cod liver oil. Give Amla-Plus vitamin C tablets, 4 per day, for protection against infection.

CHICKEN POX

Chicken pox is usually a simple illness which, in the vast majority of cases, resolves without repercussions and without any special treatment.

Vitamin A is helpful with all viral infections so an increase in the cod liver oil is appropriate during the illness.

Congaplex from Standard Process should be given, one to four capsules, four times per day—if swallowing is difficult, it can be mixed with foods like apple sauce or yogurt.

For topical itching, baking soda baths can be helpful, after which apply a paste made of baking soda to the skin. Chickweed gel or Dermarash cream from Dr. Kang Pharmacy can also help control itching and scratching.

COLIC

See Chapter 7 for a discussion of colic in infants. When baby squirms, cries or seems in distress on eating, the condition is referred to as colic. The first remedy is to hold baby upright against your shoulder and burp him after each feeding.

Gentle rubbing of baby's stomach may ease her pain. Rub gently from the lower right hand side of the abdomen up to the bottom of the rib cage, then across to the left and down, in the direction of the colon; or, put baby on your shoulder and rub her back.

Warm baths can sometimes stop a colicky episode.

Remedies include a homeopathic compound called Colic Calm Gripe Water, used according to directions. Warm chamomile oil compresses on the abdomen will often help with the acute gas and pain (see Appendix I). (Essential oils should never be given internally.) Homeopathic chamomile or chamomile tea can also often be helpful. Catnip fennel, a thick liquid preparation of concentrated herbs in a glycerin base from Nature's Sunshine, often eases colic. It can be administered as a drop on the tongue, pacifier, bottle nipple or breast.

Be sure to avoid products containing sodium bicarbonate as this will raise the natural pH of baby's stomach acid and make digestion more difficult.

The child's abdominal area should be kept warm, and her environment should be as quiet and peaceful as possible. Breastfeeding mothers should be on guard for foods they eat, which may be triggering the episodes.

Gentle chiropractic or osteopathic adjustments often work wonders for colic.

CONCUSSION

In the strict sense of the word, a concussion refers to the loss of consciousness following a head injury. If this occurs, the child needs to be seen by a physician immediately, for a thorough evaluation.

A far more common occurrence is a head injury without loss of consciousness; this is not a concussion, although it is often referred to as such. Such a trauma has an almost uniformly good prognosis and the vast majority of these children can be treated with watchful evaluation. However, if your child vomits after a head injury, he should be seen by a physician.

The child should be given bed rest in a darkened room and kept away from television and computer screens. In fact, the child may tell you that he feels like keeping his eyes closed; this is the body's way of indicating that it shouldn't process complex visual information until the brain has had a chance to recover. For the first few days after a head injury, wake the child up every three or four hours when he is sleeping to make sure he hasn't lost consciousness.

Give Traumeel, five to twenty drops in water every hour until the child is acting normally. Double the normal dose of cod liver oil and give nourishing bone broths as often as possible.

With any head injury, parents need to watch for any unexplained change in their child's mental status. If the child begins acting in a strange manner, this is a red flag and means the child should be seen by the appropriate doctors.

CONJUNCTIVITIS

Conjunctivitis, sometimes called pink eye, refers to swelling (inflammation) or infection of the membrane lining the eyelids (conjunctiva). Symptoms include itching, redness and pain in the eyes and discharge.

Conjunctivitis usually follows a cold and calls for the same treatment for colds and flu outlined in Chapter 13.

Conjunctivitis is a known side effect of vitamin A deficiency—in many studies, vitamin A status is determined by the tendency to develop conjunctivitis. Children taking cod liver oil rarely contract conjunctivitis, but if this does happen, increase the dose until well after the condition clears.

Hot chamomile compresses for five to ten minutes over the eyes, four times per day will help relieve conjunctivitis (see Appendix I). The heat and moisture act as an antiseptic and anti-inflammatory for the eyes. Ophthacare herbal eyedrops can relieve redness and hasten recovery. For infants, put a little breastmilk into the eye.

If frank pus is exuding from the eyes, the situation calls for antibiotic eyedrops. And some schools will not let children back to school unless the condition is completely cleared or they are on antibiotic eye drops. Polytrim eye drops, available by prescription, is your best choice in these cases.

CONSTIPATION

Constipation in children should never happen; when

it does, parents often attempt to treat it by adding more "fiber" to the diet—more whole grains, vegetables and fruits.

The theory that lack of fiber causes constipation comes from the work of John Burkitt, MD, who is known for first identifying a type of lymphoma common in Africa (now called Burkitt's lymphoma) and for claiming to have identified the reason traditional Africans do not suffer from constipation or other diseases of the gastrointestinal tract.

Burkitt believed that African people ate far more fiber than Europeans, who then and now are plagued with a variety of digestive disease. However, in his original papers on fiber and diseases of the gastrointestinal tract, Burkitt includes the Maasai people as one of the groups enjoying freedom from digestive and bowel disease.

The Maasai are a traditional cattle herding people in East Africa. The irony of the Maasai, which Burkitt actually noted (and then ignored), was that the Maasai don't eat any fiber at all. They only eat meat, blood and milk—and the milk is almost always cultured into a kind of yogurt. The Maasai say that plant food is for cattle.

Most people in the medical field continue to misinterpret Burkitt's research, recommending fiber for constipation, including constipation in children. But the African diet is not so much high in fiber as high in foods that have been lacto-fermented or cultured.

By necessity, the Africans were masters of the art of culturing food. Their starchy tubers are fermented and their grains are made into sour porridges and beverages. In doing so, they feed their gastrointestinal tracts a continuous supply of what we would call probiotics or beneficial bacteria.

Since Dr. Burkitt's time we have learned that it is the beneficial bacteria that are responsible for the health of the gut wall; and sloughed off bacteria make up the bulk of the stool. The fiber serves only as food for these beneficial bacteria; in fact, consumption of a lot of rough fiber can be very irritating to the intestinal tract, especially in children, and can even lead to constipation, not to mention irritable bowel syndrome (IBS) over time.

The first and most important step in treating or preventing constipation is to feed your children a steady supply of lacto-fermented foods of various sorts, such as yogurt, kefir, sauerkraut, pickles, beet kvass and so on, starting at a very young age, and daily.

Fiber-rich foods like grains should be soaked or soured in some way and most vegetables should be either fermented or thoroughly cooked to break down the fiber.

Mucilaginous foods can also help. One to two teaspoons of flax seeds soaked overnight and added to porridge will often help a child with sluggish bowels. A product called Aloe Detox from Premier Research may also be useful. Use according to the directions on the bottle. Aloe is a gentle laxative and along with the diet almost always puts the child back on the right track.

Some parents give probiotic supplements but our experience over the years confirms the observation that children who daily eat probiotic foods have less trouble than those who just take probiotic supplements.

For treating constipation in an infant, see page 149.

CROUP

Croup, which is swelling around the vocal cords, results in breathing difficulty accompanied by a "barking" cough. It is common in infants and children and can have a variety of causes. The most important thing in dealing with croup is to make sure the illness is not a rare but serious condition called epiglottitis.

With croup, the fever is low or nonexistent, and the child is not drooling or otherwise in distress. With epiglottitis, the croupy cough is accompanied by a high fever, drooling and obvious distress—a sign to take your child to the nearest emergency room. Epiglottitis is an inflammation of the tissue that covers the trachea (windpipe). It is a life-threatening condition that can cut off breathing and lead to death. It is treated with an air tube, antibiotics and anti-inflammatories—all appropriate for this rare but serious condition.

If the condition is indeed croup, the first step is to take the child into a steamy room such as a bathroom with the shower turned on as hot as possible (but don't put the child in the shower, just in the room). After this exposure to the steam, briefly take the child (warmly dressed) out in the cold air—even brief exposure to cold air often reduces the coughing. If the outdoor temperature is warm, open the door of the freezer and have the child breathe in the cold air for a few minutes. You can hold him up in your arms if necessary.

A natural remedy for croup is the medicine *Bryonia spongia* from Uriel, three to ten drops every hour until the croup subsides.

DIAPER RASH

The cure for diaper rash is to grow out of diapers! Before that is possible, the best treatment is to change the diapers as often as possible and to wash and thoroughly dry baby's genitals and bottom during changings—a hairdryer works wonders for drying the bottom, and baby will love it.

Before putting on a new diaper, rub baby's bottom well with coconut oil or with diaper cream by Weleda. In severe cases, apply high vitamin cod liver oil to the rash and surounding area.

DIARRHEA

Rudolf Steiner once pointed out that diarrhea is like coughing, simply a way to expel what we don't need. Of course, diarrhea can be a sign of a serious problem, and children in certain situations with diarrhea can die, but even if the underlying issue is a serious infection the best approach is to keep the child well hydrated with a somewhat salty bone broth, coupled with some type of "sugar" (raw honey works well), usually in herbal tea.

Keeping the child hydrated with a fast of salty broth and tea with honey is all that is needed in the vast percentage of cases of diarrhea. Give the broth just a teaspoonful at a time at first, increasing the amount as the diarrhea subsides. If the child is still nursing, then continue to hydrate with small amounts of breastmilk as tolerated. (Meanwhile, mom should pump her milk so that her supply does not diminish.)

If there is blood in the stool then a doctor should be consulted and a stool test taken for more serious infections. Likewise, if the diarrhea continues unabated and your child becomes dehydrated, take him to the emergency room where he can receive IV hydration.

Signs of dehydration include the following: sticky or dry mouth, few or no tears when crying, eyes that look sunken into the head, lack of urine or wet diapers for six to eight hours in an infant (or only a very small amount of dark yellow urine), lack of urine for twelve hours in an older child (or only a very small amount of dark yellow urine), dry cool skin, irritability and fatigue or dizziness in an older child.

GROWING PAINS

A child who wakes up in the night complaining that his legs are throbbing is suffering from "growing pains." These generally strike during two periods: in early childhood among three- to five-year-olds and, later, in eight- to twelve-year-olds.

Conventional medicine has little to offer for growing pains, but the condition is clearly a sign that the muscles are not receiving enough nutrition to keep up with the bones. The best solution is a diet with plenty of meat, fat and organ meats; pasteurized milk products should be eliminated completely. If the child consumes raw dairy products, cut back somewhat and replace dairy calories with meat calories. Cod liver oil, which supports proper and balanced growth, is a must for this condition.

HAND, FOOT AND MOUTH DISEASE

This is a viral infection caused by the same virus that causes foot and mouth disease in cattle. Symptoms include a blistering rash on the hands and sometimes on the feet, and white lesions inside the mouth, often accompanied by a moderately high fever.

This condition is usually self-limiting, lasting three to ten days, after which the child is immune to this illness for life. Follow the treatment recommended for colds and flu in Chapter 13.

HAY FEVER

The best prevention for hay fever is the general dietary principles discussed in this book, with the more stringent GAPS diet in cases accompanied by digestive issues. Raw whole milk from a local dairy is an excellent remedy. Be sure the child consumes plenty of fat at each meal—hay fever often occurs when the blood sugar drops and adequate fat keeps blood sugar levels stable. All refined sweeteners and refined carbohydrates should be eliminated.

For acute care, use local raw honey, up to one to two tablespoons, four times per day, for naturally occurring immune factors keyed to local pollen.

Freeze dried nettles from Eclectic Institute, one to two capsules two times per day, and Phytocort from Allergy Research, three capsules two to three times per day, may provide relief. Quercetin, 500 mg three times per day, may also be helpful.

Older children can be taught the NAET allergy treatment technique, a noninvasive, chemical-free method for clearing allergic triggers (see www. NAET.com).

HIVES

The best acute care natural medicine for hives is homeopathic *Apis*, usually in the 6C or 6X potency, given every hour until the hives clear. Another natural anti-allergy medicine, Antronex from Standard Process, can be used at the dose of 1-2 tablets 4 times per day until the hives clear

In addition, liposomal vitamin C, 1000 mg every hour, along with quercetin, 500 mg, three times per day, can be helpful in clearing the hives. Plenty of water (always with a pinch of salt) should be drunk to flush out the kidneys.

In boys during puberty, hives from excess testosterone sometimes occurs. In these cases, a homeopathic remedy called Skin sometimes works well.

MEASLES

Measles, also known as morbilli, is an infectious illness of the respiratory system said to be caused by a virus. Symptoms include fever, cough, runny nose, red eyes and a generalized rash. While measles can be a serious disease in children who are undernourished, in the well nourished child, it is not life-threatening.

Contrary to the pronouncements of public health officials, vaccinated children can and do get the measles—although today measles in both vaccinated and unvaccinated children is rare.

Keep the child quiet and in bed, with the blinds closed. Follow the suggestions in Chapter 13 on infectious illness, giving echinacea by Mediherb and similar herbs for immune support and *Apis belladonna* and Meteoric Iron *Prunus* for homeopathic support, using the dosage suggestions on page 228.

The high fever of measles can rapidly deplete vitamin A. Giving cod liver oil for the duration of the illness is a must. Also, feed smoothies of egg yolks and cream, and some liver paté, for additional vitamin A. Bone broth soups are of course highly appropriate.

Be sure the child goes a full day without fever before he returns to school or other activities, to ensure that the illness is thoroughly resolved.

MENINGITIS

The symptoms of meningitis are high fever, photophobia (light intolerance), stiffness in the neck and a very distressed child. There are two types of meningitis, bacterial and viral.

With some types of bacterial meningitis there is a characteristic rash and if this occurs, as with any case of suspected bacterial meningitis, the child needs urgent treatment by the closest emergency room or qualified pediatrician.

Viral meningitis is less severe, less dangerous and, after a thorough exam by a physician, can be treated in the same way as infectious illnesses (Chapter 13) with rest, cod liver oil, *Apis belladonna* and Meteoric Iron *Prunus*, using the dosage suggestions on page 228. In addition, give *Andrographis comp.* Complex from Mediherb, one tablet four times per day.

MONONUCLEOSIS (MONO)

Mononucleosis or mono, also called the "kissing disease," is a viral infection causing fever, fatigue, sore throat and swollen lymph glands, especially in the neck. It occurs most often in those age fifteen to seventeen. However, the infection may develop at any age. Mono is usually linked to the Epstein-Barr virus (EBV), but can also be caused by other organisms such as cytomegalovirus (CMV).

Mono should be treated in much the same way as the common flu and other viral diseases (see Chapter 13). It is most important that activity be restricted until the child's energy is back to normal.

An additional remedy for mono is a product called Milk Thistle 1:1 Glycetract from Mediherb, one teaspoon, twice daily to help protect the liver, which can be affected with mono.

MUMPS

Mumps is characterized by painful swelling of the salivary glands (particularly the parotid gland). Painful testicular swelling (orchitis) and rash may also occur. The symptoms are generally not severe in children. In teenage males and in adult men, complications such as infertility or subfertility are more common, although still rare in absolute terms. Obviously it is better to get the mumps as a child, rather than as an adult. Mumps in childhood confers lifelong immunity and even conventional medicine acknowledges that the disease is generally self-limiting, running its course before receding, with no specific treatment needed apart from bed rest.

Keep the child quiet and in bed, with the blinds closed. Follow the suggestions in Chapter 13 on infectious illness, giving *Apis belladonna* and Meteoric Iron *Prunus* for homeopathic support, and echinacea for immune support, using the dosage suggestions on page 228.

Swallowing is difficult so the patient will need blended soups and smoothies until the swelling subsides.

MUSCLE CRAMPS

This is a common occurrence in active children and generally needs no particular treatment except to ensure the child has adequate mineral intake and adequate hydration. Slightly salty lacto-fermented drinks such as ginger ale and beet kvass (see Recipes) will usually alleviate most cases of muscle cramps.

For a topical treatment, arnica oil can be massaged into the affected muscle. In addition, the child can be given extra magnesium in the form of Epsom salts baths before bed.

MUSCLE STRAINS AND SPRAINS

The main natural treatment for any muscle injury or trauma is arnica, probably the most popular homeopathic remedy in the world. Arnica should be part of every family's first aid kit; it comes in many forms including as a single homeopathic oral remedy, or combined with other medicines, or as a topical cream.

One excellent formulation is Traumeel drops and ointment, which can be found at most health food stores. It consists of a mixture of arnica and other appropriate wound and trauma remedies.

With the first sign of any injury, strain or sprain, give Traumeel, five to twenty drops in water every two to four hours, and rub Traumeel ointment on the affected area.

Epsom salts baths in the evening before bed will also alleviate muscle strains and sprains.

PICKINESS

A nutrient-dense weaning diet, characterized by diversity of foods, tastes and textures, is the best defense against your child becoming a picky eater. Even so, most children will develop dislikes to certain foods. If your child refuses just a handful of foods, don't force the issue. Just put a small amount of that food on her plate when you are serving it to the rest of the family and see whether she tastes it and learns to like it over time.

Many children develop pickiness about eggs, wanting them prepared in just a certain way. They may not like runny whites, for example, or seeing congealed whites in scrambled eggs. Eggs are an important food, one that should be consumed every day, so the best strategy is to cook the eggs the way your child likes them. The important thing is ensuring that your child eats eggs frequently, not forcing her to eat eggs prepared in ways she doesn't like.

Pickiness may be a sign of zinc deficiency. A good treatment is to put a nontoxic formulation of zinc oxide cream on the skin.

One cause of pickiness is consumption of fruit juice, which can take away a child's appetite. Just say no to juice, and make sure the liquids your child is getting are nutritious ones, like raw milk, bone broths and lacto-fermented beverages.

Severe pickiness, in which the child refuses all but a few foods, mostly foods based on refined carbohydrates, is a sign of gut dysbiosis. Such tendencies often go hand in hand with behavioral difficulties and call for a careful implementation of the GAPS diet (see Appendix II).

POISON OAK, POISON IVY

The best defense against poison oak or poison ivy is prevention. Children should wear long pants and long shirtsleeves when walking through the woods.

If you think your child has come in contact with poison oak or poison ivy, have him shower and wash with Tecnu soap. This is an oily soap that you leave on for several minutes; it will help remove the toxic oils from these plants. The entire body should be covered with the soap.

Tecnu is sometimes available in grocery stores and pharmacies; if not, you can order it from the internet. You should have it on hand so that you can apply the oily soap as soon as your child emerges from the woods.

If the skin breaks out in a rash, apply chickweed gel frequently. The homeopathic remedy *Rhus toxicodendron* (which is homeopathic poison ivy) will soothe itchiness. Give six pellets every few hours, or when itchiness occurs. Additional vitamin C will also help. Give four to six tablets Alma-Plus vitamin C twice daily, or even more frequently if relief is needed.

RHEUMATIC FEVER

Rheumatic fever is the feared complication of strep throat and needs pediatric consultation for any proven case.

An interesting observation about rheumatic fever is the fact that it was a common (and feared) disease in the 1920s and 1930s in this country, and then for unexplained reasons it largely disappeared, even before the widespread introduction of penicillin for the treatment of strep throat. Why this decrease occurred has been the source of much speculation in the medical literature, with no definite answers. Suffice to say, rheumatic fever, even without the use of penicillin, is exceedingly rare.

Rheumatic fever is any infection of the connective tissue that follows a bout with strep throat or scarlet fever. If any signs of rheumatic fever following strep should occur, such as fatigue, joint pains or swellings, urine issues, rapid pulse or other heart symptoms such as shortness of breath, the child should be first given the usual course of penicillin administered by a qualified physician.

For natural remedies, give the child *Andrographis Complex* from Mediherb, one tablet four times per day, extra cod liver oil, Congaplex from Standard Process, three capsules four times per day and Cardiodoron from Weleda, for heart support, twenty drops four times per day.

High-dose vitamin C therapy should also be considered, either with 4,000-10,000 mg per day of liposomal vitamin C or even high-dose IV vitamin C therapy. This would need to be coordinated with your pediatrician and adjusted depending on the age and tolerance of the child.

RUBELLA

Rubella, also known as the German measles or three-day measles, is an infection that causes a rash on the skin. Other symptoms include muscle or joint pain, bloodshot eyes and, in rare cases, bruising.

The illness presents no danger to children; however exposure of a pregnant women who has no immunity may result in birth defects. The illness is highly infectious so an afflicted child should be kept away from pregnant women. (See discussion of rubella in pregnant women on page 69.)

Keep the child quiet and in bed. Follow the suggestions in Chapter 13 on infectious illness, giving *Apis belladonna* and Meteoric Iron *Prunus* for homeopathic support, and echinacea for immune support, using the dosage suggestions on page 228.

SCARLET FEVER

Scarlet fever is a disease caused by a toxin released by the *Streptococcus* organism. The term scarlatina indicates the less acute form of scarlet fever, which is the more common form since the beginning of the twentieth century.

Until the twentieth century, scarlet fever was frequently associated with the complications from strep infections, including glomerulonephritis (a type of kidney disease) and endocarditis leading to heart valve disease, all of which were protracted and often fatal afflictions at the time.

DENTAL ISSUES: TOOTH DECAY AND CROWDED TEETH

One of the fastest growing fields in the practice of medicine is pediatric dentistry to treat skyrocketing levels of decay in toddlers and young children; even some fully breastfed babies have all their teeth come in rotten. This happens when the family diet is high in sugars and refined carbohydrates and lacking in nutrient-dense foods; it's also common when a breastfeeding mom practices a vegetarian or vegan diet.

A diet that includes raw whole milk, cod liver oil and organ meats provides the nutritional basis for strong white teeth in children. Generally. children brought up on this diet have teeth that are very resistant to decay. However, should decay occur, it's important to look first to the diet, cutting back all refined carbohydrate foods including fruit juice and strictly limiting even properly prepared whole grains. In addition to high-vitamin cod liver oil, the child should be given high-vitamin butter oil, about one-half teaspoon per day. Dr. Price used this combination in his practice to successfully treat and even reverse tooth decay. To administer, put both the high-vitamin butter oil and the cod liver oil in a small glass or mug, add hot water and stir until the butter oil is melted; then have your child gulp it down. You can also give both individually using a syringe or eye dropper. (Set the container of butter oil in simmering water so that it becomes liquid enough.) For families struggling with tooth decay in their children, a good resource is *Heal Tooth Decay* by Rami Nagel.

Brushing teeth will not prevent tooth decay, but it will give your child a clean mouth and good breath. Use a nonfluoridated brand of toothpaste. Even the FDA has warned about the dangers of fluoride in toothpaste.[3]

Like so many other branches of medicine, dentistry provides fertile opportunities for interventions of many kinds. Be prepared to just say "no" to things like fluoride treatments (which can depress thyroid function, poison enzyme pathways and cause unsightly mottling of the teeth) and tooth sealants (which leak estrogenic plastics into the mouth). If a child does have a cavity, it should be filled with a biocompatible composite material, not mercury-leaching amalgam. It is better to remove a child's tooth than to try to save it with a root canal. To find a holistic, biological dentist who understands your objections to such conventional therapies, contact the nearest chapter of the Weston A. Price Foundation, at westonaprice.org.

The diet outlined in these pages will protect against tooth decay and also, if carried out during pre-pregnancy, pregnancy and growth, should guarantee that your child will have naturally straight teeth and not need braces. However, if your child does have a narrow palate and crowded teeth, the best treatment is orthodontics that widen the palate, rather than a practice that removes teeth. For orthodontists who use palate-widening protocols, contact the American Academy of Gnathologic Orthopedics (www.aago.com) or the American Association for Functional Orthodontics (www.aafo.org). Palate widening should ideally take place when the child has his four front permanent teeth, around the age of eight or nine.

Scarlet fever or scarlatina is characterized by sore throat, fever, a bright red tongue with a "strawberry" appearance and a characteristic rash that is fine, red and rough-textured. The rash, which blanches upon pressure, usually appears twelve to seventy-two hours after the fever. It generally starts on the chest, armpits and behind the ears. It may also involve the groin.

As with other infectious illnesses, keep the child quiet and in bed. Follow the suggestions in Chapter 13 on infectious illness, giving *Apis belladonna* and Meteoric Iron *Prunus* for homeopathic support, and echinacea for immune support, using the dosage suggestions on page 228.

SCRAPES, CUTS AND BRUISES

The primary issue with scrapes, cuts and bruises is to determine whether the child needs sutures (stitches) or whether the injury will heal on its own. While this judgment call is most often made by an experienced physician, you can determine the need for sutures yourself by pulling the wound apart. If the cut is more than one-half inch deep, it will require stitches.

If the cut is more shallow or the abrasions not too deep, they can be treated at home. Carefully clean out any debris with running tepid water. Then bathe the wound in a solution of a few tablespoons of calendula tincture. Apply either calendula ointment or raw honey, both of which have antimicrobial properties. Then wrap the wound in gauze and fasten securely with surgical tape. Change the dressing daily.

The child should be given Traumeel drops, which contain arnica and other homeopathic remedies for wounds and injuries. The dose is five to twenty drops in water four times per day until the injury is healed.

SLAPPED CHEEK SYNROME

Slapped cheek syndrome is a fairly common infectious viral illness characterized by bright red cheeks. Occasionally the rash will extend over the bridge of the nose or around the mouth. In addition to red cheeks, children often develop a red, lacy rash on the rest of the body, with the upper arms and legs being the most common locations.

The rash typically lasts a couple of days and may itch; some cases have been known to last for several weeks. Patients are usually no longer infectious once the rash has appeared.

Teenagers and adults may present with a self-limiting arthritis, manifesting in painful swelling of the joints that feels similar to arthritis. Older children and adults with the disease may have difficulty in walking and in bending joints such as wrists, knees, ankles, fingers, and shoulders.

As with other infectious illnesses, keep the child quiet and in bed. Follow the suggestions in Chapter 13 on infectious illness, giving *Apis belladonna* and Meteoric Iron *Prunus* for homeopathic support, and echinacea for immune support, using the dosage suggestions on page 228. Itchy spots may be treated with chickweed gel.

Cod liver oil and nourishing bone broths will help protect against the arthritis-like side effects.

STREP THROAT

Whether or not to use penicillin for routine cases of strep throat is one of the most difficult decisions parents have to make. On the one hand, the complication of strep—rheumatic fever—is dangerous but rare. On the other hand, studies have shown that children recover from strep at the same rate whether or not they are given penicillin. Dr. Cowan has never once seen a case of rheumatic fever in his practice in spite of not giving antibiotics to hundreds of children with strep throat.

For natural remedies, treat as with rheumatic fever. Give the child *Andrographis Complex* from Mediherb, one tablet four times per day, extra cod liver oil, Congaplex from Standard Process, three capsules four times per day and Cardiodoron from Weleda, for heart support, twenty drops four times per day.

In serious cases, high dose vitamin C therapy should also be considered, either with 4,000-10,000 mg per day of liposomal vitamin C or even high dose IV vitamin C therapy. This would need to be coordinated with your pediatrician and adjusted depending on the age and tolerance of the child.

With these treatments, penicillin should not be necessary; however if the child doesn't improve in a reasonable period of time, use of penicillin is an option. It is important to note that according to school authorities, a child with strep throat who does not take penicillin must be held out from school for a full three weeks, from the onset of infection until the point when the child is not contagious.

SUNBURN

While sunlight is good for children, it is important to avoid sunburn. As summer approaches, build up exposure slowly, starting with ten minutes in the sun, and gradually increasing to thirty minutes.

Coconut oil applied topically will keep the skin moist and, according to some reports, may even encourage a tan and prevent burning. These precautions should give your child a protective tan before the hot summer months arrive.

For children who burn very easily, and for all children who are going to be in the bright sunlight for a long period of time (as on a visit to the beach), the best protection is a tee-shirt and a hat. Badger Balm natural zinc oxide sunscreen can be applied to vulnerable areas such as the cheeks and the nose.

Many have reported that the tendency to burn is lessened with a diet containing liberal amounts of saturated fat and very limited intake of polyunsaturated oils. Plentiful dietary vitamin D also seems to have this property, allowing more sun exposure before burning occurs.

If a burn should occur then aloe gel is a time honored remedy to help with healing and pain. You can use the fresh gel from leaves or one of the many aloe skin products, which should be refrigerated. The Weleda product Combudoron is also soothing for sunburns and should be in every refrigerator for this use. Apply liberally at first signs of any pain or burning.

Coconut oil is also a good topical treatment, often taking the red out overnight. In addition, for a bad sunburn, take Amla-Plus vitamin C from Radiant Life, two tablets, two times per day.

TEETHING PROBLEMS

The teeth are the hardest, most mineralized tissue of our bodies; for this reason, the process of the teeth "erupting" is often accompanied by an inflammatory process. The gums get inflamed, and this allows them to soften so the hard teeth can come through. Sometimes the inflammation of the gums expands to other tissues, such as the nose, ears, throat and lungs. This is why children sometimes get sick while they are teething. Such distress is normal and usually harmless.

When inflammation and distress are present, follow the suggestions in Chapter 13 on infectious illness, giving *Apis belladonna* and Meteoric Iron *Prunus* for homeopathic support, and echinacea for immune support, using the dosage suggestions on page 228.

For symptomatic relief of tooth or gum discomfort you can use Hyland's teething tablets; another remedy is to wrap a few frozen berries in a cheesecloth, fastened with a rubberband or twist tie, and let the child suck on these to numb her gums.

THRUSH

Thrush is an infection of the mouth caused by the candida fungus. Thrush can affect anyone, though it occurs most often in babies and toddlers, older adults and people with weakened immune systems.

If thrush occurs in a breastfed baby, the mother should dramatically decrease or eliminate her carbohydrate and sugar intake, and increase her probiotic and coconut oil intake to a high level. In most cases, this will be enough to eliminate the thrush from the infant.

For babies on our raw milk formula, increase the amount of cream in the formula and decrease lactose slightly. Be sure you are adding the probiotic powder to the formula. If baby is on solid food, increase the level of fats in the diet, add more coconut oil and limit carbohydrates until the condition clears.

A natural treatment for thrush is to rub plain yogurt or a good probiotic mixture like Biokult in baby's mouth to eliminate the infection. If this does not work, a few days of oral Nystatin may be needed, always given under a physician's supervision.

VOMITING/FOOD POISONING

Like diarrhea, vomiting is the body's way of eliminating something that is a poison. The strategy with vomiting is different from that of diarrhea; with diarrhea you want to give as much salty fluid as possible, but if your child is vomiting, then anything that comes into the stomach may produce more vomiting, which can become a vicious cycle leading to dehydration.

With vomiting, therefore, you need to keep the stomach contents below the level that will provoke vomiting. This often will mean feeding your child a teaspoon or a dropper full of fluid (tea, broth or even water) every five to thirty minutes, because to feed more rapidly will often provoke more vomiting. If vomiting persists, wait an hour and then try again. Sometimes it is helpful for the child to suck on ice chips.

So, give a dropperful, wait, and if no vomiting occurs, repeat in a few minutes. Resist the temptation to go more quickly. As the situation improves, you can decrease the interval, always making sure the vomiting doesn't return. With this technique, you can usually keep the child well hydrated and allow the infection to clear from the system.

If you know that your child is vomiting because he has swallowed something poisonous, call the poison hotline immediately. The number is 1-800-222-1222.

WHOOPING COUGH (PERTUSSIS)

This is a serious illness in children, which has been discussed in Chapter 14 of this book. In conventional medical practice, whooping cough is treated with a ten-day course of the antibiotic Erythromycin, but this is rarely needed. Dr. Cowan has treated hundreds of cases of whooping cough without antibiotics and without any serious repercussions or compromised outcomes.

The basic holistic treatment uses *Drosera Complex* from Uriel Pharmacy, three to ten drops in water alternating every two hours with *Cuprum aceticum Complex,* three to ten drops in water during the waking hours. The dosage is three drops for children age three and under, four drops for children age four and so on until ten drops for children ten and older.

Amla-Plus vitamin C can be given as well, up to four tablets twice daily, as well as *Andrographis Complex* from Mediherb, one tablet four times per day, until all the symptoms are gone.

Plaintain Spruce cough syrup from Uriel Pharmacy should be given, one tablespoon every four hours.

For a topical chest treatment, Plantain Beeswax Cough Relief Ointment from Uriel Pharmacy should be rubbed on the child's chest and back two or three times per day.

The child must be kept at a low activity level, mostly in bed during the day, even if he seems to be relatively well, as the bulk of the symptoms occur at night.

The diet should be light, mostly soup and vegetables with some coconut oil and yogurt, and butter for fats.

If pneumonia or bronchitis is threatening, give Bronchafect, 1 teaspoon 4 times per day.

Whooping cough can be a long and serious illness that taxes the reserves of any parent; it is especially frightening at night and calls upon all the spiritual reserves of the parents to continue to provide a healing space for their child. Your child really needs your strength, calm and awareness at this time. The help of a trusted physician with experience with whooping cough can be an invaluable help in this situation.

Appendix 1
Therapy Instructions

COMPRESSES

Compresses are an effective traditional treatment for a variety of conditions; they have fallen out of favor because they are time consuming and sometimes messy to administer—so much quicker to give a pill, especially in the hospital setting!

The best cloth to use is a plain white washcloth. You can also use a linen kitchen towel, folded to washcloth size, or even a piece of old diaper.

MUSTARD COMPRESS

It's best to use fresh, organic mustard seeds that you have ground yourself with a coffee grinder. Second choice would be organic ground American mustard powder, sold in the spice section of your health food store or grocery store. (British mustard powder tends to be too strong.)

Mix about one-third cup ground mustard seed with water to make a paste.

Before applying the compress to your child, it is imperative that you try it on yourself, to make sure the paste is not so hot that it will burn. We have seen blistering burns from mustard compresses. So first, put a little of the mustard paste on the inside of your wrist and leave it there for five minutes. If if burns

and blisters, add a little unbleached white flour (plus more water) to mitigate the effects of the mustard.

Once you have tested the mustard paste on yourself, apply the paste to a thin cloth, then place this over the area of the chest that has the congestion, either in front or back, with the cloth next to the skin. Cover this with a towel wrapped snugly around the chest, then wrap the child in a blanket and put him into bed. You can leave this on for two to twenty minutes depending on how hot the mustard is. The area should become slightly red but by no means burned.

After applying the compress, wash the mustard off. Then keep the child warm and covered, giving lots of sweating liquids, like elder flower tea, hot broth or hot lemon juice with honey.

CHAMOMILE COMPRESS

Make a strong chamomile tea and let it cool slightly. Dip the cloth in the tea and wring out slightly. Apply to the affected area, then cover with a towel. Leave ten to twenty minutes.

For the eyes, steep two chamomile tea bags, let cool and wring out slightly. Apply the tea bags directly to the eyes, about five minutes at a time.

ONION COMPRESS

Onions help move fluid, which is why they make us cry when they are cut open. This fluid movement is helpful in ear infections when there is a tendency for the fluid to get "stuck" in the ear.

Use an organic onion at room temperature. Cut the onion in half along its diameter, then cut two slices, one from each half. Wrap each slice of onion in gauze or cheese cloth. Apply the onion slices directly to the ears. Secure the slices by wrapping gauze or cheese cloth around the child's head and then cover the head and ears with a woolen cap.

The onion compress should be kept on as long as possible, preferably overnight. This can be a very quick and effective remedy for eliminating ear aches.

INHALATION THERAPY

Steam inhalations are mainly used for sinus and respiratory congestion.

Place a drop of essential oil (usually eucalyptus oil) or loose tea (such as chamomile flowers) in a pot of steaming water. Then carefully place your child's head over the pot, at a distance where he can breathe in the steam and still be comfortable. Great care must be taken not to burn. Drape a towel over his head. Have him slowly inhale the steam into his lungs or sinus passages.

Five to twenty minutes per session are usually enough to loosen most congestion.

BIOKULT THERAPY

An important component of the diet is the Biokult probiotic. This formulation was devised by Dr. Campbell-McBride to support gradual recolonization of the gut with beneficial bacteria. Biokult needs to be introduced gradually, otherwise it might provoke strong die-off reactions.

Start with one Biokult capsule (see Sources) per day taken in the morning before food, with a glass of warm water. If your child is very young and can't swallow pills or capsules, open the capsule and mix with water.

After three to five days, if no abnormal symptoms occur, such as nausea or diarrhea, take one capsule twice per day (the second capsule in the evening), again with warm water.

After another three to five days, if no abnormal symptoms occur, increase to two capsules in the morning and one in the evening; then after three to five days, increase to two in the morning and two in the evening.

If your child experiences nausea or diarrhea, wait three to five days after this has cleared before increasing the dose.

Continue increasing in this manner, every three to five days until reaching a maximum of four tablets in the morning and four in the evening. Continue at the maximum dose for one month and then reassess the situation. If your child has achieved the health benefits you are seeking, you can gradually reduce the dose.

Appendix II
The GAPS Diet Protocol

The Gut and Psychology Syndrome (GAPS) diet was devised by U.K. physician Dr. Natasha Campbell-McBride and described in her book *Gut and Psychology Syndrome*. It is meant to be a temporary diet that restricts sugars and starches—all disaccharides—to allow your child's intestinal tract to heal.

The diet is rich in animal foods and animal fats, and bone broths are an essential component of the protocol, as they provide healing factors to the gut. In the early stages, use "meat stocks," that is bone broths made with meaty bones and cooked only a couple of hours. As the gut heals, the patient can make the transition to long-simmered bone broths.

It is strongly recommended that patients follow the steps in the Introduction Diet, which has been designed for people with serious digestive problems and food intolerances and the behavioral disorders that often accompany these digestive problems. Once he has accomplished the steps in the Introduction Diet, your child can progress into the full GAPS diet.

In general, those who start with the Introduction Diet will be able to introduce allowed dairy foods earlier than those who go right into the full GAPS diet. Always do a sensitivity test prior to introducing the various dairy foods.

SENSITIVITY TEST

For any food to which your child might be sensitive, it is important to do a sensitivity test with that food.

Do the test at bedtime. Take a drop of the food in question (if the food is solid, mash and mix with a bit of water) and place it on the inside of your child's wrist. Let the drop dry on the skin (you can cover it with a bandaid), then let your child go to sleep.

In the morning check the spot: if there is an angry red reaction, avoid that food for a few weeks, and then try the sensitivity test again. If there is no reaction, then go ahead and introduce the food gradually, starting with a small amount.

BIOKULT THERAPY

An important component of the diet is the Biokult probiotic. This probiotic was formulated by Dr. Campbell-McBride to support gradual recolonization of the gut with specific types of beneficial bacteria. Biokult needs to be introduced gradually, otherwise it might provoke a strong die-off reaction.

Start with one Biokult capsule (see Sources) per day taken in the morning before food, with a glass of warm mineral water. If your child is very young and can't swallow pills, open the capsule and mix with water.

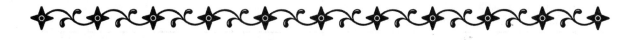

After three to five days, if no abnormal symptoms are occurring, such as nausea or diarrhea, take one capsule twice per day (the second capsule in the evening), again with warm water.

After after three to five days, if no abnormal symptoms are occurring, increase to two capsules in the morning and one in the evening; then after three to five days, increase to two in the morning and two in the evening.

If your child experiences nausea or diarrhea, wait three to five days after this has cleared before increasing the dose.

Continue increasing in this manner, every three to five days until reaching a maximum of four tablets in the morning and four in the evening. Continue at the maximum dose for one month and then reassess the situation. If your child has achieved the health benefits you are seeking, you can gradually reduce the dose.

When your child makes the transition back to a normal diet, he can discontinue the Biokult; however, this probiotic should be replaced with lacto-fermented foods, consumed on a daily basis, as a habit for life.

INTRODUCTION DIET

Depending on the severity of your child's condition he can move through this program as fast or as slowly as his progress permits. For example, you may move through Stage One in one or two days and then spend longer on Stage Two.

Following the Introduction Diet fully is essential for those suffering from diarrhea or severe constipation: it reduces symptoms quickly and speeds up the healing process in the digestive system. Even for healthy children, if you or your child gets a "tummy bug" or any other profuse diarrhea, following the Introduction Diet for a few days will clear the symptoms quickly and permanently without medication.

Those without severe digestive problems can move through the Introduction Diet quite quickly. However, do not be tempted to skip the Introduction Diet and go straight into the full GAPS Diet, because the Introduction Diet will give your child the best chance to optimize the healing process in the gut and the rest of the body.

Dr. Campbell-McBride sees many cases where skipping the Introduction Diet leads to long-term, lingering problems that are difficult to heal.

GAPS RESOURCES

Recommended books:
- *Gut and Psychology Syndrome* by Natasha Campbell-McBride
- *Breaking the Vicious Cycle* by Elaine Gottschall
- *Eat Well Feel Well* by Kendall Conrad
- *Grain-Free Gourmet* by Jodi Bager and Jenny Lass
- *Nourishing Traditions* by Sally Fallon

Yahoo groups for support, ideas and recipes:
- health.groups.yahoo.com/group/GAPSdiet/
- health.dir.groups.yahoo.com/group/healing-leakygut/
- health.groups.yahoo.com/group/gapsdiet-sf/ (for San Francisco bay area)
- health.groups.yahoo.com/group/FourfoldPatientForum/ (for Dr. Cowan's patients)

Websites:
- gaps.me
- GapsDiet.com
- gapsguide.wordpress.com
- Scdiet.com
- PecanBread.com
- BreakingTheViciousCycle.info
- Uclbs.org
- celticseasalt.com, 800-687-7258
- breakingtheviciouscycle.info
- www.nutrivene.com for Biokult, 800-899-3413

Only foods listed are allowed: your child should not have anything else. In Stage One, the most drastic symptoms of abdominal pain, diarrhea and constipation will quickly subside. If, when you introduce a new food, the diarrhea or any other digestive symptoms return, you will know that your child is not yet ready for the introduction of that food. Wait for a week and try again.

Always wait for bowel movements to normalize before moving to the next stage of the diet, and always be on the alert for food sensitivities.

If you suspect an allergy to any particular food, before introducing it, do the Sensitivity Test (page 277).

EVERY MORNING

Start the day with a cup of still mineral water or filtered water, taken with the Biokult probiotic. Make sure that the water is warm or room temperature, not cold, as cold will aggravate your child's condition.

STAGE ONE

First and foremost, introduce homemade chicken, beef or fish stock (see Recipes). In the early stages, these stocks should be cooked only for a couple of hours. Meat and fish stocks provide building blocks for the rapidly growing cells of the gut lining and they have a soothing effect on any areas of inflammation in the gut. That is why they aid digestion and have been known for centuries as healing folk remedies for the digestive tract.

Do not use commercially available soup stock granules or bouillon cubes; they are highly processed and full of detrimental ingredients such as MSG. Do not use canned or dehydrated soups, which are loaded with MSG. The key to this protocol is homemade meat stocks and bone broths, and soups made from these stocks and broths.

Chicken stock is particularly gentle on the stomach and a good choice to start with.

It is essential to use bones and joints when making your stock, as they provide the healing substances. Marrow bones should always be included when making beef stock. It is very important for your child to consume all the fat that comes off the bones and skin, as these fats are essential for the healing process. Keep giving your child warm meat stock as a drink all day, with his meals and between meals.

By the way, do not use a microwave oven for warming up the stock—microwaves destroy food. Instead use a conventional stove.

The second component in Stage One is homemade soup made with homemade meat or fish stock (see Recipes). The simplest soup is one in which a variety of any of the allowed vegetables, finely chopped, is added to the stock, along with any finely chopped meat from the bones. You can also add a little finely chopped cooked liver.

All particularly fibrous parts of vegetables need to be removed, such as skin and seeds of zucchini and squashes, stalks of broccoli and cauliflower, and any other parts that look too fibrous. Cook in the broth until the vegetables are very tender. You can serve as is, or blend all the vegetables into the soup using a handheld blender. You may add some chopped or pressed garlic. Season to taste with sea salt.

A third component is probiotic foods; it is essential to introduce these lacto-fermented foods from the beginning, starting with some sauerkraut juice or beet kvass stirred into cooled soup or stock. For Stage One, these should be made without whey (see recipes for lacto-fermented foods in Recipes).

Fermented dairy foods can be introduced at this stage if your child does not react to them in the Sensitivity Test. Homemade yogurt, kefir or buttermilk, made with whole raw milk, can be eaten plain or with a little raw honey, or stirred into cooled stock or soup. To avoid any adverse reactions, introduce these probiotic foods gradually, starting from one to two teaspoons a day for two to five days, then three to four teaspoons a day for two to five days and so on until you can add a few teaspoons of the probiotic food at every meal.

Finally, for Stage One, give ginger tea with a little honey between meals (see Recipes).

STAGE TWO

Continue with Stage One, giving bone broth soups containing vegetables, meat, marrow and small amounts of chopped liver.

You should continue with the probiotic foods, gradually increasing the amount; you can now add lacto-fermented vegetables such as sauerkraut, pickled beets or pickled turnips (made without whey) to the stocks and soups. Continue also with the probiotic dairy foods and the ginger tea.

In Stage Two we add raw organic egg yolks, preferably to every bowl of soup and every cup of meat stock. Start with one egg yolk a day and gradually increase until your child has an egg yolk with every bowl of soup.

When egg yolks are well tolerated add soft-boiled eggs to the soups (the whites cooked and the yolks still runny). If you have any concerns about egg allergy, do the sensitivity test first. There is no need to limit number of egg yolks per day, as they absorb quickly, are easy to digest and will provide your child with wonderful and most needed nutrition. Get your eggs from a source you trust: fresh, free-range and preferably soy-free.

Add stews and casseroles made with meats and vegetables. Avoid spices at this stage; just make the stew with salt and fresh herbs. A good choice is the Italian Casserole (see Recipes). The fat content of these meals must be quite high: the more fresh animal fats your child consumes, the more quickly he will recover. Add some probiotic foods to every serving, or serve them on the side.

If tolerated, increase the daily amount of homemade yogurt, kefir or buttermilk. If your child cannot yet tolerate these foods, increase the probiotic vegetables. You can continue adding sauerkraut juice and beet kvass to cooled stock and soup.

In Stage Two, you can also introduce lacto-fermented (marinated) fish (see Recipes), starting from one piece per day and gradually increasing.

Introduce ghee starting from one teaspoon per day and gradually increasing the amount. Ghee can be stirred into soups and stews. You can make your own ghee from good quality butter (see Recipes) or purchase it from a recommended source (see Sources).

STAGE THREE

Carry on with all the previous foods.

Add ripe avocado starting from one to three teaspoons and gradually increasing the amount. Avocado can be eaten plain with a little salt or added to soups.

GAPS-friendly pancakes can be added at this time (see Recipes). These pancakes are made with three ingredients: organic nut butter (almond, walnut, peanut, etc.), eggs and a piece of fresh winter squash or zucchini, peeled, de-seeded and well blended in a food processor. Fry small thin pancakes in ghee, goose fat or duck fat. Make sure not to burn them.

Eggs can be served scrambled in plenty of ghee, goose fat or duck fat. Serve them with avocado (if well tolerated) and cooked vegetables.

Cooked onion is particularly good for the digestive system and the immune system. Onion can be cooked well in duck fat or ghee.

Continue with the probiotic foods, about 1-2 tablespoons of sauerkraut or fermented vegetables with every meal, as well as fermented dairy foods as tolerated.

STAGE FOUR

Carry on with all previous foods. Stocks can be simmered longer.

Gradually add meats cooked by roasting and grilling (but not barbecued or fried). Avoid bits that are burned or too brown. Let your child eat the meat with cooked vegetables and sauerkraut (or other fermented vegetables). If the meat is not fatty enough, serve it with some ghee or duck fat.

Start adding cold pressed olive oil to the meals, starting from a few drops per meal and gradually increasing the amount to 1-2 tablespoons per meal.

Your child can now be introduced to GAPS-friendly bread, made with nuts and seeds ground into a flour (see Recipes). Start with a small piece of bread per day and gradually increase the amount. Bread should be spread with a liberal amount of ghee.

STAGE FIVE

If all the previous foods are well tolerated you can add cooked apple as an apple purée (see Recipes).

Add raw vegetables, using softer parts of lettuce and peeled cucumber. They can be served with avocado; dress with olive oil and a little vinegar or lemon juice.

Watch your child's stool to see whether the raw vegetables are being digested. As with all other types of food, start with a small amount and gradually increase if well tolerated.

After those two vegetables are well tolerated gradually add other raw vegetables, such as carrots, tomatoes and onions.

STAGE SIX

If all the introduced foods are well tolerated, try some peeled raw apple. Gradually introduce raw fruit and more honey.

THE FULL GAPS DIET

BREAKFAST CHOICES
- Eggs cooked to personal liking and served with sausages or additive-free bacon and slices of tomato and avocado. Sausages should be full fat with only herbs, salt and pepper added. Make sure that there are no commercial seasonings or MSG in the sausages.
- Scrambled eggs with sautéed mushrooms.
- Meat, fish or shellfish with cooked or raw vegetables. Dress the vegetables with lemon juice and cold pressed olive oil.
- Homemade soup with GAPS-friendly bread and butter.
- Egg frittatas.
- GAPS-friendly pancakes made with ground nuts. These pancakes are delicious with some butter and honey, or as a savory snack. If you blend some fresh or defrosted berries with honey, it will make a delicious jam to have with pancakes.
- Serve breakfast with a cup of warm meat stock or bone broth as a drink.

LUNCH CHOICES
- Homemade vegetable soup or stew in a homemade meat stock or bone broth.
- Homemade liver paté or cheese on GAPS-friendly bread.
- Avocado with meat, fish, shellfish and raw and/or cooked vegetables. Dress salad with cold pressed olive oil and lemon juice. Serve a cup of warm homemade meat stock or bone broth as a drink.
- Smoked or marinated fish with cucumber salad.

DINNER CHOICES
- One of the dishes from the lunch or breakfast choices.
- Soup made from homemade meat stock or bone broth with homemade muffin and ghee.
- Stews made from homemade meat stock or bone broth.
- Sliced roast meat with cooked vegetables dressed with plenty of butter.

DESSERT CHOICES
- Fresh fruit with homemade yogurt.
- Stewed fruit with homemade cultured cream.
- Berries blended with honey.
- Homemade ice cream made with homemade cultured cream.

GUT AND PSYCHOLOGY DIET: RECOMMENDED FOODS

Almonds, almond butter and oil
Apples
Apricots, fresh or dried
Artichoke, French
Asiago cheese
Asparagus
Aubergine (eggplant)
Bananas (ripe only, with brown
    spots on the skin)
Beans, dried white (navy), string
    beans and lima
Beef, fresh or frozen
Beets or beetroot
Berries, all kinds
Black radish
Blue cheese
Bok choy
Brazil nuts
Brick cheese
Brie cheese
Broccoli
Broth (stock), homemade, made
    from bones of poultry, beef,
    lamb, pork and fish
Brussels sprouts
Butter
Buttermilk, homemade from raw
milk
Cabbage
Camembert cheese
Canned fish, in olive oil
    or water only
Capers
Carrots
Cashew nuts, fresh only
Cauliflower
Cayenne pepper
Celeriac
Celery
Cellulose in supplements
Cheddar cheese
Cherimoya (custard apple)
Cherries
Chestnuts
Chicken, fresh or frozen
Cinnamon
Citric acid
Coconut, fresh or dried
    without sweetener or additives
Coconut milk
Coconut oil
Cod liver oil
Coffee, weak and freshly made,
    not instant
Collard greens
Coriander, fresh or dried

Cream, cultured, homemade from
    raw cream
Cucumber
Dates, fresh or dried additive-free
Dill, fresh or dried
Duck, fresh or frozen
Edam cheese
Eggplant (aubergine)
Eggs, fresh
Filberts (hazelnuts)
Fish, fresh, frozen or canned in its
    juice or oil
Game, fresh or frozen
Garlic
Ghee, homemade
Ginger root, fresh
Goose fresh or frozen
Gorgonzola cheese
Gouda cheese
Grapefruit
Grapes
Havarti cheese
Hazelnuts
Herbal teas
Herbs, fresh or dried additive-free
Honey, raw
Juices freshly pressed from
    permitted fruit and vegetables
Kale
Kefir, homemade from raw milk
Kiwi fruit
Kumquats
Lamb, fresh or frozen
Lemons
Lentils
Lettuce, all kinds
Lima beans dried and fresh
Limburger cheese
Limes
Mangoes
Meats, fresh or frozen
Melons
Monterey Jack cheese
Muenster cheese
Mushrooms
Mustard, without any non-allowed
    ingredients
Nectarines
Nut flour or ground nuts
Nutmeg
Nuts, all kinds fresh, properly
    soaked and dried
Olive oil, virgin cold-pressed
Olives without any non-allowed
    ingredients
Onions
Oranges

Papayas
Parmesan cheese
Parsley
Peaches
Peanut butter, without additives
Peanuts, soaked and dried, roasted
Pears
Peas, dried split and fresh green
Pecans
Pepper, all kinds
Peppers (green, red, and orange)
Pheasant, fresh or frozen
Pickles, without sugar or any other
    non-allowed ingredients
Pigeon fresh or frozen
Pineapples, fresh
Pork, fresh or frozen
Port du Salut cheese
Poultry, fresh or frozen
Probiotic (lacto-fermented) foods
    using any allowed vegetables
Prunes, dried without any
    additives
Pumpkin
Quail, fresh or frozen
Raisins
Rhubarb
Roquefort cheese
Romano cheese
Satsumas
Shellfish, fresh or frozen
Spices, single and pure
    without any additives
Spinach
Squash (summer and winter)
Stilton cheese
Stock, homemade, made
    from bones of poultry, beef,
    lamb, pork and fish
String beans
Swiss cheese
Tangerines
Tea, weak freshly made, not instant
Tomato juice, without additives
    except salt
Tomatoes
Turkey, fresh or frozen
Turnips
Uncreamed cottage cheese
    (dry curd)
Vinegar (apple cider); if there is
    no allergy
Walnuts
Watercress
Yogurt, homemade from raw milk
Zucchini

GUT AND PSYCHOLOGY DIET: FOODS TO AVOID

Acesulphame
Acidophilus milk
Agar-agar
Agave syrup
Algae
Aloe vera
Amaranth
Apple juice
Arrowroot
Artificial sweeteners: Nutra-
   sweet, Splenda, Equal, etc.
Aspartame
Astragalus
Baked beans
Baker's yeast
Baking powder, baking soda and
   rising agents of all kinds
Balsamic vinegar
Barley
Bean flour and sprouts
Bee pollen
Beer
Bhindi or okra
Bitter gourd
Black eye peas
Bologna
Bouillon cubes or granules
Brandy
Buckwheat
Bulgur
Burdock root
Butter beans
Buttermilk
Cannellini beans
Canned vegetables and fruit
Carob
Carrageenan
Cellulose gum
Cereals, including all breakfast
   cereals
Cheeses, processed and cheese
   spreads
Chestnut flour
Chevre cheese
Chewing gum
Chickpeas
Chickory root
Chocolate
Cocoa powder

Coffee, instant and coffee
   substitutes
Cooking oils
Cordials
Corn
Cornstarch
Corn syrup
Cottage cheese
Cottonseed
Cous-cous
Cream of tartar
Cream cheese
Dextrose
Drinks, soft
Fava beans
Feta cheese
Fish, preserved, smoked,
salted,
      breaded, canned w/ sauces
Flour, made out of grains
FOS (fructooligosaccharides)
Fructose
Fruit, canned or preserved
Garbanzo beans
Gjetost cheese
Grains, all
Gruyere cheese
Ham
Hot dogs
Ice cream, commercial
Jams and jellies
Jerusalem artichoke
Ketchup, commercial
Lactose
Liqueurs
Margarines and butter
   replacements
Meats, processed, preserved,
   smoked, and salted
Millet
Milk: animal, soy, rice, canned
   coconut milk
Milk, dried
Molasses
Mozzarella cheese
Mung beans
Neufchatel cheese
Nuts, coated or commercially
   prepared

Oats
Okra
Parsnips
Pasta of any kind
Pectin
Postum
Potato, any kind, even sweet
   potato
Primost cheese
Quinoa
Rice
Ricotta
Rye
Saccharin
Sago
Sausages, commercial
Seaweed
Semolina
Sherry
Soda (soft drinks)
Sour cream, commercial
Soy
Spelt
Starch
Sugar or sucrose of any kind
Tapioca
Tea, instant
Triticale
Turkey loaf
Vegetables, canned or preserved
Wheat and wheat germ
Whey powder or liquid
Yacon syrup
Yams
Yogurt, commercial

Gradually introduce GAPS-friendly cakes and other sweet things allowed on the diet (see Recipes). Use dried fruit as a sweetener in baking.

THE FULL GAPS DIET

Now you have reached the full GAPS diet. Getting there may take more or less time, depending on your child. Watch for bowel movements to normalize before moving to the next stage of the diet and always be on the alert for food sensitivities. Make sure your child carries on with the soups and bone broths, even when moving into the full GAPS diet.

Start the day with a glass of still mineral water or filtered water with a slice of lemon. It should be room temperature or warm, according to your child's personal preference. Take your Biokult with the water.

You may add all the other GAPS-friendly foods at this time (see list on page 282), including butter, cultured cream, cheese and shellfish. Again, test for sensitivity before adding any food you think might be problematic.

Gradually you will be able to move to a normal diet that includes carbohydrate foods like potatoes and grains like wheat, rye and oats, carefully prepared and in small amounts. Carbohydrate foods like potatoes should always be served with plenty of fat like butter. Grains need to be carefully prepared by soaking in an acidic medium. All bread should be made by genuine sourdough methods and served with plenty of butter.

You may also be able to add more natural sweeteners, raw whole milk and raw cream, always testing first to ascertain sensitivities. Likewise, you may add lacto-fermented foods made with homemade whey if your child does not show a sensitivity to whey.

Of course, all vegetable oils, refined sweeteners and processed foods should never be reintroduced as they may cause a rapid regression and ruin all your hard work administering the GAPS diet.

As you see improvements with the diet, you may gradually reduce the number of Biokult capsules. Eventually, your child will get all his probiotics from probiotic foods and will not need the Biokult any longer.

Appendix III
Recipes

This section provides a short collection of recipes appropriate for your baby, for those following the GAPS diet, and for pregnancy and lactation.

Your best resource for finding good quality ingredients, including cultures for dairy products, kombucha mushrooms, caviar and good quality mayonnaise, is the Shopping Guide produced by the Weston A. Price Foundation: http://westonaprice.org/about-the-foundation/shopping-guide.

For sources of pasture-fed animal products in your area, contact the nearest local chapter of the Weston A. Price Foundation: http://westonaprice.org/local-chapters/find-local-chapter.

Recommended books for additional recipes include:

- *Nourishing Traditions: The Cookbook that Challenges Politically Correct Nutrition and the Diet Dictocrats* by Sally Fallon, with Mary G. Enig, PhD.

- *Super Nutrition for Babies: The Right Way to Feed Your Baby for Optimal Health* by Katherine Erlich, MD, and Kelly Genzlinger, CNC, CMTA.

- *Internal Bliss—GAPS Cookbook* by Natasha Campbell-McBride, MD

RECIPES FOR BABY

EGG YOLK AND LIVER

1 pasture-fed egg, preferably soy-free
pinch sea salt
1/2 teaspoon grated raw organic liver,
    frozen for 14 days

Boil egg for 3 1/2 minutes. Place in a bowl and peel off shell. Remove egg white and discard. Yolk should be soft and warm, not hot, with its enzyme content intact. Sprinkle with a pinch of salt.

Grate liver on the small holes of a grater while frozen. Allow to warm up and stir into egg yolk.

PUREED CHICKEN LIVER
Makes about 8 Servings

1 pound pastured chicken livers, preferably soy-free
2 tablespoons lard
2 tablespoons butter, softened
1/2 cup chicken stock or filtered water
about 1/2 teaspoon sea salt

Sauté chicken livers in lard until browned. Add stock or water to the pan and boil down slightly. Process until smooth in a food processor. Add softened butter and sea salt to taste. Process until smooth. If too thick, add a little more stock or water. The "paté" should be the consistency of thick cream.

Distribute among 8 small ramekins. Cover each with plastic wrap. Refrigerate those you will use within a few days and freeze the rest. Before serving, heat by placing in a pan of simmering water.

CUSTARD FOR BABY
Makes 6 Servings

1 cup whole raw milk
1 cup heavy cream, not ultrapasteurized
1/4 cup honey or Rapadura
5 egg yolks
1 teaspoon vanilla extract

Warm milk and cream gently over a low flame. Meanwhile, beat Rapadura or honey with egg yolks. Slowly add milk and cream mixture to eggs, beating constantly. Blend in vanilla and pour into individual buttered ramekins or custard cups. Place in a pan of hot water and bake at 325 degrees for about 1 hour, or until a knife inserted into the custard comes out clean. Chill well.

SWEET POTATO CUSTARD FOR BABY
Makes 8 Servings

1 cup whole raw milk
1 cup heavy cream, not ultrapasteurized
1/4 cup honey or Rapadura
5 egg yolks
1/2 cup cooked sweet potato, mashed
1/4 teaspoon nutmeg
1/4 teaspoon cinnamon

Warm milk and cream gently over a low flame. Meanwhile, beat Rapadura or honey with egg yolks. Slowly add milk and cream mixture to eggs, beating constantly. Blend in sweet potato and spices and pour into individual buttered ramekins or custard cups. Place in a pan of hot water and bake at 325 degrees for about 1 hour, or until a knife inserted into the custard comes out clean. Chill well.

BONE MARROW CUSTARD FOR BABY
Makes 8 Servings

2 1/2 pounds beef marrow bones
    (or 1/3 cup beef marrow)
1 cup whole raw milk

4 pastured eggs or 8 yolks, preferably soy-free
1 tablespoon vanilla
3 tablespoons raw honey
1/2 teaspoon sea salt

Boil beef bones for about 10 minutes. Remove to a large bowl and allow to drain. In a medium bowl, whisk milk, eggs or egg yolks, vanilla, honey and salt.

Once marrow bones have cooled, scoop out the marrow into a small bowl. (Save the oil that has drained for use in other dishes.) Add the marrow to the custard mixture and blend with a handheld blender.

Distribute into 8 small buttered ramekins. Place in a pan containing hot water and bake at 350 degrees for 30 minutes or until set. Chill well.

BRAINS FOR BABY
Makes about 8 servings

1 set of brains (lamb, veal or beef)
1 1/2 cups sweet vegetables (parsnip, sweet potato
    and/or winter squash), roughly cut into
    1-inch cubes
stock or water for cooking
sea salt
1 egg yolk (optional)

If you can obtain brains from lamb, veal or beef, by all means prepare them for your baby. They are a wonderful food, full of nutrients, including cholesterol.

Soak brains in cold salted water (roughly 1 teaspoon per cup) for a minimum of 1 hour, or up to 24 hours, changing the water a few times.

Chop brains into 1-inch cubes. Place the brains and vegetables in a small saucepan with just enough stock or water to cover. Simmer on a gentle heat until the vegetables are soft. Remove from heat and purée with a handheld blender or food processor. Season to taste with sea salt. For added nutrition, stir through one raw egg yolk which will gently cook in the warm mixture. Distribute to individual custard cups or ramekins and cover with plastic wrap. Refrigerate or freeze for later use. To warm or thaw, set the custard cup or ramekin in simmering water.

VEGETABLE PUREE FOR BABY
Makes 4-6 servings

2 cups vegetables, such as zucchini, sweet potato
*   or carrot, roughly chopped into 1-inch pieces*
chicken or beef stock, or water
2-3 teaspoons coconut oil
2-3 egg yolks
1/2 teaspoon dulse seaweed flakes (optional)

Place the vegetables in a small saucepan and add enough stock or water to cover. Bring the liquid to a boil and simmer, with the lid on, until vegetables are soft. Remove from heat. Season to taste. If you are using dulse flakes, add them at this point. Purée using a food processor or handheld blender to reach desired consistency. Place individual servings into very clean ramekins, cover with plastic wrap and refrigerate or freeze.

To serve, heat ramekin in a bowl of hot water and add 1 egg yolk and about 1/2 teaspoon coconut oil. Mix well to make a smooth paste. The egg will gently cook and the oil should amalgamate into the mixture. Serve immediately.

CEREAL GRUEL FOR BABY
Makes 2 cups

1/2 cup freshly ground organic flour of spelt,
*   kamut, rye, barley or oats*
2 cups warm filtered water plus 2 tablespoons whey,
*   yogurt, kefir or buttermilk*
1/4 teaspoon sea salt

Mix flour with water mixture, cover and leave at room temperature for 12 to 24 hours. Bring to a boil, stirring frequently. Add salt, reduce heat and simmer, stirring occasionally, about 10 minutes. Let cool slightly and serve with cream or butter and a small amount of a natural sweetener, such as raw honey.

Note: Do not give cereals or raw honey to infants before the age of one year.

DIGESTIVE TEA FOR BABIES

about 2 cups fresh anise leaves
about 2 cups fresh mint leaves
2 quarts filtered water

This is a folk remedy for treating constipation and intestinal gas in infants.

Bring water to a boil and pour over the herbs. Let steep until water cools. Strain. Give tepid tea to baby, about 4 ounces at a time.

STOCKS (BROTHS)

CHICKEN STOCK (BROTH)
Makes 4 quarts

1 whole free-range chicken or
*   4-5 pounds bony chicken parts,*
*   such as necks, backs, breastbones and wings*
*   or the carcass of a cooked chicken*
Feet and heads from 2 chickens (optional)
cold filtered water
1/4 cup vinegar
1 large onion, peeled and coarsely chopped
2 carrots, peeled and coarsely chopped
3 celery sticks, coarsely chopped
1 bunch parsley

You can use either a whole chicken in this recipe, or chicken bones, either raw bones or bones from chicken that has already been cooked. In fact, you should never throw away chicken bones, but save them in a zip-lock bag in the freezer until you have 4-5 pounds, enough to make stock.

If you are making stock from bones, you will get lots of components of bones and joints in your stock; there is less exposure to the bones and joints when you make stock from a whole chicken, but the stock will contain lots of components of the skin, which are equally nutritious.

Place the whole chicken or chicken bones in a pot and add enough water to just cover. Add the vinegar, onion, carrots and celery. Bring to a boil, and remove scum that rises to the top. Reduce heat, cover, and simmer for 2 to 24 hours. (Use the shorter time for the early stages of the GAPS diet.) The longer you cook the stock, the richer and more flavorful it will be. About 10 minutes before finishing the stock, add the parsley.

Remove whole chicken or bones with a slotted spoon. If you are using a whole chicken, let cool and remove chicken meat and skin from the carcass. Reserve for other uses, such as chicken salads, enchiladas, sandwiches or curries. If you are making stock from the bones, remove the small amount of meat adhering to the bones. This can be cut up finely and added to soups.

Strain the stock into a large Pyrex measuring pitcher. Cool down in the refrigerator. If you want a clear stock, remove the fat that congeals on the top with a spoon, but it can be left in the stock, especially for the GAPS diet. The stock may be frozen in glass jars (filled about three quarters full) or plastic containers.

Use chicken stock for soups, sauces and gravies, or consume as is, with a little salt added, in a mug.

This recipe has many variations. You can use this method to make stock with turkey parts or a duck carcass. You can also make the stock in a slow cooker.

BEEF STOCK (BROTH)
Makes about 4 quarts

about 4 pounds beef marrow and knuckle bones
3 pounds meaty rib or neck bones
cold filtered water
1/2 cup vinegar
3 onions, peeled and coarsely chopped
3 carrots, peeled and coarsely chopped
3 celery sticks, coarsely chopped
several sprigs of fresh thyme, tied together
1 teaspoon dried green peppercorns, crushed
l bunch parsley

Place the knuckle and marrow bones in a very large pot with vinegar and cover with water. Let stand for one hour. Meanwhile, place the meaty bones in a roasting pan and brown at 350 degrees in the oven. When well browned, add to the pot along with the vegetables. Pour the fat out of the roasting pan, add cold water to the pan, set over a high flame and bring to a boil, stirring with a wooden spoon to loosen up coagulated juices. Add this liquid to the pot. Add additional water, if necessary, to just cover the bones.

Bring to a boil. A large amount of scum may come to the top, and it is important to remove this with a spoon. After you have skimmed, reduce heat and add

the thyme and crushed peppercorns.

For meat stock (for the early stages of the GAPS diet), simmer about 2-4 hours. For a rich bone broth, simmer for at least 12 and as long as 72 hours. Just before finishing, add the parsley and simmer another 10 minutes.

Remove bones with tongs or a slotted spoon. Strain the stock into a large bowl or pot. Let cool in the refrigerator. If you want a clear stock, remove the fat that congeals on the top with a large spoon, but it can be left in the stock, especially for the GAPS diet. The stock may be frozen in glass jars (filled about three quarters full) or plastic containers.

Use beef stock for soups, sauces and gravies. As with chicken stock, beef stock may be made in a slow cooker. You can use lamb bones, goat bones, pork bones or any combination. The stock may also be made in a slow cooker.

FISH STOCK (BROTH)
Makes about 3 quarts

3 or 4 whole carcasses, including heads, of
   non-oily fish such as sole, turbot,
      rockfish or snapper
2 tablespoons butter
2 onions, peeled and coarsely chopped
1 carrot, peeled and coarsely chopped
several sprigs fresh thyme
several sprigs parsley
1 bay leaf
1/2 cup dry white wine or vermouth
about 3 quarts cold filtered water

Melt butter in a large stainless steel pot. Add the vegetables and cook very gently, about 1/2 hour, until they are soft. Add wine and bring to a boil. Add the fish carcasses and cover with cold, filtered water. Bring to a boil and skim off the scum that comes to the top. Tie herbs together and add to the pot. Reduce heat, cover and simmer for at least 2 hours or as long as 24 hours. (Cook only about 2 hours for the early stages of the GAPS diet.) Remove carcasses with tongs or a slotted spoon and strain the liquid a large Pyrex measuring pitcher. Chill well in the refrigerator and remove any congealed fat. The stock may be frozen for long-term storage.

Pick off any flesh from the carcass and especially the head—the meat of the head is especially rich in vitamin A. This may be added to fish soups.

Use stock for fish soups, sauces and stews.

DAIRY FOODS

RAW MILK YOGURT
Makes 1 quart

1 quart whole raw milk
3 tablespoons plus 2 teaspoons yogurt
    (good quality store-bought
    or yogurt from the previous batch)

Place milk in a double boiler and heat to 110 degrees. Remove 2 tablespoons of the warm milk and add 1 tablespoon yogurt. Stir well and pour into a quart-sized wide-mouth mason jar. Add a further 2 tablespoons plus 2 teaspoons yogurt to the jar and stir well. Cover tightly and place in a dehydrator set at 95 degrees for 8 hours. Transfer to the refrigerator.

Please note that yogurt made from raw milk using this method will not become as solid as commercial yogurt.

RAW MILK KEFIR
Makes 2 cups

2 cups whole raw milk
1/2 cup good quality cream (optional)
1 tablespoon kefir grains or
    1 package kefir powder

If using kefir grains, place them in a fine strainer and rinse with filtered water. Place milk and optional cream in a clean, wide-mouth, quart-size mason jar. If milk is cold, place jar in a pan of simmering water until milk reaches room temperature. Add kefir grains or powder to milk, stir well and cover loosely with a cloth. Place in a warm place (65 to 76 degrees) for 12 hours to 2 days.

If using the powder, the kefir is ready when it thickens, usually within 24 hours.

If using grains, stir vigorously occasionally to re-distribute the grains. Every time you stir, taste the kefir. When it achieves a tartness to your liking, the kefir is ready. The kefir may also become thick and effervescent, depending on the temperature, incubation time and the amount of curds you use.

Pour the kefir through a strainer into another jar to remove the grains. Store in refrigerator. Use the grains to make another batch of kefir, or prepare them for storage by rinsing them well with water and placing in a small jar with about 1/2 cup filtered water. They may be stored in the refrigerator several weeks or in the freezer for several months. If they are left too long in storage, they will lose their culturing power.

RAW MILK BUTTERMILK
Makes 1 quart

1 quart whole raw milk
about 1/4 cup buttermilk culture

Buttermilk is the easiest of all the cultured milks. Place milk in a glass container, add the buttermilk culture, stir well and cover. Keep at room temperature (but not higher than 80 degrees) until the milk thickens and curdles slightly. Chill well. Reserve 1/4-1/2 cup in a separate jar in the refrigerator for the next culture.

CULTURED CREAM
Makes 1 pint

2 cups cream, preferably raw
1 tablespoon raw milk buttermilk or
    commercial crème fraiche

Place cream in a pint-sized jar. Add buttermilk or crème fraiche and stir with a fork to mix well. Cover tightly and leave at room temperature for 1-2 days. Transfer to the refrigerator. The cultured cream will last about 4 weeks well chilled.

FRESH WHEY AND YOGURT CHEESE
Makes 2 1/2 cups whey and
1 1/2 cups cream cheese

1 quart high-quality whole yogurt

Line a large strainer set over a bowl with a clean dish towel (preferably a linen towel). Pour in the yogurt, cover and let stand at room temperature overnight.

The whey will drip into the bowl and the milk solids will stay in the strainer.

At this point you have whey and a thick yogurt "cheese." This is delicious mixed with honey or maple syrup.

To make a thicker yogurt cream cheese, tie up the towel with the yogurt cheese inside, being careful not to squeeze. Tie this little sack to a wooden spoon placed across the top of a container so that more whey can drip out. When the bag stops dripping, the cheese is ready.

Store whey in a mason jar and the yogurt cheese or cream cheese in a covered glass container. Refrigerated, the cream cheese keeps for about 2 weeks and the whey for about 6 months.

You can also make this recipe using whole milk kefir or buttermilk.

CULTURED-MILK SMOOTHIE
Makes about 3 cups

1 1/4 cups wholemilk yogurt or kefir
1 ripe banana or 1 cup berries (fresh or frozen)
2 tablespoons coconut oil, melted
2 egg yolks
3-4 tablespoons maple syrup or raw honey
1 teaspoon vanilla extract (omit with berries)
pinch of nutmeg (omit with berries)

Place banana or berries in food processor or blender and process until smooth. Add remaining ingredients except melted coconut oil and process until well blended. While food processor is running, slowly pour in the coconut oil.

GHEE
Makes about 3 cups

2 pounds unsalted butter

Place the butter in a large Pyrex measuring cup and place in an oven set at 250 degrees for about 1 hour 15 minutes. The milk solids will have browned slightly and all the water evaporated off. Strain the butter though cheese cloth into a quart-sized clean glass jar. Store in the refrigerator.

LACTO-FERMENTED FOODS

LACTO-FERMENTED SAUERKRAUT
Makes 1 quart

1 medium cabbage, cored and shredded
1 tablespoon caraway seeds (optional)
1 tablespoon sea salt
4 tablespoons whey

Note: for GAPS-friendly sauerkraut, omit whey and use 2 tablespoons salt. Also, omit caraway seeds.

In a bowl, mix cabbage with optional caraway seeds, sea salt and optional whey. Pound with a wooden pounder or a meat hammer for about 10 minutes to release juices.

Place in a quart-sized, wide-mouth mason jar and press down firmly with a pounder or meat hammer until juices come to the top of the cabbage. The top of the cabbage should be at least 1 inch below the top of the jar. Cover tightly and keep at room temperature for about 3 days before transferring to cold storage. The sauerkraut may be eaten immediately, but it improves with age. It will last at least one year in the refrigerator.

LACTO-FERMENTED SAUERKRAUT JUICE
Makes 1 quart

1 cup sauerkraut, made without whey
filtered water
1 tablespoon sea salt

Lacto-fermented sauerkraut juice is a good introductory probiotic food for the GAPS diet.

Place sauerkraut, water and salt in a one-quart jar and mix well. Cover tightly and leave at room temperature 2-3 days. Transfer to the refrigerator.

LACTO-FERMENTED BEET KVASS
Makes 1 quarts

3 medium or 2 large organic beets,
  peeled and chopped up coarsely
1/4 cup whey or lacto-fermented sauerkraut juice
1 tablespoon sea salt
filtered water

For the GAPS diet, use the sauerkraut juice. For subsequent batches, you may use 1/4 cup beet kvass from the previous batch. Like the lacto-fermented sauerkraut juice, beet kvass is a good introductory probiotic food for the GAPS diet.

Place beets, whey or sauerkraut juice and salt in a quart-sized glass jar. Add filtered water to fill the container. Stir well and cover securely. Keep at room temperature for 2 days before transferring to refrigerator.

Note: Do not use grated beets in the preparation of beet tonic. When grated, beets exude too much juice resulting in a too rapid fermentation that favors the production of alcohol rather than lactic acid.

LACTO-FERMENTED BEETS
Makes 1 quart

12 medium beets
seeds from 2 cardamom pods (optional)
1 tablespoon sea salt
4 tablespoons whey
1 cup filtered water

Note: for the GAPS diet, omit the whey and use an extra 1 tablespoon salt.

Prick beets in several places, place on a cookie sheet and bake at 300 degrees for about 3 hours, or until soft. Peel and cut into a 1/4-inch julienne. (Do not grate or cut the beets with a food processor—this releases too much juice and the fermentation process will proceed too quickly, so that it favors formation of alcohol rather than lactic acid.)

Place beets in a quart-sized, wide-mouth mason jar and press down lightly with a wooden pounder or a meat hammer. Combine remaining ingredients and pour over beets, adding more water if necessary to cover the beets. The top of the beets with the covering of liquid should be at least 1 inch below the top of the jar. Cover tightly and keep at room temperature for about 3 days before transferring to cold storage.

LACTO-FERMENTED VEGETABLE MEDLEY
Makes 1 quart

1 cup cabbage, finely sliced
1 red pepper, cored, seeded and sliced
1 medium onion, peeled, quartered and sliced
1 turnip, peeled, quartered and thinly sliced
1 cup cauliflower flowers, thinly sliced
1 tablespoon parsley, chopped
4 tablespoons whey or lacto-fermented
*   sauerkraut juice*
1 tablespoon sea salt

Note: for the GAPS diet, use sauerkraut juice, not whey.

Place all the vegetables in a bowl—you chould have about 4 cups total. Toss with whey or sauerkraut juice and salt. Cover and leave one hour. Press on vegetables lightly with a wooden pounder or end of a meat hammer.

Stuff the vegetables into a quart-sized, wide-mouth mason jar. Press down with the wooden pounder or meat hammer until the juice covers the vegetables. The top of the vegetables should be at least 1 inch below the top of the jar.

Cover tightly and keep at room temperature for about 3 days before transferring to cold storage. The vegetables may be eaten immediately, but they improve with age. They will last about six months in the refrigerator.

LACTO-FERMENTED TURNIPS
Makes 1 quart

6-8 turnips, peeled
4 tablespoons whey or lacto-fermented
*   sauerkraut juice*
1 tablespoon sea salt
1 tablespoon caraway seeds (optional)

Note: for the GAPS diet, use sauerkraut juice, not whey.

Cut the turnips lengthwise and slice thinly in a food processor. Place in a bowl and toss with remaining ingredients. Let sit about one hour and then press with a wooden pounder or end of a meat hammer. Stuff into a wide-mouth, quart-size mason jar, pressing down with the pounder or meat hammer until the juices cover the turnips. The top of the turnips should be at least 1 inch below the top of the jar.

Cover tightly and keep at room temperature for

about 3 days before transferring to cold storage. The turnips may be eaten immediately, but they improve with age. They will last about six months in the refrigerator.

LACTO-FERMENTED ROOT VEGETABLES
Makes about 3 cups

2 pounds root vegetables, such as taro root,
*   yams, sweet potato or parsnips*
1 tablespoon sea salt
4 tablespoons whey or sauerkraut juice

Note: For the GAPS diet, use sauerkraut juice, not whey. This is a good recipe for babies.

Peel the root vegetables, cut into chunks and boil in filtered water until tender. Mash with salt and whey or sauerkraut juice. Place in a bowl, cover and leave at room temperature for 24 hours. Place in an airtight glass container and store in the refrigerator. This may be spread on bread or crackers like cream cheese. It also makes an excellent baby food.

SOUPS

CHOPPED VEGETABLE SOUP
Makes about 3 quarts

2 quarts chicken stock
about 3 cups finely chopped vegetables,
*   such as onion, celery, spinach, chard and*
*   cabbage*
1 cup carrots, peeled and coarsely grated
1 large tomato, seeded and chopped
1 tablespoon fresh herbs, chopped
1 tablespoon naturally fermented miso or
*   soy sauce (optional), or sea salt to taste*

This is a good soup for Stage One of the GAPS diet. Use sea salt rather than miso or soy sauce.

Bring chicken stock to a boil and remove any scum that rises to the top. Reduce to a simmer and add vegetables and herbs. Simmer until vegetables are tender. Season with 1 tablespoon naturally fermented miso or soy sauce, or with seasalt to taste.

CREAM OF VEGETABLE SOUP
Serves 6-8

2 medium onions or leeks, peeled and chopped
2 carrots, peeled and chopped
4 tablespoons butter or ghee
3 medium baking potatoes or 6 red potatoes,
*   washed and cut up*
2 quarts chicken stock or combination
*   of filtered water and stock*
several sprigs fresh thyme, tied together
1/2 teaspoon dried green peppercorns, crushed
4 zucchini, trimmed and sliced
sea salt and pepper to taste
cultured cream

Note: for the GAPS diet, omit the potatoes.

Melt butter or ghee in a large, stainless steel pot and add onions or leeks and carrots. Cover and cook over lowest possible heat for at least 1/2 hour. The vegetables should soften but not burn. Add potatoes (optional) and stock, bring to a rapid boil and skim. Reduce heat and add thyme sprigs and crushed peppercorns.

Cover and cook until the vegetables are soft. Add zucchini and cook until they are just tender—about 5 to 10 minutes. Remove the thyme sprigs. Purée the soup with a handheld blender.

If soup is too thick, thin with filtered water. Season to taste. Ladle into heated bowls and garnish with cultured cream.

CREAMY FISH SOUP
Serves 6-8

About 1 cup flaked fish meat (from head and
*   carcass of fish used in making fish stock)*
2 cups seafood, such as small shrimp, diced clams,
*   diced oysters or flaked crabmeat*
1 large onion, peeled and diced
1/4 cup bacon grease or lard
2 medium potatoes, peeled and cut
*   into 1/2-inch cubes*
1/2 cup white wine or dry vermouth
2 quarts fish stock
1 cup cultured cream
2 teaspoons dried herbs, such as tarragon or thyme
sea salt and pepper

Sauté onion in bacon grease or lard until soft. Add white wine or vermouth and bring to a boil. Add fish stock and bring to a boil, skimming off any scum that rises to the top. Add fish, seafood, potatoes and herbs. Simmer until tender. Season to taste with sea salt and pepper. Off heat, stir in cultured cream. Serve immediately.

EGGS

SCRAMBLED EGGS
Serves 1

1 pastured egg, preferably soy-free
1 pastured egg yolk, preferably soy-free
1 tablespoon cream or cultured cream
pinch salt
1 teaspoon chopped parsley or chives
1 tablespoon butter or ghee

Blend egg yolk, cream and salt with a wire whisk. Over medium heat, melt butter or ghee in a cast iron skillet. Pour in egg mix and sprinkle on chopped parsley or chives. Stir with a wooden spoon until cooked. Serve immediately with additive-free bacon or sausage.

OMELET
Serves 2

4 pastured eggs, preferably soy-free
1 teaspoon filtered water
dash tabasco sauce
1/2 teaspoon salt
2 tablespoons butter or ghee
1 medium onion, peeled, quartered and finely sliced
1 cup grated Cheddar cheese

Blend eggs, water, tabasco sauce and salt with a wire whisk. Set aside.

In a cast iron skillet, melt butter of ghee. Sauté onion in butter or ghee until browned. Pour in the egg mixture and distribute the cheese over the top.

Let the omelet cook over medium heat until the underside is browned. Do not worry if the top is not completely cooked—it will cook when you fold the omelet in half. Use a spatula to fold one side of the omelet over the other. Cook about one minute more and serve.

VEGETABLE FRITTATA
Serves 4

1 cup broccoli flowerets, steamed until tender
    and broken into small pieces
1 red pepper, seeded and cut into a julienne
1 medium onion, peeled and finely chopped
2 tablespoons butter or ghee
2 tablespoons extra virgin olive oil
6 eggs
1/3 cup cultured cream
1 teaspoon finely grated lemon rind
pinch dried oregano
pinch dried rosemary
sea salt and pepper
1 cup grated Monterey Jack or Cheddar cheese

In a cast-iron skillet, sauté the pepper and onion in 1 tablespoon each of butter or ghee and olive oil until soft. Remove with a slotted spoon. Beat eggs with cream and seasonings. Stir in broccoli, peppers and onion. Melt the remaining butter and olive oil in the pan and pour in egg mixture. Cook over medium heat about 5 minutes until underside is golden. Sprinkle cheese on top and place under the broiler for a few minutes until the frittata puffs and browns. Cut into wedges and serve.

SEAFOOD

LACTO-FERMENTED SALMON SALAD
Serves 4

1 pound fresh salmon, skinned and cut into a
    1/2-inch dice
1 small red onion, finely diced
2 teaspoons sea salt
dash tabasco sauce
1 cup fresh lime juice
2 tablespoons whey or sauerkraut juice
3 medium tomatoes, seeded and diced

1 bunch cilantro, chopped
Boston lettuce leaves
1 lime, cut into wedges

Mix lime juice with whey or sauerkraut juice, onion, salt and tabasco sauce and toss with salmon pieces. Cover and marinate in the refrigerator for at least 7 hours, and up to 24 hours, stirring occasionally. Remove from marinade with a slotted spoon and mix with tomatoes and cilantro. Serve on Boston lettuce leaves and garnish with lime wedges.

LACTO-FERMENTED TUNA SALAD
Serves 4

3/4 pound fresh tuna, cut into a 1/4-inch dice
1/4 cup lime juice
2 tablespoons whey or sauerkraut juice
1 small red pepper, seeded and diced
1/3 cup celery, diced
2 tablespoons red onion or scallions, finely diced
2 tablespoons small capers, rinsed,
*   well drained and dried with paper towels*
1 tablespoon fresh chives, chopped
1 tablespoon parsley, finely chopped
1 teaspoon fresh thyme leaves
1 tablespoon fresh basil, minced
1 tablespoon fresh lemon juice
3 tablespoons extra virgin olive oil
sea salt and pepper
Boston lettuce leaves

Mix tuna with lime juice and whey or sauerkraut juice, cover and marinate in refrigerator for 12 to 36 hours.

Lift tuna out of marinade with slotted spoon and mix with vegetables and herbs. Mix lemon juice with olive oil and toss with tuna mixture. Refrigerate, covered, for at least 1 hour. Serve on Boston lettuce leaves.

CAVIAR CANAPES
Makes about 12

1 ounce caviar
12 crispy pancakes (see recipe, page 299)
1/2 cup cultured cream
1 small red onion, peeled and very finely diced
1 tablespoon parsley, finely chopped.

Place crispy pancakes on a platter or tray. Spread each with cultured cream and put 1/3 teaspoon cav-

iar on each. Top with diced onion and a pinch of parsley.

SALMON EGGS ON TOAST
Serves 1

1 large piece sourdough bread, crusts removed
lard, bacon fat or ghee
2 tablespoons wild salmon roe
1 teaspoon fresh dill, finely chopped

Cut the bread into 4 squares or pieces. Sauté on both sides in lard, bacon fat or ghee until browned. Spread with salmon roe and sprinkle with dill.

TARAMOSALATA
(Greek Roe Spread)
Serves 12

1 pound smoked whole cod roe, casing removed
*   (available at Middle Eastern markets,*
*   often canned or in jars)*
1/2 cup cultured cream
1 clove garlic, mashed
juice of 1/2 lemon
1/4 teaspoon pepper
1/2 cup extra virgin olive oil

Use this delicious pink cream to spread on toasts, or to fill celery or endive leaves.

Place roe, cream, garlic, lemon juice and pepper in food processor and process until smooth. Using the attachment for adding oil, add the olive oil drop by drop with the motor running to form a thick, mayonnaise-like emulsion. Chill several hours.

Note: you can use 1 pound raw fish roe, casing removed, from any kind of fish, rather than smoked cod roe and add sea salt to taste. High-nutrient roe can often be obtained in season at very low cost from a good fish merchant.

SALMON SALAD
Serves 4

3 cups cooked fresh salmon, flaked with a fork
1 red onion, peeled and finely diced
1 bunch cilantro, chopped
3/4 cup good quality mayonnaise
sea salt

pine nuts or slivered almonds for garnish

Toss salmon with onion and cilantro, then mix in mayonnaise and season to taste with sea salt. Garnish with pine nuts or slivered almonds and serve with sliced tomatoes.

OYSTER FRITTERS
Makes 12

12 fresh, shucked oysters
juice of 1-2 lemons
unbleached white flour
2 cups pancake batter (page 299)
1/2 cup lard or bacon fat

Squeeze lemon on the oysters and allow to marinate about 30 minutes. Dry oysters well with paper towels. Melt the lard or bacon fat in a cast iron skillet.

Dredge each oyster in flour and then dip into the pancake batter. Fry on both sides in the lard or bacon fat. (Alternately cook the fritters on a well oiled griddle.) Drain on paper towels.

FRESH TUNA SALAD
(Salade Nicoise)
Serves 6

6 portions fresh tuna steak, about 4 ounces each
2 tablespoons extra virgin olive oil
sea salt and pepper
6 cups baby salad greens or curly lettuce
6 small ripe tomatoes, cup into wedges
6 small red potatoes, steamed until tender
1 pound cooked French beans or string beans
2 dozen small black olives
2 cups basic dressing,
1 tablespoon finely chopped parsley
1 tablespoon finely chopped chives

Brush tuna steaks with olive oil and season with sea salt and pepper. Using a heavy skillet, sauté rapidly, two at a time, for about 4 minutes per side. Set aside.

Divide salad greens between 6 large plates. Garnish with tomatoes, potatoes, beans and olives. Place tuna steaks on top of greens. Mix dressing with herbs and pour over the salad.

MEAT & ORGAN MEATS

GOURMET CHICKEN LIVER PATE
Serves 12-18

3 tablespoons butter or ghee
1 pound chicken livers
2/3 cup dry white wine or brandy
1 cup chicken or beef stock
1 clove garlic, mashed
1/2 teaspoon dry mustard
1/4 teaspoon dried dill
1/4 teaspoon dried rosemary
1 tablespoon lemon juice
1/2 stick butter (1/4 cup), softened
     or chicken or bacon fat
sea salt

Note: You can also use duck or turkey livers, or a combination.

Melt butter or ghee in a heavy skillet. Dry livers well and sauté, stirring occasionally, for about 10 minutes until livers are browned. Add brandy, stock, garlic, mustard, lemon juice and herbs. Bring to a boil and cook, uncovered, until the liquid is reduced by half. Allow to cool. Process in a food processor with softened butter or chicken or bacon fat. Season to taste with sea salt. Place in a crock or mold and chill well.

ORGAN MEAT MIXTURE
Makes 2 pounds

1 1/2 pounds fatty meat
1/2 pound heart or tongue
1/4 pound beef or chicken liver, frozen

Organ meat mixture can be used in casseroles, chile and meat loaf. This is a great way to consume organ meats. With lots of spices added to the dish, the taste of the organs is completely hidden. Some farmers prepare an organ meat blend and sell it as pet food; here is a recipe for making your own. You will need a meat grinder.

Cut the meat and heart or tongue into chunks and toss together in a bowl. Grate the liver over the meat chunks. Grind in the meat grinder. Use immediately or freeze for later use.

MEAT LOAF
Serves 6-8

2 pounds organ meat mixture (page 295)
1 medium onion, finely chopped
1 bunch parsley, finely chopped
2 pastured eggs, preferably soy-free
2 slices sourdough bread
1/2 cup raw or cultured cream
1 tablespoon sea salt
1 teaspoon back pepper
1 teaspoon Thai fish sauce
1/4 teaspoon cayenne pepper
1 small jar tomato paste

Meat loaf made with organ blend is a great food for toddlers, as well as the whole family. The meat loaf mix can be baked as a loaf, or formed as individual patties, cooked in a cast iron skillet.

Use a food processor to process the sourdough bread slices into break crumbs. Mix well with the cream, adding a little water if necessary. Let sit about 5 minutes.

Place all the ingredients except the tomato paste in a large bowl. Mix well with hands. Form into a loaf and place in a 9-by-13 pyrex pan. Add about 1 cup filtered water to the pan. Ice the top with tomato paste. Bake at 350 degrees for about 1 1/2 hours.

GAPS ITALIAN CASSEROLE
Serves about 8-10

1 shoulder of lamb or chuck roast,
*   with bone and all the fat attached*
1/2 cup ghee, duck fat, lard or other animal fat
2 cups stock (chicken, beef or mixed)
6 Italian tomatoes, cut in half and seeds removed
2 cloves garlic, peeled and chopped
4-5 pieces of zest from an organic orange
2 cups baby onions, peeled
2 turnips, peeled and quartered
sea salt and pepper
sprig of fresh rosemary
sprig of fresh thyme
2 bay leaves

Rub the meat all over with salt and pepper. Place the roast in a large oven-proof casserole with a lid. Melt the fat and brush the roast. Set casserole, uncovered, in oven at 350 degrees and roast about 1/2 hour, turning once, so the roast browns. Add the stock, tomatoes, garlic and orange zest. Bring the stock to boil on the stove and then put the casserole in the oven, set at about 250 degrees. Tie the rosemary, thyme and bay leaves together and place on top of the roast. Place the top on the pot slightly askew so steam can escape. This will allow the sauce to reduce slightly. Braise the meat for about 5-6 hours.

About 1 hour before serving, add the baby onions and turnips. Just before serving, season the sauce to taste with sea salt. Serve the roast with the vegetables and sauce.

CALVE'S LIVER
Serves 3-4

About 1 pound calve's liver, thinly sliced
1/4 cup lemon juice or vinegar
about 1/2 cup lard or bacon fat
4 medium onions, peeled and thinly sliced
about 1 cup unbleached white flour
sea salt and black pepper

The combination of vitamin A-rich liver and vitamin D-rich lard or bacon fat is a good one.

Purchase the liver already sliced, or if you have whole liver, freeze and then slice the liver when partially thawed. Cut into pieces approximately 3 inches square. Marinate (in the refrigerator) in lemon juice or vinegar for several hours.

In a heavy skillet, brown the onions in some of the bacon fat or lard. Remove from the pan, set aside and keep warm in a warm oven. Dry the liver very well with paper towels. Dredge in a mixture of flour, salt and pepper.

Over medium high heat, fry the liver slices on both sides in the skillet, adding more bacon fat or lard if necessary. Keep warm in a warm oven while frying subsequent batches. Serve with the sautéed onion.

VEGETABLES

BASIC VEGETABLES
Serves 4

about 2 cups vegetables, cut up
1/4 cup butter or ghee, melted
sea salt

You can use peeled and sliced carrots, broccoli flowerets, cauliflower pieces, strips of red or green pepper, asparagus spears, green beans (ends removed), mushrooms, onion quarters, etc., either as single vegetables or mixed. Place in the top half of a vegetable steamer and steam until tender. Transfer to a serving bowl and toss with melted butter or ghee. Season to taste with sea salt.

VEGETABLE STIR FRY
Serves 4

about 2 cups vegetables, cut up
1/4 cup lard or bacon fat
1/2 cup water
2 tablespoons naturally fermented soy sauce

As with Basic Vegetables, you can use peeled and sliced carrots, broccoli flowerets, cauliflower pieces, strips of red or green pepper, asparagus spears, green beans (ends removed), mushrooms, onion quarters, etc., either single vegetables or mixed. Melt the lard or bacon fat in a cast iron skillet. Sauté the vegetables in the skillet until lightly browned. Add water and soy sauce. Let the water boil away until the vegetables are coated with the soy sauce and fat.

SALAD DRESSINGS

BASIC SALAD DRESSING
Makes about 3/4 cup

1 teaspoon Dijon-type mustard, smooth or grainy
2 tablespoons plus 1 teaspoon raw wine vinegar
1/2 cup extra virgin olive oil
1 teaspoon expeller-expressed flax oil

Dip a fork into the jar of mustard and transfer about 1 teaspoon to a small bowl. Add vinegar and mix around. Add olive oil in a thin stream, stirring all the while with the fork, until oil is well mixed or emulsified. Add flax oil and use immediately.

This basic dressing lends itself to many variations. Suggested additions include herbs, garlic, egg yolks, raw or cultured cream, anchovies, and blue cheese or Parmesan cheese.

MAYONNAISE
Makes 1 1/2 cups

1 whole egg, at room temperature
1 egg yolk, at room temperature
1 teaspoon Dijon-type mustard
1 1/2 tablespoons lemon juice
1 tablespoon whey, optional
3/4-1 cup extra virgin olive oil or expeller-expressed
*   sesame oil or a combination*
generous pinch sea salt

Homemade mayonnaise imparts valuable enzymes, particularly lipase, to sandwiches, tuna salad, chicken salads and many other dishes and is very easy to make in a food processor. The addition of whey will help your mayonnaise last longer, adds enzymes and increases nutrient content. Use sesame oil if you find that olive oil alone gives too strong a taste. Homemade mayonnaise will be slightly more liquid than store-bought versions.

In your food processor, place egg, egg yolk, mustard, salt and lemon juice and optional whey. Process until well blended, about 30 seconds. Using the attachment that allows you to add liquids drop by drop, add olive oil and/or sunflower oil with the motor running. Taste and check seasoning. You may want to add more salt and lemon juice. If you have added whey, let the mayonnaise sit at room temperature, well covered, for 7 hours before refrigerating. With whey added, mayonnaise will keep several months and will become firmer with time. Without whey, mayonnaise will keep for about 2 weeks.

For sources of good quality ready-made mayonnaise, see the Shopping Guide of the Weston A. Price Foundation.

MEAT SALADS

CHICKEN SALAD
Serves 6

About 4 cups diced chicken meat and skin
1 cup diced celery
1/2 cup sliced green onion
1 red pepper, seeded and diced
1/4 cup parsley, finely chopped
1 cup good quality mayonnaise
1 tablespoon raw honey
1 tablespoon raw vinegar
2 tablespoons olive oil
sea salt
pine nuts or slivered almonds for garnish

Use chicken from making chicken broth with a whole chicken, and don't throw away the skin. It is the most nutritious part and can be chopped up with the chicken meat.

Cut chicken meat and skin into small pieces and toss with celery, green onion, red pepper and parsley.

Whisk the mayonnaise with the honey, vinegar and olive oil. Mix with the salad and season to taste with sea salt. Garnish with pine nuts or slivered almonds and serve with sliced tomatoes.

TACO SALAD
Serves 4

2 pounds organ meat mixture (page 295)
8 corn tortillas
about 1/2 cup lard or bacon fat
1 large yellow onion, peeled, quartered and sliced
1/2 cup chile powder
2 hearts of Romaine, chopped
4 tomatoes, seeded and diced
1 red onion, peeled, quartered and finely sliced
1/4 cup pitted black olived, sliced
1 bunch cilantro, chopped
2 avocados, peeled and cut into wedges
2 cups grated Monterey Jack
*   or mild Cheddar cheese*
1 cup cultured cream

Cut 4 of the tortillas into strips. In a heavy cast iron skillet, fry the 4 whole tortillas in some of the lard or bacon fat on both sides until crisp. Set aside. Fry the tortilla strips in the same pan until crisp, adding more lard or bacon fat if necessary. Remove with a slotted spoon and set aside.

Add more lard or bacon fat to the pan and sauté the yellow onion. Add the organ meat mixture to the pan and sauté until browned. Stir in the chile powder and mix well.

To assemble the salad, place a whole tortilla on each of 4 plates. Place chopped Romaine lettuce on the tortilla and top with meat mixture. Strew red onion, tomato, olives and cilantro on top. Garnish with avocado wedges, grated cheese and a dollop of cultured cream.

GRAINS & NUTS

BREAKFAST PORRIDGE
Serves 4

1 cup rolled oats
1 cup warm filtered water plus 2 tablespoons
*   whey, yogurt, kefir, lemon juice or vinegar*
1/2 teaspoon sea salt
1-2 cups filtered water
1 tablespoon flax seeds (optional)

Mix oats with warm water mixture, cover and leave overnight in a warm place. (Note: Those with severe milk allergies can use *lemon juice or vinegar* in place of whey, yogurt or kefir.) Bring an additional 1-2 cups water to a boil with sea salt. Add soaked oats, reduce heat, cover and simmer about ten minutes until well cooked and creamy. Meanwhile, grind optional flax seeds in a mini grinder. Remove porridge from heat, stir in optional flax seeds and let stand for a few minutes.

Serve with plenty of butter or cream and a natural sweetener like Rapadura, date sugar, maple syrup, maple sugar or raw honey. You can garnish with 1 tablespoon chopped crispy nuts or toasted pine nuts.

PANCAKES
Makes 16-20

2 cups freshly ground spelt, kamut
    or whole wheat flour
2 cups buttermilk, kefir or yogurt
2 eggs, lightly beaten
1/2 teaspoon sea salt
1 teaspoon baking soda
2 tablespoons melted butter
2 tablespoons maple syrup

Soak flour in buttermilk, kefir or yogurt in a warm place for 12 to 24 hours. Stir in other ingredients and thin to desired consistency with water. Cook on a hot, oiled griddle or in a cast iron skillet.

Serve with melted butter and maple or sorghum syrup or raw honey.

CRISPY PANCAKES
Makes about 50

These make great crackers. Use for caviar, paté, cheese, smoked salmon; or as a cookie iced with cream cheese mixed with a little honey.

Use the above recipe for pancakes, adding enough water to make a very thin batter. Cook very small pancakes on a hot oiled griddle or in a cast iron skillet.

Place pancakes on a cookie sheet and let dry in a warm oven until completely dry and crisp. Store in an air tight container.

GAPS PANCAKES
Serves 4

1/4 cup coconut flour
6 large eggs
1/2 stick (1/4 cup) butter
2 tablespoons raw honey
1/2 ripe banana
1/4 teaspoon sea salt
pinch cinnamon
pinch nutmeg

Combine all ingredients in a blender or food processor, adding the coconut flour last.

Cook pancakes on a well greased griddle or in a cast iron pan with a little ghee. Use about 1/4 cup batter per pancake. Turn after 2-3 minutes, or when bubbles appear. Cook another 1-2 minutes. Keep pancakes warm in the oven while cooking other batches.

Serve with melted butter or ghee, raw honey and additive-free sausage or bacon.

CRISPY NUTS
Makes 4 cups

4 cups raw nuts such as pecans, walnuts, cashews,
    macadamia nuts, skinless almonds or
skinless peanuts, or a mixture
1 tablespoon sea salt
filtered water

Mix nuts with salt and filtered water and leave in a warm place for at about 7-8 hours. (Note: soak cashews for 6 hours only.) Drain in a colander. Spread nuts on a stainless steel baking pan and place in a warm oven (preferably 150 degrees but no more than 170 degrees) for 12 to 24 hours, turning occasionally, until completely dry and crisp. Store in an airtight container at room temperature. (Note: walnuts should be stored in the refrigerator.)

CRISPY NUT BUTTER
Makes 2 cups

2 cups crispy nuts, such as peanuts, almonds
    or cashews
3/4 cup coconut oil
2 tablespoons raw honey
1 teaspoon sea salt

Place nuts and sea salt in food processor and grind to a fine powder. Add honey and coconut oil and process until "butter" becomes smooth. It will be somewhat liquid but will harden when chilled. Store in an airtight container in the refrigerator. Serve at room temperature.

GAPS ALMOND BREAD
Makes 1 loaf

2 1/2 cups crispy almonds
3 eggs
1/4 cup butter or coconut oil, softened

Use a food processor to process the almonds into flour. Preheat oven to 300 degrees. Grease a loaf pan with butter of coconut oil. Beat the eggs with butter or coconut oil, and gradually add the almond flour. Press the mixture into the greased loaf pan.

Bake for about an hour. Test for doneness by inserting a clean knife—it will come out clean when the bread is ready. Let it rest for at least 10 minutes before removing from the pan.

You can also do variations by adding additional ingredients, such as sliced olives, grated cheese, dried herbs like dill and rosemary, sautéed onions or even chopped dates and honey. The bread can also be cooked as individual muffins.

DESSERTS

ICE CREAM
Makes 1 quart

6 egg yolks
1/2 - 3/4 cup Rapadura, Sucanat or maple sugar
1 tablespoon vanilla extract
3 cups heavy cream, preferably raw,
*   not ultrapasteurized*

Use an ice cream maker with a double-walled canister that is kept in the freezer. Beat egg yolks with sweetener for several minutes until pale and thick. Beat in vanilla extract and cream. Prepare in the ice cream maker according to instructions. Transfer to a shallow container and store in the freezer. About five minutes before serving, remove ice cream from the freezer and allow it to soften.

Note: you may add 1 cup fruit purée and reduce the cream by 1 cup, omitting vanilla.

GAPS COOKED APPLES
Serves 4

8 organic apples
1/4 cup ghee
1/4 teaspoon ground cinnamon or nutmeg

Peel and core the apples. Place in a pan with a little filtered water. Cover and simmer the apples until soft. Add the ghee and mash with a potato masher. Stir in cinnamon or nutmeg.

GAPS COCONUT FLOUR CAKE
Serves 8

1 1/ 4cups coconut flour
1 teaspoon sea salt
1/2 teaspoon baking soda
8 large pastured eggs , preferably soy-free
2/3 cup melted grass-fed ghee
1 cup raw honey
2 tablespoon vanilla extract

Preheat the oven to 330 degrees. Grease two 8-inch cake pans and dust with coconut flour. In a large bowl, combine the coconut flour, salt and baking soda. In a medium bowl, whisk together the eggs, melted ghee, honey and vanilla extract. Blend the wet ingredients into the coconut flour mixture with a handheld mixer until thoroughly combined. Divide the batter between the two cake pans.

Bake for 35-40 minutes. Once inserted toothpick comes out dry (a few moist crumbs), cake is ready. Let cook in pan, then cool on rack. Frost after cake is cool.

GAPS FRIENDLY FROSTING
Makes about 3 cups

1 1/2 cups crispy cashews
1 cup water
2 teaspoons vanilla
7 pitted dates
 pinch of salt

Mix all ingredients in the blender on high to whip into a thick cashew cream.

BEVERAGES & TONICS

LACTO-FERMENTED GINGER ALE
Makes 2 quarts

3/4 cup ginger, peeled and finely chopped or grated
1/2 cup fresh lime juice
1/4-1/2 cup Rapadura, Sucanat or maple sugar
2 teaspoons sea salt
1/4 cup homemade whey
2 quarts filtered water

Place all ingredients in a 2-quart jug. Stir well and cover tightly. Leave at room temperature for 2-3 days before transferring to the refrigerator. This will keep several months well chilled. To serve, strain into a glass.

Ginger ale may be mixed with carbonated water and is best sipped warm rather than gulped down cold.

LACTO-FERMENTED FRUIT SODA
Makes 2 quarts

3 cups fruit, such as berries (fresh or frozen), or
*   peeled and pitted peaches or nectarines*
juice of 1 lemon
1/4 cup raw honey
2 teaspoons sea salt
1/4 cup homemade whey
about 1 1/2 quarts filtered water

Place fruit, lemon juice, honey, sea salt and whey in a food processor and blend until smooth. Strain into a 2-quart jug and add enough filtered water to fill the jug. Stir well and cover tightly. Leave at room temperature for 2 days. The brew will develop a layer on top. After 2 days, carefully pour the liquid through a strainer out from under the top layer into 2 quart-sized jars. Add enough water to fill the jars. Seal with lids very tightly and leave on the counter 1 more day.

Before transferring to the refrigerator, open the lids to let carbon dioxide escape. Transfer to the refrigerator. The fruit soda should be ready in about 1 week, but will keep in the refrigerator several months.

KOMBUCHA
Makes 1 gallon

3 quarts filtered water
1 cup white sugar
4 tea bags of organic black tea
1/2 cup kombucha from a previous culture
1 kombucha mushroom (see Sources)

Bring 3 quarts filtered water to boil. Add sugar and simmer until dissolved. Remove from heat, add the tea bags and allow the tea to steep until water has completely cooled. Remove tea bags.

Pour cooled liquid into a 4-quart pyrex bowl and add 1/2 cup kombucha from previous batch. Place the mushroom on top of the liquid. Make a crisscross over the bowl with masking tape, cover loosely with a cloth or towel and transfer to a warm, dark place, away from contaminants and insects. In about 7 to 10 days the kombucha will be ready, depending on the temperature. It should be rather sour and possibly fizzy, with no taste of tea remaining.

Transfer to covered glass containers and store in the refrigerator. If you want the kombucha to be fizzier, transfer to used glass mineral water bottles and screw cap on tightly. (Note: Do not wash kombucha bowls in the dishwasher.)

When the kombucha is ready, your mushroom will have grown a second spongy pancake. This can be used to make other batches or given away to friends. Store fresh mushrooms in the refrigerator in a glass or stainless steel container—never plastic. A kombucha mushroom can be used dozens of times. If it begins to turn black, or if the resulting kombucha doesn't sour properly, it's a sign that the culture has become contaminated. When this happens, it's best to throw away all your mushrooms and order a new clean one.

Note: White sugar, rather than an unrefined sweetener, and black tea, rather than flavored teas, give the best results. Non-organic tea is high in fluoride so always use organic tea.

MOLASSES TONIC
Serves 1

1 tablespoon molasses
1 tablespoon coconut oil
1/4 teaspoon powdered ginger
filtered water

This makes a great pick-me-up and is a good substitute for coffee.

Place all ingredients in a mug and add boiling filtered water. Stir well.

POTASSIUM BROTH
Makes 2 quarts

4 potatoes, preferably organic, well scrubbed
3 carrots, peeled and chopped
4 celery sticks, chopped
1 bunch parsley
4 quarts filtered water

Potassium broth is a great rejuvenator for those who have been sick or are recovering from childbirth.

Peel potatoes. Place peelings, carrots and celery in a pot with water. (Use peeled potatoes to make mashed potatoes.) Bring to a boil, lower heat and simmer, covered, for about 1/2 hour. Add parsley and simmer 5 minutes more. Allow to cool and strain into a 2-quart glass container. Store in refrigerator and reheat in small quantities as needed.

GINGER TEA
Makes 2 cups

1 teaspoon grated fresh ginger root
filtered water
raw honey to taste

Place ginger in a small teapot. Bring water to a boil and add it to the pot. Leave 3-5 minutes.

To serve, pour through a small strainer into a cup or mug. Stir in raw honey to taste.

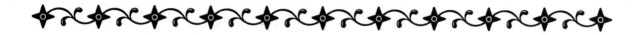

Appendix IV
Sources

FOOD RESOURCES

The Weston A. Price Foundation (WAPF): WAPF publishes a yearly shopping guide to help you find healthy foods in health foods stores and grocery stores, and by mail order. This includes liver products (liverwurst), caviar, healthy fats and oils, coconut products, unrefined salt, grain products, etc.

> http://westonaprice.org/about-the-foundation/shopping-guide
> 202-363-4394

In addition, local chapters of the Foundation can direct you to sources of pasture-based meat, eggs and raw dairy products.

> http://westonaprice.org/local-chapters/find-local-chapter
> 202-363-4394

A Campaign for Real Milk lists sources of raw milk by state.

> www.realmilk.com

REMEDY RESOURCES

Mediherb products are distributed through Standard Process; they are available through health care practitioners.
> www.mediherb.com
> 800-848-5061

Radiant Life provides all the ingredients for our whole-foods baby formula, dessicated liver, dried small whole fish and natural vitamin C (Amla-Plus C).
> www.radiantlifecatalog.com
> 888-593-8333

Standard Process makes several excellent nutritional products described in these pages. Standard Process products are available through health care practitioners. Contact them for a practitioner near you.
> www.standardprocess.com
> 800-848-5061

Uriel Pharmacy provides many herbal and homeopathic medicines recommended in these pages.
> www.urielpharmacy.com
> 866-642-2858

Weleda provides many natural skin care products.
> www.weleda.com
> 800-241-1030

INDIVIDUAL PRODUCTS

Aalgo sea vegetable baths
www.aalgo.com
sales@aalgo.com

Acidum sulfuricum e vetiolo D3 by Weleda
www.weleda.com
800-241-1030

Acupressure for easy childbirth
https://maternityacupressure.wordpress.com

Air Filter: Atmosphere Air Purifier
www.amazon.com

Aloe Detox from Premier Research, available from
www.naturalhealthyconcepts.com
866-505-7501

Aloe Vera topical products are widely available in
stores and on the Internet. Once good source is
www.aloelife.com
800-414-2563

Andrographis Complex from Mediherb
www.mediherb.com
800-848-5061

Antifertility herbs: for information, see
www.thehealthyhomeeconomist.com/
natural-birth-control-using-herbs

Antronex form Standard Process
www.standardprocess.com
800-848-5061

Apis, homeopathic formulation
www.abchomeopathy.com

Apis Belladona from Uriel Pharmacy
http://shop.urielpharmacy.com/apis-bella
donna-fever-relief-pellets-p590.aspx
866-642-2858

Apis Belladona with merciurio from Uriel Pharmacy
http://shop.urielpharmacy.com/categories.
aspx?Keyword=apis belladonna mercurius
866-642-2858

Apis-Levisticum from Uriel Pharmacy
http://shop.urielpharmacy.com/apis-
levisticum-earache-relief-pellets-p591.
aspx
866-642-2858

Arnica oil from Weleda
www.weleda.com
800-241-1030

Baby clothes, chemical free
www.safbaby.com/formaldehyde-free-
baby-and-childrens-clothing-companies

Baby Formula, commercial: Baby's Only Organic
Dairy Formula
http://www.naturesone.com/dairy/
888-227-7122

Baby Formula, homemade ingredients from
Radiant Life
www.radiantlifecatalog
888-593-8333

Baby Safe Mattress Cover
www.eves-best.com/babesafe-mattress-
covers.htm

Bifidus Bacterium supplement
www.radiantlifecatalog.com
888-593-8333

Biokult probiotic from Nutrivene
www.nutrivene.com
800-899-3413

Breast feeding aid, Lact-Aid
www.lact-aid.com
866-866-1239

Breast Pump: both small, battery-powered pumps
(for occasional use) and large, plug-in pumps (for
frequent use) are available from Medela
www.medelabreastfeedingus.com
800-435-8316

Breast Pump "horn" or shield is the part that fits
over your breast.
www.medelabreastfeedingus.com
800-435-8316

Breast Milk sharing networks:
www.humanmilkforhumanbabies.com,
www.eatsonfeets.org,
or check with a local chapter of the Weston A. Price
Foundation
http://www.westonaprice.org/get-involved/
find-local-chapter/

Bronchafect by Mediherb
www.mediherb.com
800-848-5061

Bryonia spongia from Uriel Pharmacy
http://shop.urielpharmacy.com/bryonia-
spongia-liquid-p908.aspx
866-642-2858

Butter oil, high vitamin
www.greenpasture.org
402-858-4818, Ext 1

Calendula tincture
www.localharvest.org/calendula-tincture-
calendula-officinalis-C2682

Calendula ointment or cream
www.amazon.com

Cardiodoron from Weleda
http://www.natures-source.com/product.
php?productid=1759
866-502-6789

Catalyn from Standard Process
www.standardprocess.com
800-848-5061

Catnip Fennel from Nature's Sunshine
http://www.naturessunshine.com/us/
product/catnip--fennel-2-fl-oz/sku-3195.
aspx

Chamomile, homeopathic
www.abchomeopathy.com

Chamomile tea
www.starwest-botanicals.com
800-800-4372

Chickweed Gel or Salve
http://www.amishoriginsmedicated.com/
cgi-bin/shop/pid_27.htm#Amish Origins
888-865-3771
http://chickweedhealingsalve.com/

Cod Liver Oil, fermented, high-vitamin
www.greenpasture.org
402-858-4818, Ext 1

Colic Calm Gripe Water
www.coliccalm.com
877-321-CALM

Combudoron by Weleda
www.alivepluspharmacy.com/productinfo/
Weleda_Combudoron_Gel_36g
800-578-9811

Congaplex by Standard Process
www.standardprocess.com
800-848-5061

Culturelle from Allergy Research
http://www.allergyresearchgroup.com/
Culturelle-Probiotic-30-Vegicaps-p-58.html
800-545-9960

Cuprum aceticum
www.abchomeopathy.com

Dermrash cream from Dr. Kang Formulas
http://www.drkangformulas.com/
EACHFORMULA/49.htm
800-355-3808

Dessicated Liver
www.radiantlifecatalog.com
888-593-8333

Diaper cream by Weleda
usa.weleda.com/natural-products/natural-
baby-diaper-care.aspx
800-241-1030

Diapers, cloth
www.clothdiaper.com
877-215-9004

Diapers, nontoxic disposable
    Earth's Best, www.toysrus.com
    Nature Babycare
        www.diapers.com/Nature-Babycare
    Seventh Generation
        www.seventhgeneration.com/Diapers

Diatomaceous Earth, food grade
    www.amazon.com

Drosera comp. from Uriel Pharmacy
    http://shop.urielpharmacy.com/drosera-
    comp-liquid-p926.aspx
    866-642-2858

Ear Formula Drops from Uriel Pharmacy
    http://shop.urielpharmacy.com/ear-formula-
    liquid-p928.aspx
    866-642-2858

Echinacea by Mediherb
    www.mediherb.com
    800-848-5061

Elderberry Thyme Syrup from True Botanica
    http://store.truebotanica.com/store/product/
    SRW0010/ElderberryThymeSyrup4oz.aspx
    800-315-8783

Elder Flower Tea
    www.starwest-botanicals.com
    800-800-4372

Euphrasia Complex tablets from Mediherb
    www.mediherb.com
    800-848-5061

Extra Lesson™, used widely in Waldorf schools
    www.healingeducation.org

EZ Birth Flower Essence
    http://www.healthherbsandnutrition.com/
    products/ezebirthfloweressence.htm

EZ Birth homeopathic remedy
    http://www.allaboutbirthboutique.ca/all/
    ez-birth-homeopathic-remedy.html

Fe-Max Phytosynergist Fortified Herbal Tonic from Mediherb
    www.mediherb.com
    800-848-5061

Fish, dried
    www.radiantlifecatalog.com
    888-593-8333

Floradix Iron plus herbs
    www.amazon.com
    www.vitamonshoppe.com

Folic Acid from Standard Process
    www.standardprocess.com
    800-848-5061

Glass Baby Bottles
    www.radiantlifecatalog.com
    888-593-8333

Gymnema from Mediherb
    www.mediherb.com
    800-848-5061

Hydrochloride Acid (betaine hydrochloride) from Standard Process
    www.standardprocess.com
    800-848-5061

Hylands homeopathic baby teething tablets
    http://www.hylandsteething.com/products/
    www.amazon.com

Insect Repellents: Buzz Away
    www.quantumhealth.com/productgroups/
    itchandbite.html

Lauricidin
    www.lauricidin.com
    www.amazon.com

Longvida curcumin by Nutrivene
    http://www.nutrivene.com/view_item.
    php?id=331
    800-899-3413

Magnesium Salts Baths
    www.ancient-minerals.com/products/
    magnesium-bath-salts/
    800-257-3315

Max Stress B (Max B-ND) from Premier Research
www.amazon.com

Meteoric Iron *Prunus* Immune Support Pellets from
Uriel Pharmacy
http://shop.urielpharmacy.com/meteoric-
iron-prunus-immune-support-pellets-p660.
aspx
866-642-2858

Milk Thistle 1:1 Glycetract from Mediherb, available through practitioners
www.mediherb.com
800-848-5061

Multi-vitamin from Dr. Ron's Ultrapure
http://www.drrons.com/docs-best-multi-
vitamin-mineral-antioxidant.htm
877-472-8701

NAET: Nambudripad's Allergy Elimination Techniques
wwww.naet.com

Nettles, freeze dried from Eclectic Institute
www.theherbalist.com/products/vitamin-
supplements/fresh-freeze-dried-nettle-
90-capsules-eclectic-institute.html
800-694-3727

Nettles tea
www.localharvest.org/just-nettle-tea-C8643

Ophthacare herbal eyedrops
http://www.onlineherbs.com/ophthacare-
from-himalaya-10ml.html
888-203-7804

Ox Bile (Cholacol 90) from Standard Process
www.standardprocess.com
800-848-5061

Pacifier, rubber
www.natursutten.com/

Photo-optic bilirubin-blanket
http://www.healthlinedme.com/Catalog/
Online-Catalog-Product/3107/Bili-Blanket
800-766-2027

Phytocort from Allergy Research
https://www.pureformulas.com/
phytocort-120-vegetarian-capsules-by-
allergy-research-group.html
800-383-6008

Pin-X, available in pharmacies and
www.amazon.com

Plantain Spruce cough syrup from Uriel Pharmacy
http://shop.urielpharmacy.com/
plantain-spruce-cough-syrup-p687.aspx
866-642-2858

Plantain Beeswax Cough Relief Ointment
Shop.urielpharmacy.com/plantain-beeswax-
cough-relief-ointment-p688.aspx
866-642-2858

Pleo-not homeopathic penicillin preparation from
Sanum
www.naturalhealthyconcepts.com/pleo-not-
drops-p-sanum.html
866-505-7501

Pneumotrophin by Standard Process
www.standardprocess.com
800-848-5061

Poison Hotline
800-222-1222

Probiotics for baby, Bifidus Bacterium supplement
www.radiantlifecatalog.com
888-593-8333

Pyridoxal-5-phosphate by Thorne Research
www.idealvitamins.com
800-385-1788

Quercetin from Jarrow Formulas
www.amazon.com

Rhus Tox homeopathic remedy
www.abchomeopathy.com

Rosemary Oil Bath: Dr. Haushka
www.lookfantastic.com/dr.hauschka-
rosemary-bath-150ml/10543862.html

Seagreens by Nutrivene
www.nutrivene.com/product.php?id=82
800-899-3413

Sesame Oil perles from Standard Process
www.standardprocess.com
800-848-5061

Shampoo, nontoxic for baby: Weleda Calendula baby shampoo
http://usa.weleda.com/natural-products/
natural-baby-bath-wash.aspx
800-241-1030

Spacial Dynamics® movement therapy
http://spacialdynamics.com/english
518-695-6955

Sun Screen, natural zinc oxide for baby
www.badgerbalm.com/p-372-spf-34-lightly-
scented-sunscreen.aspx

Swedish Bitters
www.swedishbitters.com/swedish-bitters-
38-alcohol-1000ml.html
www.urbanmoonshine.com
802-428-4707

Swedish Bitters, pregnancy formulation
www.urbanmoonshine.com/
product/chamomile-bitters/
802-428-4707

Tecnu soap for poison ivy, available in many stores and on the Internet
http://www.teclabsinc.com/products/poison-
oak-ivy/tecnu/
800-482-4464

Teething ring, natural rubber
http://www.natursutten.com/products/
teether-toy/teether-toy/
203-270-3797

Thorne B Complex #12
www.thorne.com/Products/Vitamins/Multi_
Bs/prd~B112.jsp
800-228-1966

Thuja-Thymus comp. pellets from Uriel Pharmacy
http://shop.urielpharmacy.com/thuja-thymus-
comp-pellets-p1509.aspx
866-642-2858

Traumeel drops and ointment
www.traumeel.com
www.amazon.com

Vermox (Mebendazole) for intestinal parasites is no longer manufactured in the U.S., but is available through your physician at some compounding pharmacies. An alternative is the over-the-counter drug Pin-X.

Vitamin B_{12} sublingual methylcobalamin tablet from Jarrow Formulas
www.amazon.com

Vitamin B_{12}-Folic Acid by Standard Process
www.standardprocess.com
800-848-5061

Vitamin C, Amla-Plus from Radiant Life
www.radiantlifecatalog.com
888-593-8333

Vitamin C, Liposomal 1000 mg from Emperical Labs
www.empirical-labs.com/product_p/
liposomalvitaminc.htm
866-948-8135

Vitamin K Drops, available to physicians from from Scientific Botanicals
www.scientificbotanicals.net
425-332-5678

Water, delivered: Mountain Valley Spring water delivers spring water in glass bottles.
www.mountainvalleyspring.com

Water Filters
www.radiantlifecatalog.com
888-593-8333

YES Essential Fatty Acid Blend
   http://www.cutcat.com/item/Y_E_S_
      Essential_Fatty_Acid_Capsules/718/pgc96
   800-497-9516

Zinc oxide cream
   www.badgerbalm.com/p-372-spf-34-lightly-
      scented-sunscreen.aspx
   Weleda Calendula Diaper Care
      http://usa.weleda.com/our-products/
      shop/calendula-diaper-care.aspx

References

INTRODUCTION

1. Spock, Benjamin. *The Commonsense Book of Baby and Child-care*. New and Revised Edition, 1968, Hawthorn Books, Inc.
2. Masterjohn C. On the Trail of the Elusive X Factor. *Wise Traditions*, the journal of the Weston A. Price Foundation, Spring 2007. http://westonaprice.org/fat-soluble-activators/x-factor-is-vitamin-k2.

CHAPTER 1
PREPARING FOR YOUR BABY

1. Masterjohn C. The Pursuit of Happiness. *Wise Traditions*, the journal of the Weston A. Price Foundation, Winter, 2008. http://westonaprice.org/mentalemotional-health/pursuit-of-happiness.
2. Zile MH and others. Function of Vitamin A in Vertebrate Embryonic Development. *J Nutr.* 2001;131:705-708.
3. Zile MH and others. Function of Vitamin A in Vertebrate Embryonic Development. *J Nutr.* 2001;131:705-708.
4. Gilbert T. Vitamin A and Kidney Development. *Nephr Dial Trans.* 2002 Sept;17(Suppl9):78-80.
5, Vitamin A's paradoxical role in influencing symmetry during embryonic development revealed. www.news-medical.net/news/2005/05/11/9979.aspx, accessed November 2, 2012.
6. Rothman KJ and others. Teratogenicity of high vitamin A intake. *NEJM.* 1995 Nov 23;333(21):1414-5.
7. Alsharif NZ and EA Hassoun. Protective Effects of Vitamin A and Vitamin E Succinate against 2,3,7,8-Tetrachlorodibenzo-p-dioxin (TCDD)-Induced Body Wasting, Hepatomegaly, Thymic Atrophy, Production of Reactive Oxygen Species and DNA Damage in C57BL/6J Mice. *Basic & Clinical Pharmacology & Toxicology.* 95 (2004) 131-138.
8. Russell RM. The vitamin A spectrum: from deficiency to toxicity *Am J Clin Nutr.* 71 (2000) 878-84.
9. Masterjohn, C. Vitamin A On Trial: Does Vitamin A Cause Osteoporosis? *Wise Traditions*, the journal of the Weston A. Price Foundation, Winter 2005/Spring 2006. www.westonaprice.org/fat-soluble-activators/vitamin-a-on-trial.

10. Aikawa H and others. Relief effect of vitamin A on the decreased motility of sperm and the increased incidence of malformed sperm in mice exposed neonatally to bisphenol A. *Cell Tissue Res.* 2004;315(1):119-24.
11. Rothman KJ and others. Teratogenicity of high vitamin A intake. *N Engl J Med.* 1995;333:1369-73.
12. Werler MM and others. Teratogenicity of high vitamin A intake. *N Engl J Med.* 1996;334:1195-1197.
13. Werler MM and others. Teratogenicity of high vitamin A intake. *N Engl J Med.* 1996;334:1197.
14. Martínez-Frías ML and Salvador J. Epidemiological aspects of prenatal exposure to high doses of vitamin A in Spain. *Eur J Epidemiol.*1990;6(2):118-123.
15. Shaw GM and others. High maternal vitamin A intake and risk of anomalies of structures with a cranial neural crest cell contribution. *Lancet.*1996;347:899-900.
16. Mills JL and others. Vitamin A and birth defects. *Am J Obstet Gynecol.* 1997;177(1):31-6.
17. Mastroiacovo P and others. High vitamin A intake in early pregnancy and major malformations: a multicenter prospective controlled study. *Teratology.*1999;59(1):7-11.
18. Thureen PJ and Hay WW. *Neonatal Nutrition and Metabolism: Second Edition.* Cambridge University Press, 2006, page 26.
19. Joshi S and others. Differential effects of fish oil and folic acid supplementation during pregnancy in rats on cognitive performance and serum glucose in their offspring. *Nutrition.* 2004;20(5):465-72.
20. Stene LC and others. Use of cod liver oil during pregnancy associated with lower risk of Type I diabetes in the offspring. *Diabetologia.* 2000;43(9):1093-8.
21. Hyppönen E and others. Intake of vitamin D and risk of type 1 diabetes: a birth-cohort study. *Lancet.* 2001 Nov 3;358(9292):1500-3.
22. Olafsdottir AS and others. Relationship between dietary intake of cod liver oil in early pregnancy and birthweight. *BJOG.* 2005 Apr;112(4):424-9.
23. Helland IB and others. Maternal supplementation with very-long-chain n-3 fatty acids during pregnancy and lactation augments children's IQ at 4 years of age. *Pediatrics.* 2003 Jan;111(1):e39-44.

24. Zeisel SH. The fetal origins of memory: the role of dietary choline in optimal brain development. *J Pediatr.* 2006;149:S131-S136.

25. *Ibid.*

26. Long C and Alterman T. Meet Real Free-Range Eggs. *Mother Earth News.* October/November 2007.

27. Masterjohn C. Precious Yet Perilous: Understanding the Essential Fatty Acids. *Wise Traditions*, the journal of the Weston A. Price Foundation, Fall, 2010.www.westonaprice.org/know-your-fats/precious-yet-perilous.

28. Centers for Disease Control and Prevention (CDC). Food-borne Active Surveillance Network (FoodNet) Population Survey Atlas of Exposures. Atlanta, Georgia: U.S. Department of Health and Human Services, Centers for Disease Control and Prevention, 2006-2007. cdc.gov/foodnet/surveys/Food-NetExposureAtlas0607_508.pdf.

29. Beals T. Those Pathogens, What You Should Know. *Wise Traditions*, the journal of the Weston A. Price Foundation, Summer 2011. www.realmilk.com/real-milk-pathogens.html.

30. Flynn D. Still Too Many Raw Oyster Deaths in Gulf States. *Food Safety News.* November 22, 2011,www.foodsafetynews.com/2011/11/still-too-many-raw-oyster-deaths/, accessed November 3, 2012.

31. Raw Milk, What the Scientific Literature Really Says: A Response to Bill Marler, JD. Prepared by the Weston A. Price Foundation. http://realmilk.com/documents/ResponsetoMarlerListofStudies.pdf , accessed November 22, 2012.

32. A Campaign for Real Milk, Powerpoint presentation prepared by the Weston A. Price Founation. http://realmilk.com/ppt/index.html.

33. Ho KJ and others. The Masai of East Africa: Some unique biological characteristics. *Arch Path.* 1971;91:387-410.

34. *Interpretive Summary* – Listeria Monocytogenes *Risk Assessment*, Center for Food Safety and Applied Nutrition, FDA, USDHHS, USDA, Sept. 2003, page 17.

35. Cdc-foodborne-illness-report-1973-2005.pdf.

36. Fritz R and others. Listeriosis outbreak caused by acid curd cheese "Quargel," Austria and Germany 2009. *Eurosurveillance.* Volume 15, Issue 5, 04 February 2010.

37. Price, WA. *Nutrition and Physicial Degeneration.* 1945. Published by the Price-Pottenger Nutrition Foundation.

38. A Campaign for Real Milk, Powerpoint presentation prepared by the Weston A. Price Foundation. http://realmilk.com/ppt/index.html.

39. Riedler J and others. Exposure to farming in early life and development of asthma and allergy: a cross-sectional survey. *Lancet.* 2001 Oct 6;358(9288):1129-33; Perkin MR and DP Strachen. Which aspects of the farming lifestyle explain the inverse association with childhood allergy? *J Allergy Clin Immunol.* 2006 Jun;117(6):1374-81; Waser M. Inverse association of farm milk consumption with asthma and allergy in rural and suburban populations across Europe. *Clinical & Experimental Allergy.* 2007 May;37(5):661-70; Loss G. The protective effect of farm milk consumption on childhood asthma and atopy: The GABRIELA study. *Journal of Allergy and Clinical Immunology.* Volume 128, Issue 4 , Pages 766-773. e4, October 2011.

40. Rajakumar K. Infantile scurvy: a historical perspective. *Pediatrics.* 2001;108(4):E76.

41. *The History of Randleigh Farm.* p 215. http://www.realmilk.com/documents/Randleigh-page215.pdf.

42. Gregory JF. Denaturation of the folacin-binding protein in pasteurized milk products. *J Nutr.* 1982, 1329-1338.

43. Ford JE and others. Influence of the heat treatment of human milk on some of its protective constituents. *J Pediatrics.* Jan 1977, 29-35.

44. *The History of Randleigh Farm.* p 215. http://www.realmilk.com/documents/Randleigh-page215.pdf.

45. Said HM and others. Intestinal uptake of retinol: enhancement by bovine milk beta-lactoglobulin. *Am J Clin Nutr.* 1989;49:690-694; Runge FE and R Heger. Use of microcalorimetry in monitoring stability studies. Example: vitamin A esters. *J Agric Food Chem.* 2000 Jan;48(1):47-55.

46. Hollis BW and others. Vitamin D and its metabolites in human and bovine milk. *J Nutr.* 1981;111:1240-1248; Yang MC and others. Evidence for beta-lactoglobulin involvement in vitamin D transport in vivo--role of the gamma-turn (Leu-Pro-Met) of beta-lactoglobulin in vitamin D binding. *FEBS Journal.* 2009 2251-2265.

47. Ford JE and others. Influence of the heat treatment of human milk on some of its protective constituents. *J Pediatr.* 1977;90(1):29-35.

48. Wheeler SM and others. Effect of processing upon concentration and distribution of natural and iodophor-derived iodine in milk. *J Dairy Sci.* 1983;66(2):187-95.

49. Vegarud GE and others. Mineral-binding milk proteins and peptides; occurrence, biochemical and technological characteristics. *Br J Nutr.* 2000 Nov;84 Suppl 1:S91-8.

50. Caustic Commentary, *Wise Traditions*, the journal of the Weston A. Price Foundation, Winter 2005-Spring 2006; http://westonaprice.org/caustic-commentary/caustic-commentary-winter-2005-spring-2006.

51. Masterjohn C. On the Trail of the Elusive X Factor. *Wise Traditions*, the journal of the Weston A. Price Foundation, Spring 2007. http://westonaprice.org/fat-soluble-activators/x-factor-is-vitamin-k2.

52. *Ibid.*

53. Hibbeln JR and others. Maternal seafood consumption in pregnancy and neurodevelopmental outcomes in childhood (ALSPAC study): an observational cohort study. *Lancet.* 2007 Feb 17;369 (9561):578-85.

54. What's In Your Mouth. . . Mercury Fillings Smoking Teeth, www.youtube.com/watch?v=o2VCen1vCMY, accessed November 3, 2012.

55. Rowland IR. Tissue content of mercury in rats given methylmercuric chloride orally: influence of intestinal flora. *Arch Environ Health.* May 2001;35:3, 155-160.

56. Masterjohn C. Glutathione 101, Part 1: Cysteine Misbehaves, But Glutathione Saves. www.westonaprice.org/blogs/cmasterjohn/tag/glutathione/, accessed November 3, 2012.

57. Rees WD and others. Sulfur amino acid metabolism in pregnancy: the impact of methionine in the maternal diet. *J Nutr.* 2006;136(6 Suppl):1701S-1705S.

58. Liao YJ and others. Deficiency of glycine N-methyltransferase results in deterioration of cellular defense to stress in mouse liver. *Proteomics Clin Appl.* 2010;4(4):394--406; Yang CP and others. Characterization of the neuropsychological phenotype of glycine N-methyltransferase-/- mice and evaluation of its repsonses to clozapine and sarcosine treatments. *Eur Neuropsychopharmacol.* 2012;22(8):596-606.

59. Rees WD and others. Sulfur amino acid metabolism in pregnancy: the impact of methionine in the maternal diet. *J Nutr.* 2006;136(6 Suppl):1701S-1705S.

60. Guarner F and Malagelada JR. Gut flora in health and disease. *Lancet.* February 2003 361 (9356): 512–9; Shanahan F. The host-microbe interface within the gut. *Best Pract Res Clin Gastroenterol.* December 2002 16 (6): 915–31.

61. Boscia F. Silencing or knocking out the Na(+)/Ca(2+) exchanger-3 (NCX3) impairs oligodendrocyte differentiation. *Cell Death Differ.* 2012 Apr;19(4):562-72.

62. Robertson AF. Reflections on Errors in Neonatology III. The "Experienced" Years, 1970 to 2000. *Journal of Perinatology.*

(2003) 23, 240–249.

63. Enig MG. *Trans Fatty Acids in the Food Supply, A Comprehensive Report Covering 60 Years of Research, 2nd Edition*.1995. Enig & Associates, Bethesda, MD.

64. Fields M. The Severity of Copper Deficiency in Rats is Determined by the Type of Dietary Carbohydrate. *Proc Soc Exp Bio Med*. 1984, 175:530-537.

65. Earles J. Sugar-Free Blues: Everything You Wanted to Know About Artificial Sweeteners. *Wise Traditions*, the journal of the Weston A. Price Foundation, Winter 2003. www.westonaprice.org/modern-foods/sugar-free-blues.

66. Mercola J. The Potential Dangers of Sucrolose (Splenda). http://www.redicecreations.com/specialreports/sucralose.html, accessed November 3, 2012.

67. Advisory Committee on Novel Foods and Processes, Committee Paper for Discussion, Effect of GM Soya on Newborn Rats (Nov. 2005), www.bioeticanet.info/omg/transgeREC.pdf,accessed November 3, 2012.

68. Ho MW. Transgenic pea that made mice ill. *Science in Society*. 29, 28-29, 2006.

69. Ho MW. GM ban long overdue. Dozens ill & five deaths in the Philippines. *Science in Society*. 29, 26-27, 2006.

70. French experts very disturbed by health effects of Monsanto GM corn. *GMWatch*. 23 April 2004. www.gmwatch.org.

71. Pusztai A and others. Genetically modified foods: Potential human health effects. *Food Safety: Contaminants and Toxins*. (J P F D'Mello ed.), Scottish Agricultural College, Edinburgh, CAB International, 2003.

72. Fares NH and El-Sayed AK. Fine structural changes in the ileum of mice fed on dendotoxin-treated potatoes and transgenic potatoes. *Natural Toxins*. 1998, 6, 219-33; Cummins J and MW Ho. Bt is toxic. *ISIS News 7/8*, February 2001, ISSN: 1474-1547 (print), ISSN: 1474-1814 (online) http://www.i-sis.org.uk/isisnews.php Agricultural Biotechnology 2006, www.ISAAA.org.

73. Novotny E. Animals avoid GM food, for good reasons. *Science in Society*. 21, 9-11, 2004.

74. Séralini, GE and others. Long term toxicity of a Roundup herbicide and a Roundup-tolerant genetically modified maize. *Food and Chemical Toxicology*. Volume 50, Issue 11, November 2012, Pages 4221–4231.

75. Fallon S. Dirty Secrets of the Food Processing Industry. www.westonaprice.org/modern-foods/dirty-secrets-of-the-food-processing-industry, accessed November 3, 2012.

76 Fallon S and Enig MG. Tragedy and Hype: Third International Soy Symposium. http://westonaprice.org/soy-alert/tragedy-and-hype,accessed November 3, 2012.

77. Flynn KM and others. Effects of genistein exposure on sexually dimorphic behaviors in rats. *Toxicol Sci*. 2000 Jun;55(2):311-9.

78. Names of ingredients that contain processed free glutamic acid (MSG). (Last updated February, 2011),www.truthinlabeling.org/hiddensources.html, accessed November 3, 2012.

79. Pregnancy and Adrenal Fatigue. www.anneshealthplace.com/blog/2010/10/pregnancy-and-adrenal-fatigue, accessed November 3, 2012.

80. Pope S. The Dangers of Microwave Cooking. www.thehealthyhomeeconomist.com/dangers-of-microwave-cooking.

81. http://westonaprice.org/local-chapters/find-local-chapter.

82. Plapp FW. Perilous Pathways: Environmental Chemicals and Environmental Illness, A Major Role for Vitamin A. *Wise Traditions*, the journal of the Weston A. Price Foundation, Fall, 2002, www.westonaprice.org/environmental-toxins/perilous-pathways; Stohs and others. Effects of BHA, d-alpha-tocopherol and retinol acetate on TCDD-mediated changes in lipid peroxidation, glutathione peroxidase activity and survival. *Xenobiotica*. Vol. 14 No. 7 (1984) 533-7; Masterjohn C. Dioxins in Animal Foods: A Case for Vegetarianism? *Wise Traditions*, the journal of the Weston A. Price Foundation, Fall, 2005. www.westonaprice.org/environmental-toxins/dioxins-in-animal-foods.

83. Harvey RA and others. *Lippincott Illustrated Reviews: Biochemistry: 3rd Edition*. Lippincott Williams & Wilkins. Baltimore, Philadelphia. 2005, p 73.

84. Ahlbom IC and others. Review of the epidemiologic literature on EMF and Health. *Environmental Health Perspectives*. December 2001, 109 (Suppl 6): 911–33; See Michelozzi P and others. Childhood leukemia near a high-power radio station in Rome, Italy. *American Journal of Epidemiology*. 2002 155 (12): 1096–103; Draper G and others. Childhood cancer in relation to distance from high voltage power lines in England and Wales: a case-control study. *BMJ*. June 2005 330 (7503): 1290; Fews AP and others. Corona ions from power lines and increased exposure to pollutant aerosols. *International Journal of Radiation Biology*. December 1999 75 (12): 1523–31.

85. Ashok A and others. Effect of cell phone usage on semen analysis in men attending infertility clinic: an observational study. *Fertility and Sterility*, 2008. www.clevelandclinic.org/reproductiveresearchcenter/docs/agradoc239.pdf, accessed November 3, 2012.

86. www.smartmeterdangers.org/;www.earthcalm.com/emf-dangers-2/smart-meter-radiation-risks/, accessed November 3, 2012.

87. Pellon, R and others. *Drug-Induced Nutrient Depletion Handbook*. 2001. Lexi-Comp. pg 467-471.

88. Kelly P and others. Unmetabolized folic acid in serum: acute studies in subjects consuming fortified food and supplements. *Am J Clin Nutr*.1997;65(6):1790-5.

89. Tamura T, and Picciano MF. Folate and human reproduction. *Am J Clin Nutr*. 2006;83(5):993-1016.

90. Yajnik CS. Vitamin B_{12} and folate concentrations during pregnancy and insulin resistance in the offspring: the Pune Maternal Nutrition Study *Diabetologia*. Jan 2008;51(1):29-38.

91. Why Fathers Really Matter. *New York Times*. Sept 8, 2012.

CHAPTER 2
NUTRITION FOR FETAL DEVELOPMENT

1. North K and Golding J. A maternal diet in pregnancy is associated with hypospadias. *BJU Int*. 2000, 35, 107-113.

2. Barker DJP. The origins of the developmental origins theory. *J Intern Med*. 2007;261:412-417.

3. Barker DJP. Fetal nutrition and cardiovascular disease in later life. *British Medical Bulletin*. 1997;53(1):96-108.

4. Tegethoff M and others. Stress during Pregnancy and Offspring Pediatric Disease: A National Cohort Study. *Reprod Fertil Dev*. 2007;19:53-63.

5. Barker DJP. Fetal nutrition and cardiovascular disease in later life. *British Medical Bulletin*. 1997;53(1):96-108.

6. Brooks AA. Birth weight: nature or nurture? *Early Human Dev*. 1995;42(1):29-35.

7. Godfrey K and others. Maternal nutrition in early and late pregnancy in relation to placental and fetal growth. *BMJ*. 1996;312:410.

8. Olafsdottir AS and others. Relationship between dietary intake of cod liver oil in early pregnancy and birthweight. *BJOG*. 2005;112(4):424-9.

9. Tamura T and Picciano MF. Folate and human reproduction. *Am J Clin Nutr*. 2006;83(5):993-1016.

10. Thureen PJ and Hay WW. *Neonatal Nutrition and Metabolism: Second Edition.* Cambridge University Press, 2006, p 26.

11. Price, WA. *Nutrition and Physical Degeneration*, published by the Price-Pottenger Nutrition Foundation, 1945.

12. Biesalski HK and Nohr D. Importance of vitamin A for lung function and development. *Mol Aspects Med.* 2003;24:431-440.

13. Panel on Micronutrients, National Academy Press (2000). pp 82-61.

14. Devereux G. Early life events in asthma--diet. *Pediatr Pulmonol.* 2007;42(8):663-73.

15. Hoogenboezem T and others. Vitamin D metabolism in breast-fed infants and their mothers. *Pediatric Research.* 1989; 25: 623-628).

16. Devereux G. Early life events in asthma--diet. *Pediatr Pulmonol.* 2007;42(8):663-73.

17. Feldman D and others. V*itamin D: Second Edition.* 2005; 803-810.

18. Hyppönen E and others. Intake of vitamin D and risk of type 1 diabetes: a birth-cohort study. *Lancet.* 2001 Nov 3;358(9292):1500-3.

19. Pfluger P and others. Vitamin E: underestimated as an antioxidant. *Redox Rep.* 2004;9(5):249-54.

20. Berkner KL. The vitamin K-dependent carboxylase. *Annu Rev Nutr.* 2005; 25: 127-49.

21. Howe KM and others. Severe cervical dysplasia and nasal cartilage calcification following prenatal warfarin exposure. *Am J Med Genet.* 1997;71(4):391-6.

22. *Ibid.*

23. Lioka H and others. A study on the placental transport mechanism of vitamin K$_2$ (MK-4). *Asia Oceania J Obstet Gynaecol.* 1992;18(1):49-55.

24. *Ibid.*

25. Innis SM. Dietary (n-3) fatty acids and brain development. *J Nutr.* 2007;137:855-859.

26. Mock DM. Marginal biotin deficiency is teratogenic in mice and perhaps humans: a review of biotin deficiency during human pregnancy and effects of biotin deficiency on gene expression and enzyme activities in mouse dam and fetus. *J Nutr Biochem.* 2005;16(7):435-7.

27. http://lpi.oregonstate.edu/infocenter/vitamins/biotin, accessed November 3, 2012.

28. Durance TD. Residual Avid in Activity in Cooked Egg White Assayed with Improved Sensitivity. *J Food Sci.* 1991;56(3):707-709.

29. Tamura T and Picciano MF. Folate and Human Reproduction. *Am J Clin Nutr.* 2006;83(5):993-1016.

30. *Ibid.*

31 Kelly P and others. Unmetabolized folic acid in serum: acute studies in subjects consuming fortified food and supplements. *Am J Clin Nutr.* 1997;65(6):1790-5.

32. Zeisel SH. The fetal origins of memory: the role of dietary choline in optimal brain development. *J Pediatr.* 2006;149:S131-S136.

33. *Ibid.*

34. *Ibid.*

35. Oberlander TF. Prenatal exposure to maternal depression, neonatal methylation of human glucocorticoid receptor gene (NR3C1) and infant cortisol stress responses. *Epigenetics.* 2008 Mar-Apr;3(2):97-106.

36. Jiang X and others. Maternal choline intake alters the epigenetic state of fetal cortisol-regulating genes in humans. *FASEB J.* 2012 Aug;26(8):3563-74.

37. Rees WD. Sulfur amino acid metabolism in pregnancy: the impact of methionine in the maternal diet. *J Nutr.* 2006;136(6 Suppl):1701S-1705S.

38. Sturman JA. Taurine in development. *Physiol Rev.*73(1), 119-147, Jan 1, 1993.

39. Lin B and others. Alteration of acidic lipids in human sera during the course of pregnancy: characteristic increase in the concentration of cholesterol sulfate *Journal of Chromatography B.* 704, 99–104, 1997.

40. Geier DA and others. A prospective study of transsulfuration biomarkers in autistic disorders. *Neurochem Res.* 34(2) 386-393, 2009; Seneff S and others. Might cholesterol sulfate deficiency contribute to the development of autistic spectrum disorder? *Medical Hypotheses.* 8, 213–217, 2012.

41. Côté F and others. Maternal serotonin is crucial for murine embryonic development. *Proc Natl Acad Sci U S A.* 2007 Jan 2;104(1):329-334.

42. German JB and Dillard CJ. Saturated fats: a perspective from lactation and milk composition. *Lipids.* 2010;45(10):915-23.

43. Bilbo SD and Tsang V. Enduring consequences of maternal obesity for brain inflammation and behavior of offspring. *FASEB J.* 2010;24(6):2104-15.

44. Smedts HP and others. Maternal intake of fat, riboflavin and nicotinamide and the risk of having offspring with congenital heart defects. *Eur J Nutr.* 2008;47:357-65.

45. Aaltonen J and others. Impact of maternal diet during pregnancy and breastfeeding on infant metabolic programming: a prospective randomized controlled study. *Eur J Clin Nutr.* 2011;65:10-19).

46. Khoury J and others. Effect of a cholesterol-lowering diet on maternal, cord, and neonatal lipids, and pregnancy outcome: a randomized clinical trial. *Am J Obstet Gynecol.* 2005;193(4):1292-301.

47. Khoury J and others. Effects of an antiatherogenic diet during pregnancy on markers of maternal and fetal endothelial activation and inflammation: the CARRDIP study. *BJOG.* 2007;114(3):279-88; Khoury J and others. Effect of a cholesterol-lowering diet during pregnancy on maternal and fetal Doppler velocimetry: the CARRDIP study. *Am J Obstet Gynecol.* 2007;196(6):549.e1-7.

48. Bo S and others. Dietary fat and gestational hyperglycaemia. *Diabetologia.* 2001;44:972-8.

49. Wang Y and others. Dietary variables and glucose tolerance in pregnancy. *Diabetes Care.* 2000. 23:460-4.

50. Radesky JS and others. Diet during early pregnancy and development of gestational diabetes. *Pediatr Perinat Epidemiol.* 2008;22(1):47-59; Ley SH and others. Effect of macronutrient intake during the second trimester on glucose metabolism later in pregnancy. *Am J Clin Nutr.* 2011;94:1232-40).

51. Tovar A and others. The impact of gestational weight gain and diet on abnormal glucose tolerance during pregnancy in Hispanic women. *Matern Child Health J.* 2009;13(4):520-30).

52. Martins AP and Benicio MH. Influence of dietary intake during gestation on postpartum weight retention. *Rev Saude Publica.* 2011;45(5):870-7.

53. Hui A and others. Lifestyle intervention on diet and exercise reduced excessive gestational weight gain in pregnant women under a randomised controlled trial. *BJOG.* 2012;119(1):70-7.

54. Phelan S. Randomized trial of a behavioral intervention to prevent excessive gestational weight gain: the Fit for Delivery Study. *Am J Clin Nutr.* 2011;91:373-80)

55. Ilic S. Comparison of the effect of saturated and monounsaturated fat on postprandial plasma glucose and insulin concentration in women with gestational diabetes mellitus. *Am J Perinatol.* 1999;16(9):489-95.

CHAPTER 3
A HEALTHY PREGNANCY

1. Burkhard A. Pregnancy and Celiac Disease. www.celiaccen-tral.org/research-news/Celiac-Disease-Research/134/vo-bid--2030/, accessed November 4, 2012.
2. Anjum N. Maternal celiac disease autoantibodies bind directly to syncytiotrophoblast and inhibit placental tissue transgluta-minase activity. *Reprod Biol Endocrinol.* 2009 Feb 19;7:16.
3. Gedgaudas N. Do You Have Pyroluria? www.primalbody-primalmind.com/?p=398,accessed November 4, 2012.
4. Smith C and others. Pregnancy outcome following women's participation in a randomised controlled trial of acupuncture to treat nausea and vomiting in early pregnancy. *Complement Ther Med.* 2002 Jun;10(2):78-83.
5. Carlsson C and others. Manual acupuncture reduces hyper-emesis gravidarum: a placebo-controlled, randomized, single-blind, crossover study. *Journal of Pain and Symptom Management.* October 2000;20(4):273-279.
6. Einarsson JI and others. Sperm exposure and development of preeclampsia. *American Journal of Obstetrics and Gynecology.* May, 2003, 188(5):1241–3; Robertson SA and others. Seminal "priming" for protection from pre-eclampsia-a unifying hypothesis. *Journal of Reproductive Immunology.* August, 2003 59(2): 253–65.
7. Koelman CA and others. Correlation between oral sex and a low incidence of preeclampsia: a role for soluble HLA in seminal fluid? *Journal of Reproductive Immunology.* March, 2006 46(2):155–66.
8. Jefferson T and others. Vaccines to prevent influenza in healthy adults http://summaries.cochrane.org/CD001269/vaccines-to-prevent-influenza-in-healthy-adults, accessed November 4, 2012.
9. www.marchofdimes.com/baby/birthdefects_rh.html, accessed November 4, 2012; Lubusky M and others. Prevention of Rh (D) alloimmunization in Rh (D) negative women in pregnancy and after birth of Rg (D) positive infant, Mendeley. Vol 71 Issue 3 Pgs 173-179. 2006; Moise K. Management of Rhesus Alloimmunization in Pregnancy. *Obstetrics & Gynecology* (ACOG). Vol 112 No 1. Jul 2008.
10. Ayoub DM and Yazbak FE. Influenza Vaccination during Pregnancy: Advisory Committee on Immunization Practices. *J Am Physicians and Surgeons.* Summer 2006 11(2):41-47.
11. Folkes JB and others. American Institute of Ultrasound in Medicine consensus report on potential bioeffects of diagnostic ultrasound: executive summary. *J Ultrasound Med.* 2008 Apr;27(4):503-15.
12. Samuel E. Fetuses can hear ultrasound examinations. *New Scientist.* December 2001.
13. Edwards MJ. Apoptosis, the heat shock response, hyperthermia, birth defects, disease and cancer. Where are the common links? *Cell Stress & Chaperones.* 1998 3(4):213-20.
14. Newnham JP and others. Effects of frequent ultrasound during pregnancy: a randomised controlled trial. *Lancet.* 1993 342(Oct.9), 887-891.
15 Campbell JD. Case-control study of prenatal ultrasonography exposure in children with delayed speech. *Canadian Medical Association Journal.* 1993 149(10), 1435-1440.
16. Ewigman BG and others. Effect of prenatal ultrasound screening on perinatal outcome. RADIUS Study Group. *N Engl J Med.* 1993 Sept 16;329:821-7; Lefebre ML and others. A randomized trial of prenatal ultrasonographic screening: impact on maternal management and outcome. RADIUS (Routine Antenatal Diagnostic Imaging with Ultrasound) Study Group. *Am J Obstet Gynecol.* 1993 Sept 15;169:483-9.
17. Devi PU. Effect of fetal exposure to ultrasound on the behavior of the adult mouse. *Radiat Res.* (QMP) 1995 141(3), 314-7.
18. Hande MP and Devi PU. Teratogenic effects of repeated exposures to X-rays and/or ultrasound in mice. *Neurotoxicol Teratol.* (NAT) 1995 17(2), 179-88.
19. Barnett SB. The sensitivity of biological tissue to ultrasound. *Ultrasound Med Biol.* 1997;23(6):805-12.
20. Dalecki D and others. Hemolysis in vivo from exposure to pulsed ultrasound. *Ultrasound Med Biol.* 1997;23(2):307-13.
21. Stanton MT. Diagnostic ultrasound induces change within numbers of cryptal mitotic and apoptotic cells in small intestine. *Life Sci.* 2001 Feb 16;68(13):1471-5.
22. http://chriskresser.com/natural-childbirth-iib-ultrasound-not-as-safe-as-commonly-thought, accessed November 4, 2012.
23. And ES and others. Prenatal exposure to ultrasound waves impacts neuronal migration in mice. *Proceedings of the National Academy of Sciences.* 2006 103: 12903-12910.
24. Questions about Prenatal Ultrasound and the Alarming Increase in Autism. www.whale.to/a/questions9.html, accessed November 4, 2012.
25. *Healthy from the Start.* 1999. The Pew Charitable Trusts (Environmental Health Commission). www.pewtrusts.com/pdf/hhs_healthy_from_start.pdf, quoted from http://www.midwiferytoday.com/articles/ultrasoundrodgers.asp, accessed November 4, 2012.
26. Bianchi DW. Genome-Wide Fetal Aneuploidy Detection by Maternal Plasma DNA Sequencing. *Obstetrics & Gynecology.* May 2012 - Volume 119 - Issue 5 - p 890–901
27. Edwards MJ and others. Effects of heat on embryos and foetuses. *Int J Hyperthermia.* 2003 May-Jun;19(3):295-324.
28. Milunsky A and others. Maternal heat exposure and neural tube defects. *JAMA.* 1992 268(7):882-885.
29. Alfirevic Z and others. Doppler ultrasound of fetal blood vessels in normal pregnancies. http://summaries.cochrane.org/CD001450/doppler-ultrasound-of-fetal-blood-vessels-in-normal-pregnancies, accessed November 4, 2012.
30 Ponder S. Gestational diabetes can have long-term effects on mother, infant. Mywesttexas.com: *West Texas Living.* February 23, 2012. www.mywesttexas.com/life/article_99995307-3bfb-5c00-8ed6-83789c7c3944.html#ixzz28ePmV6FO, accessed November 4, 2012.
31. Current Trends Rubella Vaccination During Pregnancy -- United States, 1971-1981 www.cdc.gov/mmwr/preview/mmwrhtml/00001154.htm, accessed November 4, 2012.
32. Butler H. Rubella in Babies & Pregnant Women, http://www.whale.to/m/butler2.html,accessed November 4, 2012.
33. *The Dr. Brewer Pregnancy Diet.* drbrewerpregnancydiet.com, accessed November 4, 2012.

CHAPTER 4
YOUR BABY IS BORN

1. Price W. *Nutrition and Physical Degeneration*, published by the Price-Pottenger Nutrition Foundation, 1945.
2. Childbirth in Early America. www.digitalhistory.uh.edu/historyonline/childbirth.cfm,accessed November 4, 2012.
3. Revolutionary Changes in Childbirth. http://reflectionsinhindsight.wordpress.com/tag/martha-ballard/, accessed November 4, 2012.
4. Price W. *Nutrition and Physical Degeneration*, published by the Price-Pottenger Nutrition Foundation, 1945, page 380.
5. New York Academy of Medicine, Committee on Public Health Relations: *Maternal Mortality in New York City: A Study of All Puerperal Deaths, 1930-1932.* New York: The Academy,

1933.

6. Rooks J and others. Outcomes of Care in Birth Centers: The National Birth Center Study. *New England Journal of Medicine.* 321:1804-1811, (December 28), 1989.

7. Odent M. Is the Participation of the Father at Birth Dangerous? www.midwiferytoday.com/articles/fatherpart.asp, November 4, 2012.

8. Bromberger P and others. The influence of intrapartum antibiotics on the clinical spectrum of early-onset group B streptococcal infection in term infants. *Pediatrics.* Aug 2000; 106: 244-250).

9. Babies are born dirty, with a gutful of bacteria. *New Scientist.* April 14, 2012, http://www.newscientist.com/article/mg21428603.800-babies-are-born-dirty-with-a-gutful-of-bacteria.html, accessed November 4, 2012.

10. http://www.homeopathyforwomen.org/birthing.htm, accessed November 4, 2012.

11. Goer H, When Is My Baby Due? http://www.ivillage.com/when-baby-due/6-a-129259, accessed November 4, 2012.

12. Freeman ME and others. Prolactin: Structure, Function, and Regulation of Secretion. *Physiol Rev.* 2000;80(4):1523-1631.

13. Gimpl G and Fahrenholz F. The Oxytocin Receptor System: Structure, Function, and Regulation. *Physiol Rev.* 2001;81(2):629-83.

14. Reisine T and Bell GI. Molecular Biology of Opioid Receptors. *TINS.* 1993;16(12):506-10.

15. Barnes PJ. Beta-adrenergic receptors and their regulation. *Am J Respir Crit Care Med.* 1995;152:838-60.

16. Combs GF. *The Vitamins: Fundamental Aspects in Nutrition and Health: Fourth Edition.* London, UK: Academic Press, 2012. pp. 244-5.

17. Michaluk A and Kochman K. Involvement of copper in female reproduction. *Reprod Biol.* 2007;7(3):193-205.

18. Bousquet-Moore D and others. Peptidylglycine alpha-amidating monooxygenase and copper: a gene-nutrient interaction critical to nervous system function. *J Neurosci Res.* 2010;88(12):2535-45.

19. Mousa SA and others. Subcellular Pathways of Beta-Endorphin Synthesis, Processing, and Release from Immunocytes in Inflammatory Pain. *Endocrinology.* 2004; 145(3):1331-41.

20. BRENDA: The Comprehensive Enzyme Information System. EC 3.4.21.94 proprotein convertase 2. www.brenda-enzymes.org/php/result_flat.php4?ecno=3.4.21.94 Accessed July 8, 2012.

21. Thony B and others. Tetrahydrobiopterin biosynthesis, regeneration and functions. *Biochem J.* 2000;347(Pt 1):1-16.

22. Harvey RA and Ferrier DR. *Lippincott's Illustrated Reviews: Biochemistry.* Baltimore, MD: Lippincott Williams & Wilkins. 2001.

23. Qiu Y and others. Cholesterol regulates micro-opioid receptor-induced beta-arrestin 2 translocation to membrane lipid rafts. *Mol Pharmacol.* 2011;80(1):210-8.

24. BRENDA. The Comprehensive Enzyme Information System. DNA-directed RNA polymerase. www.brenda-enzymes.org/php/result_flat.php4?ecno=2.7.7.6. Accessed July 8, 2012.

25. Rush J and others. The effects of whirlpools baths in labor: a randomized, controlled trial. *Birth.* 1996 Sep;23(3):136-43

26. Thöni A and others. Water birthing: retrospective review of 2625 water births. Contamination of birth pool water and risk of microbial cross-infection. *Minerva Ginecol.* 2010 Jun;62(3):203-11

27. Water Birth—A Near-Drowning Experience. www.neonatologie.ugent.be/waterbirth.pdf, accessed November 4, 2012.

28. Buckley SJ. Ecstatic Birth. http://www.mothering.com/pregnancy-birth/ecstatic-birth-the-hormonal-blueprint-of-labor?page=0,0.

29. Hannah ME and others. Planned caesarean section versus planned vaginal birth for breech presentation at term: a randomised multicentre trial. Term Breech Trial Collaborative Group. *Lancet.* 2000 (356:1375-1383).

30. Helsten C and others. Vaginal breech delivery: is it still an option? *Eur J Obstetrics & Gynecology Reproductive Biology.* 2003 Dec 10;111(2):122-8.

31. Molkenboer JF and others. Birth weight and neurodevelopmental outcome of children at 2 years of age after planned vaginal delivery for breech presentation at term. *Am J Obstetrics and Gynecology.* 2006 Mar;194(3):624-9.

32. Alran S. and others. Differences in management and results in term-delivery in nine European referral hospitals: descriptive study. *Eur J Obstetrics & Gynecology Reproductive Biology.* 2002 Jun 10;103(1):4-13.

33. Kumari AS and Grundsell H. Mode of delivery for breech presentation in grandmultiparous women.*International J Gynecology & Obstetrics.* 2004 Jun;85(3):234-9.

34. Noraihan MN. An Audit of Singleton Breech Deliveries in a Hospital with a High Rate of Vaginal Delivery. *Malays J Med Sci.* 2007 January; 14(1): 28–37.

35. Wagner M and Wagner MG, 1994, *Pursuing the Birth Machine,* 1st ed. French's Forest, Australia, James Bennett Pty Ltd.

36. Screening for Intrapartum Electronic Fetal Monitoring,http://www.uspreventiveservicestaskforce.org/uspstf/uspsiefm.htm, accessed November 4, 2012.

37. Otto SJ and others. Increased risk of postpartum depressive symptoms is associated with slower normalization after pregnancy of the functional docosahexaenoic acid status. *Prostaglandins Leukot Essent Fatty Acids.* 2003 Oct;69(4):237-43.

CHAPTER 5
NEWBORN INTERVENTIONS

1. Hutton EK and Hassan ES. Late vs early clamping of the umbilical cord in full-term neonates: systematic review and meta-analysis of controlled trials. *JAMA.* 2007 Mar 21;297(11):1241-52.

2. *Ibid.*

3. Morley GM. How the Cord Clamp Injures Your Baby's Brain. www.whale.to/a/morley1.html, accessed November 4, 2012.

4, Windle WF. Brain damage by asphyxia at birth *Scientific American.* 1969 Oct;221(4):76-84.

5. Klebanoff MA. The Risk of Childhood Cancer after Neonatal Exposure to Vitamin K. *N Engl J Med.* Sept 23, 1993; 329:905-908.

6. Cohain J. The Myth of A Safer Hospital Birth for Low Risk Pregnancies. www.gentlebirth.org/archives/lateClamping.html, accessed November 4, 2012.

7. Bower B. Cry-Babies Demonstrate "Sweet" Dispositions. *Science News.* Vol 138 No 15, Oct 13, 1990.

8. Harrison D and others. Efficacy of sweet solutions for analgesia in infants between 1 and 12 months of age: a systematic review. *Archives of Disease in Childhood.* 2010 95:406-413.

9. Johnston CC and others. Routine sucrose analgesia during the first week of life in neonates younger than 31 weeks' preconceptional age. *Pediatrics.* 2002 Sep;110(3):523-8.

10. Pope S. The Scary Side of Synagis, http://www.thehealthyhomeeconomist.com/the-scary-side-of-synagis/. Accessed October 13, 2012.

11. http://en.wikipedia.org/wiki/Circumcision.

12. *Ibid.*

CHAPTER 6
VACCINATIONS

1. Ferrie JP and Troesken W. *Death and the City: Chicago's Mortality Transition. 1850-1925.* Working Paper 11427. www.nber.org/papers/w11427.

2. Channick R. More asthma inhalers going to school: New state law eliminates need for doctor's written permission. *Chicago Tribune.* October 1, 2012.

3. Hewitson L and others. Influence of pediatric vaccines on amygdala growth and opioid ligand binding in rhesus macaque infants: A pilot study. *Acta Neurobiol Exp.* (Wars) 2010;70(2):147-64.

4. Dr. Andrew Moulden (Interview): What You Were Never Told About Vaccines. http://vactruth.com/2009/07/21/dr-andrew-moulden-interview-what-you-were-never-told-about-vaccines/,accessed November 4, 2012.

5. Claridge S. Unvaccinated Children are Healthier. http://www.whale.to/ias1992study.pdf,accessed November 4, 2012.

6. Kemp T and others. Is infant immunization a risk factor for childhood asthma or allergy? *Epidemiology.* 1997 Nov; 8(6), 678-80.

7. Cristensen I and others. Routine vaccinations and child survival: follow up study in Guinea-Bissau, West Africa. *British Medical Journal.* 2000, 321: 1435-8.

8. McKeever TM and others. Vaccination and Allergic Disease: A Birth Cohort Study. *American Journal of Public Health.* June 2004, Vol 94, No. 6, pp 985-989.

9. http://healthimpactnews.com/2011/new-study-vaccinated-children-have-2-to-5-times-more-diseases-and-disorders-than-unvaccinated-children/, accessed November 4, 2012.

10. Blaylock RL. What They Don't Tell You About Vaccination Dangers Can Kill You or Ruin Your Life. www.whale.to/a/blaylock34.html, accessed November 4, 2012.

11. Reactions/Conditions.http://www.novaccine.com/reactions-conditions/, accessed November 4, 2012.

12. Blaylock RL. Vaccination Dangers Can Kill You or Ruin Your Life. http://articles.mercola.com/sites/articles/archive/2004/05/12/vaccination-dangers.aspx, accessed November 4, 2012.

13. Blaylock, RL, The Deadly Impossibility of Herd Immunity Through Vaccination. http://www.vaccinationcouncil.org/2012/02/18/the-deadly-impossibility-of-herd-immunity-through-vaccination-by-dr-russell-blaylock/, accessed November 4, 2012.

14. "The whole trend goes in a direction where a way will finally be found to vaccinate bodies so that these bodies will not allow the inclination towards spiritual ideas to develop and all their lives people will believe only in the physical world they perceive with the senses. Out of impulses which the medical profession gained . . . from the consumption they themselves suffered. . . people are now vaccinated against consumption, and in the same way they will be vaccinated against any inclination towards spirituality. This is merely to give you a particularly striking example of many things which will come in the near and more distant future in this field. . . the aim being to bring confusion into the impulses which want to stream down to earth after the victory of the spirits of light." Steiner R. Lecture: Fall of the Spirits of Darkness, Lecture 13. The Fallen Spririts' influence in the World, Dornach, 27, October, 1917; "A longing will arise (and become) general opinion: Whatever is spiritual, whatever is of the spirit, is nonsense, is madness! Endeavours to achieve this will be made by bringing out remedies to be administered by inoculation just as inoculations have been developed as a protection against diseases, only these inoculations will influence the human body in a way that will make it refuse to give a home to the spiritual inclinations of the soul. People will be inoculated against the inclination to entertain spiritual ideas. Endeavours in this direction will be made; inoculations will be tested that already in childhood will make people lose any urge for spiritual life." Lecture 3, *Secret Brotherhoods and the Mystery of the Human Double: Seven Lectures.* November 1917.

15. Specific Vaccines, http://www.novaccine.com/specific-vaccines/, accessed November 4, 2012.

16. Maciej J and others. Multiple mechanisms are involved in the biliary excretion of acetaminophen sulfate in the rat: role of MRP2 and BCRP1. *The American Society for Pharmacology and Experimental Therapeutics.* 2005 Vol. 33, No. 8, 1158–1165.

17. Li, XM. Efficacy and mechanisms of action of traditional Chinese medicines for treating asthma and allergy. *Journal of Allergy and Clinical Immunology.* (Feb 2009;123(2):297-306.

18. Flöistrup H. Allergic disease and sensitization in Steiner school children. *J Aller Clin Immunol.* 2006 Jan 117(1):59-66.

CHAPTER 7
NOURISHING YOUR BABY

1. Takemura Y and others. Relation between Breastfeeding and the Prevalence of Asthma: The Tokorozawa Childhood Asthma and Pollinosis Study *American Journal of Epidemiology.* July 2001;154(2):115-119.

2. Sears MR and others. *Lancet.* Sept 21, 2002, New Zealand, breastfed *Lancet.* Sept 21, 2002.

3. Male C and others. Prevalence of iron deficiency in 12-mo-old infants from 11 European areas and influence of dietary factors on iron status (Euro-Growth study). *Acta Paediatrics.* May 2001;90(5):492-8.

4. Hardell L and Dreifaldt AC. Breast-feeding duration and the risk of malignant diseases in childhood in Sweden. *European Journal of Clinical Nutrition.* March 2001;55(3):179-85.

5. Wefring KW and others. Nasal congestion and earache--upper respiratory tract infections in 4-year-old children. *Tidsskr Nor Laegeforen.* April 30, 2001;121(11):1329-32.

6. Neifert MR. Prevention of breastfeeding tragedies. *Pediatric Clinics of North America* noted that many breastfed babies suffer from failure-to-thrive and dehydration (April 2001;48(2):273-97.

7. Gillman MW and others. Risk of overweight among adolescents who were breastfed as infants. *JAMA.* May 16, 2001;285(19):2461-7.

8. Temboury MC. Influence of breastfeeding on the infant's intellectual development. *Pediatric Gastroenterology and Nutrition.* Jan 1994;18(1):32-36; Kramer MS. Breastfeeding and Child Cognitive DevelopmentNew Evidence From a Large Randomized Trial. *Archives of Diseases of Children.* September 2001;85(3):183-188; Agostini C. Breastfeeding duration, milk fat composition and developmental indices at 1 year of life among breastfed infants. *Prostaglandins, Leukotrines and Essential Fatty Acids.* February 2001;64(2):105-109.

9. *Nutrition During Pregnancy and Lactation.* National Academy of Sciences, Washington, DC 1992.

10. Price-Pottenger Nutrition Foundation *Health Journal.* Winter 1999, 23(4):5-8)

11. Labbok MH and Hendershot GE. Does Breastfeeding Protect Against Malocclusion? An Analysis of the 1981 Child Health Supplement to the National Health Interview Survey. *Journal of Preventive Medicine.* 1987;3(4): 227-232.

12. Adamiak, E. Occlusion Anomalies in Preschool Children in Rural Areas in Relation to Certain Individual Features. *Czas Stomat.* 1981;34:551-5.

13. Boyd, MR. Oral-Digital Habits of Childhood: Thumb Sucking. *Practitioner's Guide to Evidence-Based Psychotherapy.* 2006, pp 718-725.

14. Hennart PF and others. Lysozyme, lactoferrin, and secretory immunoglobulin A content in breast milk: influence of duration of lactation, nutrition status, prolactin status, and parity of mother. *Am J Clin Nutr.* 1991 Jan;53(1):32-9.

15. Filteau SM and others. Breast milk immune factors in Bangladeshi women supplemented postpartum with retinol or beta-carotene. *AJCN.* 1999 69(5):953-958.

16. Price WA. Vitamins in Immunity and Growth. *Journal of the American Dental Association.* May 1930.

17. Anderson NK and others. Dietary fat type influences total milk fat content in lean women. *J Nutr.* 2005;135:416-421).

18. Teter BB and others. Milk fat depression in C57Bl/6J mice consuming partially hydrogenated fat. *J Nutr.* 1990;120:818-824.

19. Anderson NK and others. Dietary fat type influences total milk fat content in lean women. *J Nutr.* 2005;135:416-421.

20. Personal communication, Mary G. Enig, PhD.

21. Koletzko B and others. Long chain polyunsaturated fatty acids (LC-PUFA) and perinatal development. *Acta Paediatrics.* April 2001;90(4):460-4.

22. Chen ZY. Breast milk fatty acid composition: a comparative study between Hong Kong and Chongqing Chinese. *Lipids.* 1997;32(10):1061-1067.

23. Garg ML and others. *FASEB Journal.* 1988, 2:4:A852; Oliart Ros RM and others. Meeting Abstracts. *AOCS Proceedings.* May 1998:7, Chicago, IL.

24. Jensen RG. Lipids in human milk. *Lipids.* December 1999;34(12):1243-1271.

25. Reddy S and others. The influence of maternal vegetarian diet on essential fatty acid status of the newborn. *European Journal of Clinical Nutrition* May, 1994;48(5)358-368.

26. Personal communication, Kim Rodriguez, MS, RD, LD.

27. Lukas R. Influence of organic diet on the amount of conjugated linoleic acids in breast milk of lactating women in the Netherlands *British Journal of Nutrition.* 2007 97:735-743.

28. Filer LJ. Relationship of nutrition to lactation and newborn development. *Nutritional impacts on women.* 1977, pp 151-159.

29. Hoppu U. Breast milk--immunomodulatory signals against allergic diseases. *Allergy.* April 2001;56 suppl 67:23-6.

30. Greer FR. Do breastfed infants need supplemental vitamins? *Pediatric Clinics of North America.* April 2001;48(2):415-23.

31. Balogun FA. *Biological Trace Element Research.* 1994:471-479.

32. Packard VS. *Human Milk and Infant Formula.* 1982.

33. Lovelady C and others. Effect of energy restriction and exercise on vitamin B_6 status of women during lactation. *Medicine and Science in Sports and Exercise.* 2001;33:512–518.

34. Fischer LM and others. Choline intake and genetic polymorphisms influence choline metabolite concentrations in human breast milk and plasma. *Am J Clin Nutr.* 92: 336-346, 2010.

35. Rabin RC. Vitamin D Deficiency May Lurk in Babies. *New York Times.* August 26, 2008.

36. Fallon S and Enig MG. Vitamin A Saga. *Wise Traditions*, the journal of the Weston A. Price Foundation. Winter 2001. www.westonaprice.org/fat-soluble-activators/vitamin-a-saga.

37. Stoltzfus RJ and Underwood BA. Breast-milk vitamin A as an indicator of the vitamin A status of women and infants. *Bull World Health Organ.* 1995; 73(5): 703–711.

38. Strobel M and others. The importance of beta-carotene as a source of vitamin A with special regard to pregnant and breast-feeding women. *Eur J Nutr.* 2007 Jul;46 Suppl 1:11-20.

39. Vitamin B_{12} deficiency in the breast-fed infant of a strict vegetarian. *Nutr Rev.* May 1979;37(5):142-144.

40. Dórea JG. Magnesium in Human Milk. *JACN.* 2000 19(2):210-219.

41. Semba RD and Delange F. Iodine in human milk: perspectives for infant health. *Nutr Rev* 2001;59(8):269-278; Milk Secretion and Composition. *Neonatal Nutrition and Metabolism.* 2006.

42. Enig MG. *Trans Fatty Acids in the Food Supply, A Comprehensive Report Covering 60 Years of Research, 2nd Edition.*1995. Enig & Associates, Bethesda, MD.

43. Naturally Occurring Trans Fats. http://www.tfx.org.uk/page62.html, accessed Nov 4, 2012.

44. Setchell KD and others. Exposure of infants to phyto-oestrogens from soy-based infant formula. *Lancet.* July 5, 1997;350:23-27.

45. Vadas P and others. Detection of peanut allergens in breast milk of lactating women. *JAMA.* April 4, 2001;285(13):1746-8.

46. Elander G and Lindberg T. Short mother-infant separation during first week of life influences the duration of breastfeeding. *Acta Paediatr Scand.* 1984;73:237–40.

47. Brazelton TB. Psychophysiologic reactions in the neonate. II. Effects of maternal medication on the neonate and his behavior. *J Pediatr.* 1961;58:513–8.

48. Crowell MK and others. Relationship between obstetric analgesia and time of effective breast feeding. *J Nurse Midwifery.* 1994;39:150–6.

49. Vestermark V. Influence of the mode of delivery on initiation of breast-feeding. *Eur J Obstet Gynecol Reprod Biol.* 1991;38:33–8.

50. Hartley BM and O'Connor ME. Evaluation of the "Best Start" breastfeeding education program.*Arch Pediatr Adolesc Med.* 1996;150:868–71.

51. Chen DC. Stress during labor and delivery and early lactation performance. *Am J Clin Nutr.* 1998;68:335–44.

52. Yamauchi Y and Yamanouchi I. Breastfeeding frequency during the first 24 hours after birth in full-term neonates. *Pediatrics.* 1990;86:171–5.

53. Victora CG and others. Pacifier use and short breastfeeding duration: cause, consequence, or coincidence? *Pediatrics.* 1997;99:445–53.

54. Fride E and others. Critical role of the endogenous cannabinoid system in mouse pup suckling and growth. *European Journal of Pharmacology.* Volume 419, Issues 2–3, 11 May 2001, pp 207–214.

55. http://kellymom.com/health/baby-health/bfhelp-tonguetie, accessed November 4, 2012.

56. Personal communication, Lindy Woodard, MD, Pediatric Alternatives, October, 2012.

57. Semba RD and others. Maternal vitamin A deficiency and mother-to-child transmission of HIV-1. *Lancet.* 1994 Jun 25;343(8913):1593-7.

58. Breast Milk Kills HIV and Blocks Its Oral Transmission in Humanized Mouse. http://www.sciencedaily.com/releases/2012/06/120614182751.htm, accessed November 4, 2012; Newly Discovered Breast Milk Antibodies Help Neutralize HIV. http://www.sciencedaily.com/releases/2012/05/120522152653.htm accessed November 4, 2012.

59. Breastfeeding and Lyme Disease. http://kellymom.com/bf/can-i-breastfeed/illness-surgery/lyme-disease/, accessed November 4. 2012.

60. Phend C. Probiotics Prevent GI Infection in Premature Infants. http://www.medpagetoday.com/OBGYN/Pregnancy/5627, accessed November 4, 2012.

61 Probiotics help extremely premature infants gain weight. http://phys.org/news191912597.html, accessed November 4, 2012.

62. Infant colic significantly reduced with supplementation of *Lactobacillus reuteri Protectis*. http://biogaia.com/study/infant-colic-significantly-reduced-supplementation-lactoba-cillus-reuteri-protectis, accessed November 4 2012.

63. N Baumslag and Michels DL. *Milk, Money and Madness: The Culture and Politics of Breastfeeding.* 1995.

64. *Ibid.*

65. Simone CJ. Prolactin in Animal Experimentation *J. Clin. Chem. Clin. Biochern.*Vol. 23, 1985, pp. 423-431. http://edoc.hu-berlin.de/oa/degruyter/cclm.1985.23.7.423.pdf, accessed November 4, 2012.

66. FDA Poisonous Plant Database. http://westonaprice.org/im-ages/pdfs/fdasoyreferences.pdf, accessed November 4, 2012.

67. Teter BB and others. Milk fat depression in C57Bl/6J mice consuming partially hydrogenated fat. *J Nutr.* 1990;120:818-824.

68. Carlsen SM and others. Mid-pregnancy androgen levels are negatively associated with breastfeeding. *Acta Obstet Gynecol Scand.* 2010;89(1):87-94.

69. Dioxins in Food Chain Linked to Breastfeeding Ills.http://esciencenews.com/sources/science.daily/2009/06/09/dioxins.in.food.chain.linked.to.breastfeeding.ills, accessed November 4, 2012.

70. Neifert MR and others. Pediatrics. 1985 Nov;76(5):823-8. Lactation failure due to insufficient glandular development of the breast. *Pediatrics.* Nov 1985;76 (5):823-828.

71. Sołtyski J and others. A case of megaloblastic anemia in an 11-month-old infant fed with goat milk *Pediatr Pol.* 1996 Aug;71(8):709-11.

CHAPTER 8
BRINGING UP BABY

1. Blackwell, PL. Infants & Young Children: The Influence of Touch on Child Development: Implications for Intervention. *Infants and Young Children.* July 2000 - Volume 13 - Issue 1

2. Schwartz J. Baby DVDs, videos may hinder, not help, infants' language development. www.washington.edu/news/archive/id/35898, accessed November 4, 2012.

3. Real Diaper Association, Diaper Facts. www.realdiaperasso-ciation.org/diaperfacts.php, accessed November 4, 2012.

4. Warner, J. *Perfect Madness: Motherhood in the Age of Anxiety,* 2006.

5. Hays, S. *Cultural Contradictions of Motherhood,* 1998.

6. Birkenhead P. Cribs vs. Beds: Parenthood's all-out war. www.salon.com/2010/07/02/cribs_v_beds_parenting_wars/, accessed November 4, 2012.

7. Scheibner V. Medical Research on SIDS and Epidemics. http://www.vierascheibner.org/in-dex.php?view=article&catid=47%3Acot-deaths-sids&id=73%3Avaccinations-part-i-medical-research-on-sids-and-epidemics-&option=com_content&Itemid=58.

8. Baniel A. *Kids Beyond Limits: The Anat Baniel Method for Awakening the Brain and Transforming the Life of Your Child With Special Needs.* 2012.

9. Havas M. Health Canada needs to issue warning about Wireless Baby Monitors. http://www.magdahavas.com/health-can-ada-needs-to-issue-warning-about-wireless-baby-monitors/, accessed November 4, 2012.

10. Burrows P and Griffiths P. Do baby walkers delay onset of walking in young children? *Br J Community Nurs.* November 2001, 7(11):581–6.

11. The Dangers of Baby Walkers. http://consults.blogs.nytimes.com/2010/02/22/the-dangers-of-baby-walkers/, accessed November 4, 2012.

12. Rovers MM and others. Is pacifier use a risk factor for acute otitis media? A dynamic cohort study. *Fam Pract.* 2008 Aug;25(4):233-6.

13. Bessa CF and others. Prevalence of oral mucosal alterations in children from 0 to 12 years old. *J Oral Pathol Med.* 2004 Jan;33(1):17-22.

14. Moon RY and others. Pacifier use and SIDS: evidence for a consistently reduced risk. *Matern Child Health J.* 2012 Apr;16(3):609-14.

15. McDonald TA. A perspective on the potential health risks of PBDEs. *Chemosphere.* 46 (2002) 745–755.

16. *Ibid.*

17. Price WA. *Nutrition and Physical Degeneration*, published by the Price-Pottenger Nutrition Foundation, 1945.

18. Elizabeth Plourde, PhD, *Sunscreens Biohazard: Treat as Hazardous Waste.* 2011.

19. *Ibid.*

20. Bacteria That Can Increase Intelligence. http://medicmagic.net/bacteria-that-can-increase-intelligence.html , accessed November 4, 2012.

21. Toilet Training. http://en.wikipedia.org/wiki/Toilet_training, accessed November 4. 2012.

22 Caffey J. On the Theory and Practice of Shaking Infants. *American Journal of the Disease of Children.* 124, 161 – 169, (1972).

23. Frompovich C. Bone Density Test Can Disprove Shaken Baby Syndrome: http://www.vaccinationcouncil.org/2012/02/05/bone-density-test-can-disprove-shaken-baby-syndrome-by-catherine-frompovich/, accessed November 4, 2012.

24. Caffey J. The Whiplash Shaken Baby Syndrome: Manual Shaking by the Extremities With Whiplash-Induced Intracranial and Intraocular Bleedings, Linked With Residual Permanent Brain Damage and Mental Retardation. *Pediatrics.* 54, 396 – 403 (1974).

25. Seeley MB. Unexplained Fractures in Infants and Child Abuse:The Case for Requiring Bone-Density Testing Before Convicting Caretakers. http://lawreview.byu.edu/articles/1325789487_13Seeley.FIN.pdf, accessed November 4, 2012.

26. Pourcyrous M and others. Primary immunization of premature infants with gestational age <35 weeks: Cardiorespiratory complications and C-reactive protein responses associated with administration of single and multiple separate vaccines simultaneously. *J Pediatrics.* 2007:151, p.171; Lowry CA. Identification of an immune-responsive mesolimbocortical serotonergic system: Potential role in regulation of emotional behavior. *Neuroscience.* Volume 146, Issue 2, 11 May 2007, Pages 756–772.

CHAPTER 9
NOURISHING A GROWING CHILD

1. Chantry CJ and others. Full Breastfeeding Duration and Risk for Iron Deficiency in U.S. Infants. *Breastfeeding Medicine.* June 2007, 2(2): 63-73.

2. Lozoff B and others. Preschool-aged children with iron deficiency anemia show altered affect and behavior. *J Nutr.* 2007 Mar;137(3):683-9.

3. Percival M. *Infant Nutrition*. Health Coach System. 1995.

4. Tye JG and others. Differential expression of salivary (Amy1) and pancreatic (Amy2) amylase loci in prenatal and post natal development. *Journal of Genetics*. 1976 13:96-102.

5. Sanderson IR and Walker WA. *Development of the Gastrointestinal Tract*. p 262.

6. Jensen, RG, Lipids in Human Milk. *Lipids*. 1999;34:1243-1271.

7. *Ibid*.

8. Chen ZY. Breast milk fatty acid composition: a comparative study between Hong Kong and Chongqing Chinese. *Lipids*. 1997;32(10):1061-1067.

9. Fallon S. Be Kind to Your Grains. January, 2000. www.westonaprice.org/food-features/be-kind-to-your-grains, accessed November 4, 2012.

10. Persson LA and others. Are weaning foods causing impaired iron and zinc status in 1-year-old Swedish infants? A cohort study. *Acta Paediatr*. 1998; 87(6): 618-22.

11. Krebs, N. Research in Progress. Beef as a first weaning food. *Food and Nutrition News*. 1998; 70(2):5.

12. Krebs NF. Dietary zinc and iron sources, physical growth and cognitive development of breastfed infants. *J Nutr*. 2000;130:358S-360S.

13. Shattock P and Whiteley P. Biochemical aspects in autism spectrum disorders: updating the opioid-excess theory and presenting new opportunities for biomedical intervention. Autism Research Unit, University of Sunderland, UK, 2002.

14. Radas P and others. Daily bingeing on sugar repeatedly releases dopamine in the accumbens shell. *Neuroscience*. Volume 134, Issue 3, 2005, pp 737-744.

15. Evidence of MSG Toxicity. http://evidenceofmsgtoxicity.blogspot.com/, accessed November 4, 2012.

16. Engelmann MD and others. The influence of meat on non-heme iron absorption in infants. *Pediatr. Res*. 1998a;43:768-7.

17. Makrides, M and others. A randomized controlled clinical trial of increased dietary iron in breast-fed infants. *J Pediatr*. 1998; 133(4): 559-62; Engelmann, M and others. Meat intake and iron status in late infancy: an intervention study, *J Pediatr Gastroenterol Nutr*. 1998; 26(1): 26-33.

18. Jalla S and others. Comparison of zinc absorption from beef vs iron fortified rice cereal in breastfed infants. *FASEB J*. 1998;12:A346(abs.).

19. Engelmann MD and others. Meat intake and iron status in late infancy: an intervention study. *J. Pediatr Gastroenterol Nutr*. 1998b;26:26-33; Westcott JL and others. Growth, zinc and iron status, and development of exclusively breastfed infants fed meat vs cereal as a first weaning food. *FASEB J*. 1998;12:A847(abs.); Birch LL and K Grimm-Thomas. Food acceptance patterns: children learn what they like. *Pediatr Basics*. 1996;75:2-6.

20. Lifshitz F and Moses N. Growth failure. A complication of dietary treatment of hypercholesterolemia. *AJDC*. 1989 May;143:537-542).

21. Dagnelie PC and others. Nutritional status of infants aged 4 to 18 months on macrobiotic diets and matched omnivorous control infants: a population-based mixed-longitudinal study. II. Growth and psychomotor development. *Eur J Clin Nutr*. 1989 May;43(5):325-38.; Dagnelie PC and others. Increased risk of vitamin B_{12} and iron deficiency in infants on macrobiotic diets. *Eur J Clin Nutr*. 1989 Oct;50(4):818-24.

22. Makrides M. Nutritional effect of including egg yolk in the weaning diet of breastfed and formula-fed infants: a randomized controlled trial. *Am J Clin Nutr*. June 2002 (Vol. 75, No. 6, 1084-1092.

23. Krebs NF. Dietary zinc and iron sources, physical growth and cognitive development of breastfed infants. *J Nutr*. 2000;130:358S-360S.

24. Modi N. Sodium intake and preterm babies. *Arch Dis Child*. 1993 July; 69(1 Spec No): 87–91; http://www.nutraingredients-usa.com/Research/Salt-supplements-aid-premature-baby-development, accessed November 4, 2012.

25. Smith MM and Lifshitz F. Excess Fruit Juice Consumption as a Contributing Factor in Nonorganic Failure to Thrive. *Pediatrics*. Mar 1994;93(3):438-443.

26. Masterjohn C. Precious Yet Perilous: Understanding the Essential Fatty Acids. *Wise Traditions*, the journal of the Weston A. Price Foundation, Fall, 2010.www.westonaprice.org/know-your-fats/precious-yet-perilous.

27. Lozoff B and others. Iron-Fortified vs Low-Iron Infant Formula Developmental Outcome at 10 Years. *Arch Pediatrics Adoles Dev*. Mar 2012, Vol 166, No. 3.

28. Sazawal S and others. Effects of routine prophylactic supplementation with iron and folic acid on admission to hospital and mortality in preschool children in a high malaria transmission setting: community-based, randomised, placebo-controlled trial. *Lancet*. 2006 367: 133–143.

29. Wen W and others. Parental medication use and risk of childhood acute lymphoblastic leukemia. *Cancer*. 2002 Oct 15;95(8):1786-94.

30. Ionnatti LL and others. Iron supplementation in early childhood: health benefits and risks. *Am J Clin Nutr*. December 2006 vol. 84 no. 6 1261-1276.

31. Salonen JT and others. High stored iron levels are associated with excess risk of myocardial infarction in eastern Finnish men. *Circulation*. 1992 Sep;86(3):803-11).

32. Ozsvath DL. Fluoride and environmental health: a review. Earth and Environmental Science. *Reviews in Environmental Science and Biotechnology*. Volume 8, Number 1 (2009), 59-79.

33. Canedy D. Toothpaste a Hazard? Just Ask the F.D.A. *New York Times*. March 24, 1998. http://www.nytimes.com/1998/03/24/us/toothpaste-a-hazard-just-ask-the-fda.html?pagewanted=all&src=pm, accessed November 4, 2012.

34. Overview: Infant Formula and Fluorsis. http://www.cdc.gov/fluoridation/safety/infant_formula.htm, accessed November 4, 2012.

35. Choi AL and others. Developmental fluoride neurotoxicity: a systematic review and meta-analysis. *Environ Health Perspect*. 2012 Oct;120(10):1362-8.

CHAPTER 10
FROM BIRTH TO ADULTHOOD

1. Liedloff J. *The Continuum Concept: In Search of Happiness Lost*. 1986.

2. Curriculum Research. curriculumresearch.blogspot.com/2006/10/sex-education.html, accessed November 4, 2012.

CHAPTER 11
CHILD SPACING AND BIRTH CONTROL

1. Price WA. *Nutrition and Physical Degeneration*. Published by the Price-Pottenger Nutrition Foundation, 1945, page 323.

2. Malinowski B. *The Sexual Life of Savages*. 1987.

3. Njoh AJ. *Tradition, Culture And Development in Africa: Historical Lessons for Modern Development Planning*. Ashgate Publishing Company, 1988.

4. Personal communication, Anna Yekhanina, Moscow, Russia, January, 2010.

5. Family planning: Get the facts about pregnancy spacing.www. mayoclinic.com/health/family-planning/MY01691/, accessed November 4, 2012.

6. New Findings on Birth Spacing: Three to Five Years is the Optimal Interval. www.rhcatalyst.org/site/ PageServer?pagename=Programs_Birth_Spacing_Optimal_ Interval, accessed November 4, 2012.

7. Zhu BP and others. Effect of the interval between pregnancies on perinatal outcomes. *NEJM*. 1999;340(8):589-594.

8. Strobel M and others. The importance of beta-carotene as a source of vitamin A with special regard to pregnant and breast-feeding women. *Eur J Nutr.* 2007 Jul;46 Suppl 1:11-20).

9   Cheslack-Postava K and others. Closely spaced pregnancies are associated with increased odds of autism in California sibling births. *Pediatrics.* 2011 Feb;127(2):246-53.

10. FAQ Sheet: Frequently Asked Questions on Breastfeeding and Maternal Health, http://pdf.usaid.gov/pdf_docs/PNACS875. pdf,accessed November 16, 2012; Hornstra G. Essential fatty acids in mothers and their neonates. *Am J Clin Nutr.* 2000 May;71(5 Suppl):1262S-9S.

11. Sulloway FJ. Birth Order and Intelligence.*Science.* 22 June 2007: 1711-1712.

12. Thompson A. Study: Older Siblings Have Higher IQs. http:// www.livescience.com/1651-study-older-siblings-higher-iqs. html, accessed November 4, 2012.

13. Goleman D. Spacing of Siblings Strongly Linked to Success in Life. *New York Times*. May 28, 1985.

14. Pellon R and others. *Drug-Induced Nutrient Depletion Handbook.* 2001. Lexi-Comp. pg 470-471.

15. *Ibid.*, p 467.

16. Personal communication, Natasha Campbell-McBride.

17. Campbell-McBride N. *The Gut and Psychology Syndrome: Natural Treatment for Autism, Dyspraxia, A.D.D., Dyslexia, A.D.H.D., Depression, Schizophrenia*, 2010.

18. Grant. E. *Sexual Chemistry: Understanding Our Hormones, the Pill and HRT*. 1996.

19. Singer K. *Honoring Our Cycles*. 2006.

20. Schaefer O. When the Eskimo Comes to Town. *Nutrition Today*. November-December 1971, p. 16.

CHAPTER 12
THE ILLNESSES OF CHILDHOOD

1. Fever: New View Stresses Its Healing Benefits. *New York Times*. December 28, 1982.

2. Schulman CI. The effect of antipyretic therapy upon outcomes in critically ill patients: a randomized, prospective study. *Surgical Infection*. 2005 Winter; 6(4):369-75.

3. Williams LK and others. The relationship between early fever and allergic sensitization at age 6 to 7 years. *J Allergy Clin Immunol.* 2004 Feb;113(2):291-6.

4. Chen Q and others. Fever-range thermal stress promotes lymphocyte trafficking across high endothelial venules via an interleukin 6 trans-signaling mechanism. *Nature Immunology.* 2006:1299-1308.

5. Hoption Cann SA and others. Dr. William Coley and tumour regression: a place in history or in the future. *Postgraduate Med.* 2003 79:672-680; Hobohm U. Fever therapy revisited. *British Journal of Cancer.* 2005; 92:421-425.

CHAPTER 13
STRATEGIES FOR INFECTIOUS DISEASE

1. Keith I and Block MD. Immune System Effects of Echinacea, Ginseng, and Astragalus: A Review. *Integr Cancer Ther.* September 2003 vol. 2 no. 3 247-267.

CHAPTER 14
EARS, NOSE & THROAT

1. Glasziou P and others. Antibiotics for acute otitis media in children. Cochrane Review. *The Cochrane Library*, issue 3. Oxford, England: Update Software, 2000.

2. Grens K. Whooping cough vaccine fades in pre-teens: study. *Reuters.* April 3, 2012. http://www.reuters.com/article/2012/04/03/us-whoopingcough-idUSBRE8320TM20120403,accessed November 16, 2012.

3. Spike in whooping cough cases alarms CDC. *Arizona Daily Star.* July 20, 2012. http://azstarnet.com/news/science/health-med-fit/spike-in-whooping-cough-cases-alarms-cdc/article_bed87aa3-4f21-5f97-b618-7e5368fd92a4.html, accessed November 17, 2012.

4. Pertussis --- United States, 1997--2000, http://www.cdc.gov/ mmwr/preview/mmwrhtml/mm5104a1.htm, accessed November 17, 2012.

5. Personal communication, Maureen Diaz, October 11, 2012.

CHAPTER 15
ALLERGIES, ASTHMA & ECZEMA

1. Margellos-Anast H and others. Improving asthma management among African-American children via a community health worker model: findings from a Chicago-based pilot intervention. *J Asthma.* 2012 May;49(4):380-9. Epub 2012 Feb 21.

2. Riedler J and others. Exposure to farming in early life and development of asthma and allergy: a cross-sectional survey. *Lancet.* 2001 Oct 6;358(9288):1129-33; Perkin MR and Strachan DP. Which aspects of the farming lifestyle explain the inverse association with childhood allergy? *J Allergy Clin Immunol.* 2006 Jun;117(6):1374-81; Perkin MR. Unpasteurized milk: health or hazard? *Clinical and Experimental Allergy* 2007 May; 35(5) 627-630. Loss G and others. The protective effect of farm milk consumption on childhood asthma and atopy: the GABRIELA study. *Journal of Allergy Clin Immunol.* 2011 October 128(4):766-773.e4).

3. Wen MC. Efficacy and tolerability of anti-asthma herbal medicine intervention in adult patients with moderate-severe allergic asthma. *J Allergy & Clin Immunol.* 2005 Sept 116(3):517-524).

CHAPTER 16
NEUROLOGICAL DISORDERS

1. Autism. http://en.wikipedia.org/wiki/Autism, accessed October 25, 2012.

2. Campbell-McBride N. *The Gut and Psychology Syndrome: Natural Treatment for Autism, Dyspraxia, A.D.D., Dyslexia, A.D.H.D., Depression, Schizophrenia.* 2010.

3. Newport MT. *Alzheimer's Disease, What If There Was a Cure: The Story of Ketones.* 2011.

4. Masterjohn C. The Pursuit of Happiness. *Wise Traditions*, the journal of the Weston A. Price Foundation, Winter, 2008. http://westonaprice.org/mentalemotional-health/pursuit-of-happiness.

5. Seyfried TN. The restricted ketogenic diet: an alternative treatment strategy for glioblastoma multiforme, treatment strategies. *Brain and Spinal Cord Cancer.* July 2011; Schmidt M and others. Effects of a ketogenic diet on the quality of life in 16 patients with advanced cancer: a pilot trial. *Nutr Metab.* 2011; 8:54; Klement RJ. Is there a role for carbohydrate restriction in the treatment and prevention of cancer? *Nutrition and Metabolism.* 2011, 8:75.

6. Goldsworthy A. How Electromagnetically Induced Cell Leakage May Cause Autism. http://citizensforsafetechnology.org/How-Electromagnetically-Induced-Cell-Leakage-May-Cause-Autism,6,1013, accessed November 17, 2012.

CHAPTER 17
REMEDIES FOR THE ILLNESSES OF CHILDHOOD

1. Yancy WS and others. Improvement of gastroesophogeal reflux disease after initiation of a low-carbohydrate diet: five brief case reports. *Alternative Therapies.* 2001 Nov, Vol 7, No 6, 120 116-119.

2. Abdel-Rahman A and others. Subchronic dermal application of N,N-diethyl m-toluamide (DEET) and permethrin to adult rats, alone or in combination, causes diffuse neuronal cell death and cytoskeletal abnormalities in the cerebral cortex and the hippocampus, and Purkinje neuron loss in the cerebellum. *Exp Neurol.* 2001 Nov;172(1):153-71.

3. CFR - Code of Federal Regulations Title 21. http://www.accessdata.fda.gov/scripts/cdrh/cfdocs/cfCFR/CFRSearch.cfm?fr=355.50.

Index

Recipe Index

Other Titles from NewTrends Publishing

Nourishing Traditions: The Cookbook that Challenges Politically Correct Nutrition and the Diet Dictocrats
by Sally Fallon with Mary G. Enig, PhD
> Now a classic, this best-selling cookbook re-introduced the principles of traditional diets to the western world.

The Nourishing Traditions Cookbook for Children
by Suzanne Gross and Sally Fallon Morell, illustrations by Angela Eisenbart
> All the principles of *Nourishing Traditions*, beautifully illustrated for children.

The Fourfold Path to Healing
by Thomas S. Cowan with Sally Fallon and Jaimen McMillan
> The companion to *Nourishing Traditions*; traditional diets and wholistic therapies applied to a wide range of medical conditions.

Honoring Our Cycles
by Katie Singer
> Natural family planning without hormonal drugs; includes cycle charts.

Performance without Pain
by Kathryne Pirtle
> A simplified, *Nourishing Traditions* program for those with serious health problems.

The Whole Soy Story
by Kaayla T. Daniel, PhD, CCN
> The dark side of America's favorite health food.

The Untold Story of Milk
by Ron Schmid, ND
> A history of the campaign to demonize raw milk, Nature's perfect food

The Yoga of Eating
by Charles Eisenstein
> An approach to eating that embodies both common sense and spiritual insight.

A Life Unburdened
by Richard Morris
> An inspiring journey and practical guide to weight loss through traditional whole foods. 2008 Eric Hoffer Award Winner.

newtrendspublishig.com
(877) 707-1776
customerservice@newtrendspublishing.com
Case Discounts Available

About the Authors

Sally Fallon Morell, MA is founding president of the Weston A Price Foundation (www.westonaprice.org) and founder of A Campaign for Real Milk (realmilk.com).

Mrs. Fallon Morell lectures extensively around the world on issues of health and nutrition and is the nation's number one spokesman for nutrient-dense diets for pregnant women and growing children. She is a prolific writer of numerous articles and books and serves as editor of *Wise Traditions in Food, Farming and the Healing Arts*, the quarterly journal of the Weston A. Price Foundation.

In 1996, Mrs. Fallon Morell published the best-selling *Nourishing Traditions* (with Mary G. Enig, PhD), the cookbook that launched her career in alternative health.

Fallon Morell resides in Washington, DC with her husband Geoffrey Morell. She is the mother of four grown children.

Thomas S. Cowan, MD, discovered the work of the two individuals who would have the most influence on his career while teaching gardening as a Peace Corps volunteer in Swaziland, South Africa. He read *Nutrition and Physical Degeneration* by Weston Price, and a fellow volunteer explained the arcane principles of Rudolf Steiner's biodynamic agriculture. These events inspired him to pursue a medical degree. Cowan graduated from Michigan State University College of Human Medicine in 1984. After his residency in Family Practice at Johnson City Hospital in Johnson City, New York, he set up an anthroposophical medical practice in Peterborough, New Hampshire. Dr. Cowan relocated to San Francisco in 2003.

Dr. Cowan has served as vice president of the Physicians Association for Anthroposophical Medicine and is a founding board member of the Weston A. Price Foundation. He is the principal author of the book, *The Fourfold Path to Healing*, published in 2004 by New Trends Publishing. He writes the "Ask the Doctor" column in *Wise Traditions in Food, Farming and the Healing Arts*, the Foundation's quarterly magazine, and has lectured throughout the United States and Canada. He has three grown children and currently practices medicine in San Francisco where he resides with his wife, Lynda Smith Cowan.

Dr. Cowan sees patients at his office in San Francisco and does long-distance consultations by telephone. He also gives lectures and presentations across the country.